T0299935

Routledge Revivals

Sharing Child Care in Early Parenthood

Originally published in 1987, Malcolm Hill examines the different ways in which parents share responsibility for looking after their pre-school children with other people, whether members of their social networks, formal groups or paid carers. He also looks at the reasons parents give for choosing and changing their particular arrangements. In this way he provides insights into a range of ideas which ordinary members of the public have about children's needs; the rights and responsibilities of mothers and fathers; and how children think and feel.

Marked differences are described in the social relationships of families and in notions about who is acceptable as a substitute carer for children, in what circumstances and for what purpose. Several of these contrasts are linked to attitudes and life-conditions which are affected by social class.

The book identifies possible consequences for individual children's social adaptability resulting from these patterns of care. It suggests that people working with the under-fives could profit from adapting their activities and services to children's previous experiences of shared care and families' differing expectations about groups for children.

Sharing Child Care in Early Parenthood

Malcolm Hill

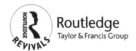

Routledge
Taylor & Francis Group

First published in 1987
by Routledge & Kegan Paul Ltd

This edition first published in 2023 by Routledge
4 Park Square, Milton Park, Abingdon, Oxon, OX14 4RN

and by Routledge
605 Third Avenue, New York, NY 10017

Routledge is an imprint of the Taylor & Francis Group, an informa business

© 1987 Malcolm Hill

All rights reserved. No part of this book may be reprinted or reproduced or utilised in any form or by any electronic, mechanical, or other means, now known or hereafter invented, including photocopying and recording, or in any information storage or retrieval system, without permission in writing from the publishers.

Publisher's Note
The publisher has gone to great lengths to ensure the quality of this reprint but points out that some imperfections in the original copies may be apparent.

Disclaimer
The publisher has made every effort to trace copyright holders and welcomes correspondence from those they have been unable to contact.

A Library of Congress record exists under ISBN: 0710204973

ISBN: 978-1-032-43811-5 (hbk)
ISBN: 978-1-003-37000-0 (ebk)
ISBN: 978-1-032-44023-1 (pbk)

Book DOI 10.4324/9781003370000

Sharing Child Care in Early Parenthood

MALCOLM HILL

Department of Social Policy and
Social Work, University of Edinburgh

ROUTLEDGE & KEGAN PAUL
London and New York

First published in 1987 by
Routledge & Kegan Paul Ltd
11 New Fetter Lane, London EC4P 4EE

Published in the USA by
Routledge & Kegan Paul Inc.
in association with Methuen Inc.
29 West 35th Street, New York, NY 10001

Phototypeset in Linotron Century, 10/12 pt
by Input Typesetting Ltd
and printed in Great Britain
by T. J. Press, Padstow, Cornwall

© Malcolm Hill 1987

No part of this book may be reproduced in
any form without permission from the publisher
except for the quotation of brief passages
in criticism

Library of Congress Cataloging in Publication Data

Hill, Malcolm.
  Sharing child care in early parenthood.

  Bibliography: p.
  Includes index.
  1. Child care—Great Britain—Case studies.
2. Child development—Great Britain—Case studies.
3. Child rearing—Great Britain—Case studies.
4. Social classes—Great Britain—Case studies.
5. Sex role—Great Britain—Case studies.
I. Title.
HQ778.7.G7H55 1987   649'.1'0941   87–4475

British Library CIP Data also available

ISBN 0–7102–0497–3

'Three is a delightful age'
GESELL, *1951*

Contents

Tables

Figures

Acknowledgments

This research concerns a number of families who were willing to help by talking to me about themselves and their children. I am very grateful for their openness and co-operation, which provided the raw material for the study.

The research on which the work described in this book was based, was originally carried out for a doctoral thesis. Therefore, I would also like to thank my supervisors, Dr John Triseliotis and Professor Adrian Sinfield. They were encouraging and tolerant as my ideas emerged and shifted direction. Their comments contributed stimulation and realism, both of which have been welcome.

At various stages of the research, I have had helpful discussions with the following people: Professor Michael Anderson, Tom McGlew, Lynn Jamieson, Kathryn Backett, Neil Fraser, Nita Brown and Martin Hughes (Edinburgh University); Willem van der Eycken (then at Southlands College, Wimbledon); Albert Osborn (CHES, Bristol); Jenny Haystead (Scottish Council for Research in Education, Edinburgh); Peter Moss (Thomas Coram Foundation, London); Elsa Ferri (National Children's Bureau, London); Joyce Watt (University of Aberdeen); Professor Christopher Turner (University of Stirling); Professor Rudolf Schaffer (University of Strathclyde); and Sarah Cunningham-Burley (Aberdeen MRC Medical Sociology Unit, later at the Usher Institute, Edinburgh). To all of them, I am very thankful. I have also received interesting suggestions and documents by correspondence from Steven Duck and Janet Finch (University of Lancaster); Martin Richards (University of Cambridge); Jacqueline Tivers (University of Surrey); Nigel Beail (Wakefield Health Authority) and James Swift (University of Wurzburg). For technical advice about the use of the Edinburgh University computer, I am much indebted to David Goda, Eric Hanley, James McGeldrick and John Murieson.

Access to research subjects in the social sciences is often difficult and this study was no exception. Therefore, after I had travelled up several blind alleys, I was very appreciative of the assistance of Dr Helen Zealley (Community Medicine Specialist) who opened the way for me to approach relevant families, following her negotiations on my behalf with the Lothian Health Board. I am grateful for the Board's agreement for me to obtain names and addresses from their birth register.

This research was made possible by a three-year grant from the Social Science Research Council. Nonetheless, considerable financial sacrifice was necessary and I am grateful to my wife for her unquestioning willingness to share that with me. In addition, she and others shared care of my daughter in the first four years of her life and this enabled me to follow my interest in what arrangements other families make at comparable periods in their lives.

Notes

1 References in the text to books, articles or papers are given as follows: (Author, Year of Publication) e.g. (Smith, 1979). When there is a quotation from a work of reference, then the page number is indicated too: e.g. (Smith, 1979: 16). When more than one reference is cited at the same time, these are given in alphabetical order which sometimes differs from the date order. Full details of all references are given in the bibliography. Some organisations with long names are specified in the text by their initials only, such as EOC and CPRS. Their complete names are placed at the beginning of the bibliography.

2 In the interests of clarity, details of statistical associations are not recorded fully in the text. Instead, the significance level of the particular correlation or cross-tabulation is given. This expresses the probability that an association between two features might have arisen by chance. The lower the probability, the more likely it becomes that an association is not coincidental. Statisticians conventionally use the letter 'p' to designate probability and it is expressed as a decimal. Thus, 0.1 represents a one in ten chance, 0.01 a one in a hundred chance, and so on. For simplicity, five bands of significance levels have been used, i.e.:

$p < 0.1$ a suggestive relationship
$p < 0.05$ a significant relationship
$p < 0.02$ a significant relationship
$p < 0.01$ a highly significant relationship
$p < 0.001$ a highly significant relationship

In most cases the chi-square test was used to establish statistical significance. In a few instances where there were continuous variables the Pearson correlation coefficient (r) was used.

3 Quotation marks are used for the following:
   (a) A verbatim excerpt from a book or article
   (b) A verbatim excerpt from an interview
   (c) A key concept which is being introduced or a term
       which is applied in a special sense (e.g. 'local',
       'protective')
   The context should make clear which purpose applies.
   Brackets within a quotation indicate that part of what was
   said has been omitted or summarised for the sake of brevity
   or lucidity.
4 Tables in the text are referred to by a dual number which
   indicates the chapter to which the table applies and its order
   within that chapter. For instance, Table 4.2 is the second
   table of chapter 4.
5 The children and adults referred to in this book have been
   given names to make them more vivid and to reduce
   repetition of phrases like 'one child did this, another did
   that'. *All the names are false*, so that the identity of the real
   people concerned may be preserved. Likewise, occasionally
   a fact which might identify someone, like their job or a
   key location, has been altered to something comparable.
   Otherwise all the details given are accurate and quotations
   are taken verbatim from actual conversations.

1 *Introduction*

This book is about the circumstances which lead parents to leave their young children in the care of someone else. A convenient term to describe this is 'sharing care'. It includes any situation where a child who lives with one or both parents spends time apart from them both. Since most children spend more time with their mothers than with their fathers, it is in practice more often women than men who arrange alternative care outside the nuclear family.

During the course of my research on this topic, I arrived by appointment one evening to talk to a couple about their daughter. The mother was putting the children to bed so her husband welcomed me. He was very friendly and chatted briefly about his work as a taxi-driver. Once I was comfortably seated in their front room he asked me a question which these opening paragraphs seek to answer: 'What's the point of doing this research about children? Ordinary people never get to hear about it. They just do what comes naturally – they don't read books.' He doubted whether they would have much to say in the interview. He also thought that what they did have to say would be of little value or interest to anybody else. As it happens, I departed into the night over four hours later after an exhausting but fascinating discussion to which he had made a major contribution.

Yet, in spite of this eventual loquaciousness, his opening question needs to be responded to. Many people don't read books much at all. Most adults have probably learnt about bringing up children mainly from their own experience or from watching and talking to others who are raising or have raised children. On the other hand, publications about baby and child care by professionals and other presumed experts are undoubtedly popular, even though the tone and nature of the advice given by different people and at different times has often been contradictory (Hardyment, 1983; Rapoport *et al.*, 1977). The current work is not about the do's and don'ts of being a mother or father. By and large it describes what happens and does not offer an ideal version of what should happen. It analyses what parents say about what they do and why. That should be of intrinsic interest. In all societies the ways in which children are reared are crucial for the transmission of the past and the creation of the future. Normally parents have a central role, especially in early childhood, but other people too play parts in children's lives, to widely differing extents and presumably with significant consequences. Over the course of the last hundred years or so professional wisdom and lay views have tended to agree that the earliest years of childhood are crucial for the individual's development. More recently it has been acknowledged that later experiences and events may modify or even reverse a person's life prospects but clearly those initial foundations remain important.

Sharing care has specific implications since it is the mirror image of parental care. What difference does it make if young children are always with at least one of their parents, away from them both once a week or spend time apart every day? Are parents prompted by similar situations to share care or do they do so for very different reasons? What are the values and beliefs which guide people in deciding who they will trust to look after their child? How does children's previous experience of shared care affect them when they start to attend school or a pre-school group? More widely, in what ways do children's experiences of being looked after by other people fit with other aspects of their family life and of their contacts with the outside world? These are some of the themes with which we shall be concerned.

The original purpose of the study was an academic one but since it is about 'ordinary people' and their everyday activities and relationships it is hoped that it may be of wider interest, particularly amongst practitioners (those who work with pre-school children and/or their parents) or indeed anyone with a special concern for families and young children. Before a child is five years old parents have wide discretion as to the frequency and timing with which they share care, with whom and for what reasons, subject to the resources they have available. Yet outside their own circle of contacts they may know little about what other people do or think about these matters. It will be shown that to some extent most people do as the opening quotation suggested: they do 'what comes naturally' in the sense of sharing care in a manner which appears to them to be straightforward, obvious or normal. But in other ways there is nothing natural or inevitable about parents' arrangements for their children. For a start there is a great variety of ways in which parents may distribute the time their children spend with themselves and other people. That is true even in a city like Edinburgh, where the research took place, though the cultural diversity is much less than in other parts of urban Britain. Parents are influenced by diverse social backgrounds and ideas. They live in many kinds of social and physical environments. Furthermore people have different assumptions about what is typical, right or desirable as regards the care of children. Often they may be unsure or change their views in response to events or as a result of experience.

The research explored some of the circumstances and perceptions which influence the varied ways in which parents arrange for their children to stay with other people. There was no attempt to define in advance what such arrangements might consist of. Thus it was not just about 'day care', or 'working mothers', or 'pre-school groups', which have been the usual categories that have been investigated in the past. Instead the study embraced any instance of shared care which occurred for whatever reason, either deliberately or incidentally, at any time. Shared care includes evening and overnight care as well as daytime care. It was hoped that keeping an open mind about the nature and boundaries of the topic would increase our knowledge of young children's everyday experience. This approach can also shed light on the manner in which people manage their adjustment to the responsibilities, constraints and opportunities of parenthood. That may have consequences not only for the children personally, but also for the wider social and economic relationships of all members of the family. In this way, the study was as much about people's informal networks as about 'official' child care. This perspective helps us to understand the contexts in which services for pre-school children are needed and used. It brings some sociological understanding to bear on a matter which has traditionally been almost exclusively left to the more individualistic approach of child psychology.

Most previous research on the care of young children had concentrated either on mothers (especially mothers and infants) or on situations where children were absent from their mothers for considerable periods, as in nurseries. Comparatively little was known about more intermediate and commonplace arrangements. Recently, psychologists have turned their attention to fathers and even brothers and sisters, although usually considered in isolation (Dunn, 1983; McKee and O'Brien, 1982; Parke, 1981). Very little is known about young children's wider relationships outside the family, except of course for everyone's not inconsiderable observations from their own lives (O'Donnell, 1983). Sociologists have written theoretically about childhood (Dreitzel, 1973; Jenks, 1982), but only rarely have they studied empirically the lives of real children below school age (Denzin, 1977; Furstenberg, 1985). Our systematic knowledge comes therefore largely from observational studies in psychology, general surveys and a limited number of service-oriented investigations. By these means a fair amount of information has been gathered about the pre-school care of children in groups (particularly in nurseries) but this has not been understood as part of children's overall life experience at home and outside (Bronfenbrenner, 1979).

For a long time two main considerations dominated expert thinking about shared care. On the one hand there was an overriding concern about possible emotional damage which might be done to children. This linked to the strong and persistent belief that young children need to be with their mothers as much as possible. This applied particularly to infants. On the other hand, benefits have been perceived to arise from involvement in pre-school groups at least after the age of three. Amongst the benefits of these which have been put forward are educational improvements and compensation for disadvantages in children's home life. Opinions about this are affected by views about the role of government as well as about families and children. Some people see pre-school facilities as essential or desirable. Others see them as a luxury or believe that they foster the abnegation of parental (i.e. maternal) duties. Even those with similar opinions about the value of pre-school groups may differ over the priority they think should be given to them from public funds.

In recent years this whole subject has acquired a special relevance and topicality as a result of the feminist critiques of conventional family and child care patterns (Finch and Groves, 1983; New and David, 1985). This means that it is no longer adequate to consider children's needs narrowly in relation to what mothers ought to do (either directly or through participation in pre-school arrangements). It is necessary to examine the responsibilities and rights of men and women, parents and others, in relation to the care of our children. Although the focus of the present discussion is with 'external' sharing (i.e. by people other than parents), this will be shown to interact in important ways with what might be called 'internal' sharing between parents. Whatever stance is taken about the right way or ways to balance the interests of children, women and men, there is no doubt that the issue of shared care is a central one.

In the remainder of this chapter, I shall examine briefly what previous research has revealed about the nature of shared care. That is followed by a brief sketch of the main issues involved in relevant social policy discussions. Finally, the rationale and methods of the present study will be presented to show how it sought to map out and connect some parts of the terra incognita in this area of knowledge.

The extent and nature of shared care

It is convenient to deal separately with non-official and official shared care arrangements. The latter are those which are publicly provided or regulated, such as day nurseries and childminding. By convention, most writers also include nursery schooling and playgroups as forms of day *care*, because these all look after children in the absence of their parents although their primary purpose is to offer social and/or educational experiences for the child (Taylor *et al.*, 1972). Much less is known about non-official than official forms of care but these are much more important for the great majority of children under three. Scant information exists about how the two forms of care affect each other.

From the few investigations which have asked parents about shared care within their networks it is clear that by the age of two the majority of children have stayed away from their parents at some time. They are most likely to stay with relatives and less commonly with neighbours or parents' friends (Douglas and Blomfield, 1958; GHS, 1979; Rosser and Harris, 1965). It is not often made explicit but most of the people who are referred to as carers are women. Sharing care seems to occur *on average* more often for middle-class children than working-class children and perhaps more frequently for boys than girls (Allan, 1979; Honey, 1973).

The information available about why and how people share care with relatives, friends and neighbours is very sketchy, except for those arrangements made in connection with mothers' work. It has been an oft-repeated preconception even among experts that childminding is the 'principal form of looking after children of working mothers' (Bruner, 1980: 27). But all the evidence shows that when both parents work then care of the children by relatives (especially grandparents) and by parents themselves is consistently more common than either childminding or nursery care (Moss, 1976; Thompson and Finlayson, 1963; Yudkin and Holme, 1963). This discrepancy between beliefs and reality stems from the fact that people tend to visualise such mothers as working full-time. In reality the vast majority of those with young children work part-time. All the recent increase in the number of mothers of under-fives who are working is accounted for by part-time arrangements (Moss, 1980).

About two thirds of all children will have attended some form of official group at some point by the time they reach the age of five (Osborn *et al.*, 1984; van der Eycken *et al.*, 1979). The attendance rate is lower at any fixed point in time when between one quarter and one third of children under five are estimated to have a place (Bone, 1977). The two forms of official care attended by easily the largest numbers of children are playgroups and nursery schools. (To avoid repetition nursery schools will be taken to include nursery classes which are attached to primary schools.) As a result of both increased provision and a decline in the birth rate, the percentage of children going to one or the other of these doubled during the 1970s, although the absolute increase in places was smaller (GHS, 1979; SED, 1980). All these forms of care usually restrict entry to children aged at least three years (occasionally two and a half), so that most of those children who attend any kind of daily group facility do so for one or two years immediately before they start school.

Unlike nursery schools and playgroups, childminding and day nurseries provide places for children for a full day (roughly 9–5) and cater for those aged under as well as over three. They are used by far fewer families. It is generally agreed that official statistics about the number of children looked after by childminders are misleading because many minders do not notify their local authorities and registers also usually include some people who are no longer minding (Jackson, 1971; Yudkin, 1967). There is less consensus about the true numbers of children cared for by minders. Estimates vary enormously from 100,000 (J. Tizard *et al.*, 1976) to 300,000 (Jackson, 1975). Whatever the real figure may be, it seems clear that it is much larger than the number of children who attend day nurseries (26,000). Both taken together make up quite a small proportion of all the children aged under five in Britain of over 3½ million (CPRS, 1978).

How far does the actual usage of different care forms correspond with what people want? Again this question has been asked almost exclusively in relation to official services. The geographical distribution of facilities is irregular and so the variations in what is available may well affect people's perceptions of what they want (Blackstone, 1971; Packman, 1968). Even so, there is evidence that on a national as well as a local scale, parents' expressed desire for some kind of daytime care outside their network represents twice as many families as are currently using such services (Bone, 1977; Moss and Plewis, 1976). The greatest discrepancy between supply and demand occurs when children are aged two (Table 1.1).

It is little use knowing about the levels of demand for care if the reasons for it are not understood. Some important survey

Table 1.1 *Usage and desire for day care at different ages*

Age	Usage	Desire
All under-fives	32% (46%)	64% (64%)
0–1	4% (6%)	20% (17%)
1–2	8% (12%)	41% (44%)
2–3	19% (43%)	72% (73%)
3–4	47% (72%)	87% (90%)
4–5	72% (80%)	90% (91%)

All the numbers are percentages of those interviewed. The figures given first are from Bone's national study (1977), while those in parentheses refer to the study by Moss and Plewis (1976) in three areas of London. Note that the London usage figures are considerably higher, but the desire rates are almost identical.

reports have largely ignored the reasons why people want day care, which conveys the impression of a uniform large demand for the same thing. As it happens, parents' needs and wishes are more complex than this. Demand for pre-schooling has been explained in terms of rising female employment, reduced network support and increased social or expert pressures (Leach, 1979; J. Tizard *et al.*, 1976). In fact, mothers' employment is an important factor for only a small minority of those wanting group care. Most parents say they want group care for their children's social or educational benefit. They want opportunities for them to be stimulated, play, make friends and prepare for school (Blatchford *et al.*, 1982; Haystead *et al.*, 1980).

It is helpful to place our understanding of these current British patterns in context by reflecting on the range of shared care arrangements and attitudes which have existed at other times and in other cultures. In most societies the care of children is provided mainly by females. Usually mothers are the prime carers, as in Britain (Barry and Paxson, 1971). On the other hand, our society appears unusual in stressing the constant companionship of the mother before the age of three. It has also been unique in establishing formal groups of children in narrow age bands after they are three years old under the supervision of people previously unknown to them, though this pattern has now spread widely. In most other societies there is ready access by young children to a much broader range of adults and also to older children as playmates and carers (Blurton-Jones, 1974; Smith, 1980; Weisner and Gallimore, 1977). In non-industrial societies it appears to be quite normal for women to do productive work soon after childbirth. They carry the infant while working, stay close to the home or entrust care of the child to other people – usually close kin (Dahlberg, 1981; Oakley, 1974a; Schapera, 1971). Among many peoples sharing care appears to occur earlier, more frequently and for more extended periods than is generally the case in Britain (Dunn and Kendrick, 1982; Tizard and Tizard, 1971). Such patterns were apparently also more prevalent in Europe in the Middle Ages than they are nowadays (Aries, 1971; Hunt, 1970).

The implications of sharing care

Only three sorts of shared care have been closely examined to determine what their consequences may be. These are separations from mothers in unfamiliar surroundings; arrangements made by working mothers; and children in group care. The main concern has been with possible emotional difficulties these situations may cause for the child. That choice of topics is not neutral; it results from worries which many people have that sharing care may be harmful for children. Important though that issue is, it does mean that little attention has been given to the effects of different ways of sharing care on the adults concerned or what may be their wider social and societal implications.

In the 1950s and 1960s, much of the thinking about shared care was dominated by the idea that young children need to have a unique attachment to one person (normally their mother) and by the notion that infants and toddlers lack interest in interaction with children of the same age. The idea was promulgated that separation of a child from his or her mother for all but the briefest periods was likely to have *by itself* harmful long-term effects on the child. John Bowlby became famous for applying the term 'maternal deprivation' as a general explanation for the ill-effects of such varied phenomena as 'broken homes', poor quality care in large institutions and short separations from a mother-figure in an experimental setting (Ainsworth, 1962, 1965; Bowlby, 1965, 1969, 1973). The theory of maternal deprivation was sometimes used by others in ways that the authors later disclaimed or qualified. However, at the time, Bowlby's writings made it clear that he regarded all but very brief, occasional absences from the mother as undesirable. His narrow concentration on the mother-child relationship failed to take into account adequately the role and importance of fathers let alone children's wider family and social networks. It has since become clear that the interpretations put on the evidence at that time reflected prevailing views about motherhood and that alternative explanations are possible. More careful reviews of the relevant research have subsequently shown that the reported damage to children in some kind of substitute care usually resulted from unloving, unstimulating or very inconsistent care rather than separation or loss per se (Rutter, 1980a; Schaffer, 1977). The children to whom the term *maternal* deprivation was applied had been deprived not only of their mothers but also of their fathers, brothers, sisters and many features of a normal home life. It must be borne in mind, though, that even now the body of relevant and carefully controlled research remains small and not conclusive (Silverstein, 1981). Even when substantial damage from prolonged deprivation of normal parenting does occur, the prospects for the child can still be much improved even after the age of five by placing him or her in a suitable adoptive family (Kadushin, 1970; Tizard, 1977). In any case, although inferences were in fact applied to less extreme situations, conclusions about gross deprivation have little bearing on briefer separations from parents in everyday life. Moreover, distress arising from short separations can occur with any familiar person, not just mothers (Lamb, 1976; Schaffer and Emerson, 1964). It is now recognised that children have a range of needs which can perhaps be met by a single person, but also by a number of people in combination (Lewis and Feiring, 1978; Schaffer, 1985). Indeed, older babies and toddlers have a propensity to form attachments to several people who are familiar and responsive to them (Smith, 1979; Schaffer and Emerson, 1964). Nor are children under three uninterested in others of the same age, as has sometimes been suggested by misapplying findings about parallel play and cognitive egocentricity. In fact they show great interest in playing with their peers from infancy onwards. This is accompanied by adept observational, turn-taking and interactive skills, albeit naturally of a different kind and speed from those of older children (Becker, 1977; Corsaro, 1981; Cox, 1980).

Much of the more specific research on the effects of shared care has been prompted by an assumption or fear that mothers' employment outside the home (unlike fathers') harms young children. There are several reasons why it is unwise to generalise about this. Mothers who work do so for very different length of time and with a wide array of care forms, so no simple comparison with non-working mothers is possible. In addition there are outside factors which can both influence the decision for a mother to work and affect the child. In particular, when working mothers were fewer they included a higher proportion of those with material or social difficulties. Therefore they were more likely to have children with problems whether they worked or not. Nearly all more recent comparisons between working and non-working mothers which allow for these external influences have refuted earlier reports about the apparent bad effects of mothers' work (Davie *et al.*, 1972; Etaugh, 1974; Hoffman, 1979).

Another widespread belief is that it is wrong for young children to spend much time in nursery groups apart from their parents, especially before three years of age. Attempts to test if that is really the case have also proved fraught with methodological difficulties: nurseries and other kinds of group are diverse in their nature, hours and age span. Furthermore, it is difficult to assess whether features associated with attendance are caused by that experience or result from family or other circumstances which may lead to attendance. Even then, interpretation of effects can be difficult and subjective. What one person sees favourably as independence may be viewed less happily as non-conformity by another (Webb, 1977).

The immediate effects of entry to group care seem to be short-lived. Some children are upset when starting but more typical is temporary watchful passivity which soon gives way to sociable participation (McGrew, 1972a, 1972b; Schwartz *et al.*, 1974). With regard to longer term consequences, Glass concluded as long ago as 1947 that group care causes no problem in itself compared with home care, when differences in family circumstances are allowed for. This finding has been reaffirmed many times (e.g. Harper, 1978; Rubenstein *et al.*, 1981). Group care does not appear to lessen children's trust in their mothers, but can mean that the child has additional people as sources of comfort (Caldwell, 1973; Kagan, 1979). It has also been shown to help children's social skills and capacity to make friends from an early age (Cornelius and Denney, 1975; Rubin, 1980). It seems that primary school entrants who have been to nursery school tend to be more confident and independent than others, but may also be more restless (Morsbach *et al.*, 1981; Thompson, 1975; Widlake, 1971). However, the differences are not large, perhaps because other relevant experience in the comparison groups, notably playgroup attendance, has not always been taken into account.

Just when the concern about the emotional effects on pre-school children of non-maternal care was at its height, a contrary notion gained support that they might benefit cognitively from special groups, at least after they were three years old. New educational methods and rather simplified interpretations of research evidence appeared to show that major teaching inputs in pre-school groups could have lasting intellectual benefits (Clark, 1967). It was soon realised that some of the claims made for this had been exaggerated. Thorough reviews by Bronfenbrenner (1975) and Tizard (1974) clearly demonstrated that substantial immediate gains in language and intelligence can occur but the effect soon dissipates. Moreover, the advantages of very early schooling accrue mainly to those from disadvantaged backgrounds or with low initial ability levels. The impact of pre-school education on the later intellectual performance of children with at least average ability appears to be minimal. More lasting improvements can result if the child's family are systematically involved and if extra educational inputs persist throughout the school career (Halsey, 1980; Rutter, 1980b; Woodhead, 1976).

Whilst research about day centres has in the main failed to support common prejudices, some of the empirical work relating to childminding has upheld the negative public image.

Worrying instances of poor and even dangerous physical conditions have been observed. A considerable number of minders in poor inner city areas apparently offer limited stimulation and responsiveness. Many children stay only a short while and may experience one or more changes of minder (Jackson and Jackson, 1979; Mayall and Petrie, 1977, 1983). Fortunately, two recent studies by Bryant *et al.* (1980) and Shinman (1981) give a more balanced picture. These researchers described minders as being in the main warm-hearted women with strong local ties. They offered good everyday experience to the children they looked after. Carefully controlled research from Germany suggests that for children in disadvantaged circumstances it can be more beneficial to have supplemantary care from publicly supported and trained minders than to remain with their mothers nearly all the time (Gudat and Permien, 1980; Swift, 1982).

The availability and organisation of day care options

Scientific and expert knowledge such as we have just briefly looked at has only a partial and often indirect influence on the ideas and actions of the representatives, officials and lobby groups who seek to determine the actual policies affecting shared care. The next few sections will deal together with both the activity of policy making/implementation and commentaries on those actions. These are what Pinker (1971) has called the 'institutional' and 'intellectual' aspects of social policy respectively. Most policy discussion has looked at day care in the narrow sense of that which is officially provided or regulated. This occurs even when authors begin with definitions which cover sharing care in its widest sense (e.g. Fein and Clarke-Stewart, 1973; Tizard, 1976). Nonetheless, official policy often rests on implicit assumptions that care of pre-school children should be carried out primarily or even exclusively by the 'community' rather than by publicly provided facilities (Land and Parker, 1978). Consequently it is pertinent to look at how far existing services do in fact fit with families' wishes and their capacities to make the child care arrangements they want from within their own networks and neighbourhoods (Barnes and Connelly, 1978; Parker, 1974). Several

full historical analyses of official policy developments exist so
it is unnecessary to repeat a chronological account here (see,
for example, J. Tizard *et al.*, 1976; van der Eycken, 1977).
Instead, there will be an examination of the ways in which
policy actions and inaction influence the availability of
different forms of shared care to different kinds of people. This
will be followed by a brief analysis of the main influences on
public policy and proposed strategies for future policy.

During the last one hundred years there have been fluctuations and inconsistencies in the extent to which public or
'government' participation in child care before the age of five
has been seen as legitimate, desirable or affordable. There has
also been uncertainty about the extent to which pre-school
facilities should be concerned with health, education or welfare
functions. Day nurseries began as a health service facility
located mainly in inner city areas. The number of places was
considerably expanded in both World Wars to facilitate the
contribution of working mothers to the war effort. However,
many were closed or converted soon afterwards. Provision of
day nursery places is now very limited and access to them is
largely restricted to those in special categories, such as children in single parent families or who are 'at risk'. They are
now run by social work departments. In contrast, there has
been a substantial expansion in nursery schooling. This
occurred under the aegis of yet a third department (education).
However, developments have often been largely segregated
from mainstream educational provision for older children.
Local authorities do have a legal power to make provision for
under-fives but there is no duty to do so as there is with respect
to the over-fives. Since there is no obligation to guarantee
nursery school places when parents want them they are
restricted to children aged three plus, uneven in geographical
coverage and variable in attendance hours. In 1967 the
Plowden Report espoused an ideal of meeting the demand
for places everywhere, though not necessarily for the hours
wanted. This principle was accepted in the Government White
Papers of 1972. However, as in the past, there was only a brief
commitment to growth before retrenchment occurred (Penn,
1982; Whitbread, 1972).

Services provided through central or local government are

often available in other forms. It is important to understand how such alternatives supplement or substitute for public provision and to examine the influence of government policies on this non-public arena (Titmuss, 1976). The shortfall in public provision for the under-fives has fostered the expansion of a vigorous voluntary sector. The rapid expansion of the playgroup movement since the 1960s has been a remarkable example of the development of mutual-aid. Beginning as an attempt by parents to provide the pre-school experience the state was failing to offer, playgroups subsequently established a distinctive identity and philosophy which emphasises participation by mothers in the organisation and day to day running of the groups (Crowe, 1973). Some have been set up and run by charitable bodies and private individuals, however. In the last decade a more radical form of self-help has arisen in the form of community nurseries. These vary in form but are usually run partly or completely by groups of local parents. They offer full-day care for children from an early age and seek to provide a multi-purpose community resource (Garvey, 1974; Sutton, 1981).

Very little is known about private nurseries, schools and playgroups, especially as they are not differentiated from voluntary playgroups in official records. Doubt has been expressed about the quality of care in some private nurseries given that the fees are too low to pay for adequate staffing (EOC, 1978). Apparently, new private schools and classes have opened to meet demand as cutbacks in the public sector have occurred (Clark, 1978). Childminding is also usually arranged and paid for privately. It constitutes the main form of full-day care available for children of all ages and has little rationing of access except by cost. From a parental viewpoint, minding often calls for a large percentage of income, but for the minder the fees provide small financial rewards for long hours without customary employment benefits. Therefore, some people have sought to redefine minding as skilled work with entitlements to better pay, training and contracts (Hannon, 1978; Jackson and Jackson, 1979).

By and large workplace day care has not figured promi-nently in British policy discussions compared with places like Eastern Europe, China or even the United States. In the whole of Britain there are fewer than one hundred creches provided by employers and these are mostly for children over two (Day, 1975; Hermann and Komlosi, 1972; Kessen, 1975; Moss, 1978). Perhaps even more crucial to shared care options is the extent of co-operation between employers and both parents in organising their time to fit with child care needs. Rare examples of this are job sharing and job twinning (Rapoport and Rapoport, 1976, 1978). In Sweden there is considerable support for either or both parents of infants to work part-time (Karre, 1973; Lijlestrom, 1978). The tax and allowance system ('fiscal welfare') can also affect parents' decisions about how they share care. In Britain, unlike the United States, child care expenses are not normally deductible from taxable income but they can be allowed for in Supplementary Benefit payments (Allbeson and Douglas, 1982; EOC, 1979; Zigler and Gordon, 1982).

Until the 1970s the non-public sectors of day care were either ignored by governments or else simply made subject to local authority regulation without any kind of positive assistance. Recently there have been attempts to provide limited moral and in some cases financial support. This has applied particularly to childminding and playgroups which have been seen as low-cost alternatives to public day care. There have only been piece-meal local initiatives, however. In any case properly supported projects are not cheap (Willmott and Challis, 1977; Phillips, 1976).

It is evident that Britain lacks the coherent organisation of pre-school care which can be found in some other countries (OECD, 1975). This can be seen either as a healthy diversity of choice or a restrictive fragmentation of services. Partly out of some dissatisfaction with the previous lack of co-ordination, there has been a trend in the last decade towards both a common range of functions offered by different services and closer co-operation between them. Functional convergence is illustrated by the attempts within all the care forms to provide a more comprehensive and skilled service (Ferri, 1978; Moss, 1978). Increasingly, attempts have been made to foster co-operation between different forms of daytime care which remain separate but have interdependent functions (Watt, 1976). Many commentators believe this should be taken further by allocating responsibility for all pre-school care to one government department, usually education. This could enable the provision of a non-divisive service which is available to everyone for the hours they want, without stigma and including a teaching component for the children. Recently, Scotland's most populous region has accepted just such a plan (Strathclyde, 1985). For similar reasons, some voluntary agencies and local authorities have made operational changes and provide a range of services in a single 'combined centre' (Hughes *et al.*, 1980). Ideally these should be able to meet every child's needs, whether it be for physical care, social interaction or educational experience, for short periods or longer periods. In practice such centres have encountered difficulties because of the differing traditions, beliefs and work conditions of the staff (Ferri *et al.*, 1981, 1982).

Challis (1980) has argued forcibly that organisational issues should be set aside whilst efforts are made to clarify agreed aims for day care. Unfortunately, views about what arrangements can or should be made for young children and their parents are so diverse, emotionally charged and at times incompatible that a clear consensus is improbable.

Influences on policy and ideas embodied in policy

Government policy in the day care field has been affected by a number of demographic, economic and social factors. These have operated in association or in conflict with ideas about the nature of children, the family and state intervention. Fluctuations in the number of under-fives has affected allocation of resources and modified their per capita impact (SWSG, 1976; Osborn, 1981b). The steady rise in the paid employment of mothers coupled with the concentration of most work opportunities outside the home has been widely perceived as a major pressure for more non-maternal care. Both World Wars witnessed temporary transformations in the government's willingness to expand group care places so that more women could work (Ferguson and Fitzgerald, 1954). Wartime insecurity and separations may have contributed to the emphasis which was placed in the post-war periods on nuclear family attachments (Crowe, 1973; Fletcher, 1973). Last but not least, the country's poor economic performance has repeatedly led to reversals in group care expansion programmes.

Differing assumptions about what children and mothers can or should do have resulted in opposing ideas about the value of non-maternal care in its various forms. Young children have often been portrayed as vulnerable, indifferent to social interaction and unable to cope emotionally or cognitively with different environments, especially before the age of three (Baers, 1954; Hassenstein, 1974; Pringle, 1975; Schmutzler, 1976). In official pronouncements about day care it has been repeatedly asserted that public services should be confined to children with special needs or in special circumstances. These have been accompanied by admonitions that young children should ordinarily be at home and should be there with their mother (Hadow, 1933; Fonda, 1976). Critics of such traditional wisdom put forward an alternative view that interaction with peers and with non-parent adults can enhance social and practical competence in children more than exclusive mothering (Fein and Clarke-Stewart, 1973; Lewis and Rosenblum, 1975; Liegle, 1974). It has been remarked that efforts to confine mothers to the home are motivated mainly by economic convenience and result in the suppression of women's rights and talents (Hughes et al., 1980; Murray, 1975). Feminists argue that both mothers and children can benefit from extensive alternative experience, whilst men should take more responsibility for child care which could make their lives more fulfilling too (Hagen, 1973; Land, 1978).

Policy in relation to sharing care often concerns the division of responsibility between the family and wider society as represented by central and local government. Officially provided day care services have been regarded variously as supportive of parental fulfilment; the guarantor of good quality care; the basis of proper intellectual development in the child; and the prerequisite for wider parental choice (Rapoport et al., 1977; TUC, 1977). But others have seen state provision as undermining family responsibility and expropriating family functions (Coote and Hewitt, 1980; Lasch, 1977; Mount, 1982; Wicks, 1983). Berger and Berger (1983:205) argue that women should ideally prefer to devote themselves full-time to their children but if they choose to work 'they should not expect

public policy to underwrite and subsidise their life-plans'. Such
a view ignores men's responsibilities for their children and is
inconsistent with society's investment of time and money in
girls' education. It leaves out of account that the public has
an interest in maximising individuals' range of choices and
reducing the stress which full-time motherhood brings in
many cases. Ideals of nuclear family privacy and extended
family obligation have been used to justify minimal intervention by society, except to buttress those unfortunate
enough to be without available kin (Land and Parker, 1978).
Within such implicit models of family life are assumptions
about 'the centrality of family obligations in determining life-
styles of women, especially wives' and of the secondary importance of women's attachment to the labour market (Finch and
Groves, 1980:501). Thus, 'community', 'family' or 'parental
responsibility' often act as code phrases for women's duty.

The strong commitment to expansion of nursery schooling
in the 1970s after a long period of inactivity was prompted by
beliefs that this would be an investment in the future generation. There was a renewed and overoptimistic faith that early
entry to the education system could not only lead to cognitive
benefits, but could also have a wider role in tackling deprivation (Chazan, 1973; Roby, 1973). Such ideas also provided
the fertile soil without which the playgroup movement, germi-
nated by a letter to the *Guardian*, might never have blossomed. Following disappointment that pre-schooling does not
by itself lead to prolonged changes, it seems more realistic
to cherish its intrinsic short-term merits and attractions for
children regardless of whether there are long-term educational
benefits or not.

The main day care policy strategies

These diverse influences have led to government policies which
have been inconsistent from one time to another and uneven
in their local impact. Consequently, they have been reproved
for opposite reasons by different people. For example Leach
(1979) denounced what she believes to be government's
excessive substitution for parental responsibility whilst
Hughes *et al.* (1980) deplored what they believe has been inad-

equate supplementation to parental care. In order to summarise the various goals and attitudes espoused by both proponents and critics of government policies it is useful to draw on the outline made by Rein (1976) of three main frameworks for action which he discerned in social policy. These are differentiated according to their main target – individuals, institutions or power systems (Table 1.2). Of course, particular policy statements or practical actions may combine elements of more than one framework.

The individualist 'child welfare' view is most long-standing and has been most influential. It suggests that there are limited resources which should therefore be devoted particularly to those in special circumstances (Chaplin, 1975; Pringle and Naidoo, 1975). It is argued that mothers should be encouraged to look after children most of the time, although playgroups are acceptable for short periods after the child is aged three (Leach, 1979; Wilby, 1980). Proponents of an individualist strategy do want some wider changes, but more in terms of societal values than service provision. It is argued that motherhood embracing full responsibility for a child should remain central but be portrayed more realistically and less glamorously. Moreover, it should be accorded high status as a vital function for society. In this way being a 'full-time' mother would become more attractive with more achievable expectations and greater self-esteem. The preferred policy option from the individualist perspective consists of high child care allowances to enable mothers to stay home without financial strain.

In contrast to the mainly educational and fiscal elements of an individualist strategy an institutional framework for action entails the extension of publicly funded child care services. A common aim is to achieve a level of provision which is both universal and comprehensive, i.e. open to all free of charge and offering a wide range of functions (Hughes *et al.*, 1980; TUC, 1977). What parents want should be the only criterion of access, rather than ability to pay or expert judgments of need. To meet demand in this way would involve much expense. In times of recession, there has been reluctance to commit public money to something which has a precarious value in that its worth for individuals and society at large

Table 1.2 Policy strategies and sharing care

Policy action framework	Description	Roughly equivalent shared care strategy	Desired outcome
INDIVIDUALIST	Favours small-scale support by government to individuals deemed to be unable to cope. The majority are assumed to be able to make satisfactory arrangements individually.	TRADITIONAL OR CHILD WELFARE APPROACH	Selective public day care services for the needy, e.g. single parents, children at risk. 'Low-cost alternatives' may be encouraged, too.
INSTITUTIONAL	Supports expansion of communal services, sometimes accompanied by changes in their form or administrative structures.	UNIVERSAL PUBLIC SERVICES	Comprehensive public services available free on demand, particularly in the form of combined centres.
STRUCTURAL	Proposes basic transformation in the arrangements of people's influence and command over resources.	RADICAL OR FEMINIST	Social changes in access to finance and care forms. OR Redistribution of child care between women and men.

Adapted from Rein (1976).

remains controversial (Clark, 1956; Uttley, 1980). Some people support childminding rather than pre-school group care as an institution to be strengthened. Minders are seen to provide personalised care embedded in everyday life in the community (Davidson, 1970; Emlen, 1973). Likewise, financial and other help has been advocated for playgroups and community nurseries as a means of consolidating or expanding their contribution of more intimate care arrangements and neighbourhood co-operation.

The most prominent 'structural' changes suggested in the day care field entail reallocation of power, resources of opportunities between women and men. Whereas an 'individualist' approach seeks to raise the status of women as equal in worth to men *but different*, structural change would confer on women equal *and identical* rights to those of men. For some this necessitates an array of services such as home makers and in particular widely available day care centres open for long hours and with an early age of entry (Challis, 1974; Clarke-Stewart, 1982). Such strategies have been attempted in countries like Cuba, China and the USSR. They have had some limited success in facilitating greater female participation in the labour market (Stone, 1981; Williams and Winston, 1980). Such policies are only superficially egalitarian if care is simply transferred from one set of women (mothers) to another set (female carers). A more substantial transformation would be to alter attitudes and work organisation so that both women and men are equally available to their young children (Lecoultre, 1976; Mayo, 1977).

The present study

The foregoing discussion has revealed that policy has been based on apparently confident assumptions which are made about what parents actually do and what they want with regard to sharing care. Yet empirical knowledge about this is far from complete. In particular, little is known about less formal arrangements which are made within family networks or how these fit in with parents' usage and appraisals of organised groups. Several writers have regretted the lack of knowledge about non-group care and its impact on child and adult relationships, work patterns and neighbourhood functioning (Belsky and Steinberg, 1978; Schorr, 1974; Tizard, 1974). These then are the aspects which the current study concentrated on. Furthermore it sought to place shared care in the wider context of families' overall social contacts. In this way sharing care would not be considered in isolation from the rest of people's lives. Indeed, it could act as a means of illuminating some of the processes and structures of family life.

The theoretical basis for the research is described in more detail elsewhere (Hill, 1984). Insights were gained from more than one school of thought in sociology, psychology and anthropology. Each one of these could have provided a satisfactory overall framework in itself to handle some important features of sharing care. Yet each would also have difficulty in dealing with other vital aspects so it was preferred to blend elements from several perspectives to arrive at a more complete picture.

An important influence on the research was the interpretive approach which has become popular in sociology partly as a reaction to quantitative or 'scientific' methods which are seen as too deterministic and abstracted from the complexity of real life (Bell and Newby, 1977; Wright Mills, 1970; Wrong, 1961). Consequently, instead of trying to obtain outside measures of behaviour, emphasis is placed on how people themselves describe and explain what they are doing or have done. In relation to marriage and parenthood, the task of the researcher becomes one of understanding and categorising family members' accounts to identify the main kinds of ways in which they differ or are similar. Parents' views are not regarded as fixed or predetermined but as evolving through exposure to common-sense ideas, general knowledge and the media. More particularly, people's perceptions of family life are modified in the light of discussion with and observation of other parents. Watching and interacting with children, especially your own, is also a major opportunity for developing ideas too, of course (Backett, 1982; Berger and Kellner, 1965; La Rossa and Wolf, 1985). Important though this approach is, it has tended to leave out of the picture the structural and environmental influences which have been the bread and butter of more traditional sociology. In psychology, too, external real-life influences on children have often been ignored, this time because of the concern to carry out studies under experimental conditions or observe children in specific contexts, notably day care centres. An ecological perspective is a useful corrective to these biases. For instance Bronfenbrenner (1977, 1979) and Belsky and Steinberg (1978) have suggested a framework applicable to day care which takes account of the mutual interaction amongst the contexts of household, network, neighbourhood, work and class (Table 1.3). Recently, too, psychologists have tried to rectify earlier descriptions of parent-child interaction as a largely one-way process by emphasising that children are active not passive participants in what happens in families. Their general temperament and character as well as their specific actions can affect how their parents behave. That may be as important as parents' influences on children (Lerner and Spanier, 1978b; Sameroff, 1975a, 1975b).

Exchange and network theories give more specific insights into the social aspects of parents' choices of carers and relationships with them. Understanding the relationship between parents and carers was assisted by seeing this as a form of social exchange (Befu, 1977; Ekeh, 1974; Pinker, 1979). Sharing care is in one sense a service concerning which people have different expectations as to how far it is necessary or desirable to 'give' something to the carer in return for looking after the child, whether in cash, by a reciprocal service or in some other way. Carers are already part of or else become members of a family's social network. Theories about networks have focused on the nature of the linkages between network members, as much if not more so than the purpose or content of the relationship itself. Of particular relevance to the present topic was the key insight of Bott (1957) that there is a mutual interaction of relationships within families and between family members and people outside. She made a specific hypothesis that the extent to which a couple's network members know each other varies systematically according to the degree of segregation of marital roles. In the following decade this hypothesis was put to the test by several other people, but thereafter her more general insight about the connection between the inner and outer aspects of family relationships was lost sight of as mathematical analyses of network structures were carried out in isolation from research

Table 1.3 *The four ecological systems of child development*

System	Definition	Description	Example relating to day care
MICROSYSTEM	A person's immediate setting	The pattern of roles and activities and interpersonal relationships experienced in a particular setting	Adult models or age groupings in different day care settings
MESOSYSTEM	Interrelations between two or more settings in which a developing person participates	The prime mesosystems are home and day care, and family and work	Influences on parents of care-takers, or on parental roles of shared parenting
EXOSYSTEM	One or more settings, in which the person is not active, but in which there are events that affect or are affected by him	The processes by which outer settings influence the child or family	Effects on day care of work, marital relationship and functioning of the neighbourhood
MACROSYSTEM	The consistencies in the lower order systems which are present at the level of culture and subculture	This is the level at which beliefs, ideology and public policy impinge	Impact on day care of societal attitudes to care of children, family functions and women's roles

Adapted from Bronfenbrenner (1979) and Belsky and Steinberg (1978).

into marital or parent-child relationships. Yet a cardinal issue for a study of sharing care seems to be the way in which decisions are made distributing child care between husband and wife, on the one hand, and between the parents and other people, on the other. This ties in with feminist criticisms of conventional approaches to studying and theorising about families. These have illuminated the differential impact of parenthood on men's and women's satisfactions and choices. No current study of family life should remain untouched by this perspective. Consequently it is vital to acknowledge the distribution between men and women of both the tasks and responsibilities involved in primary and shared care. These have major implications for the experiences and opportunities of men, women and children (Morgan, 1975; Roberts, 1981).

It followed from these diverse theoretical influences that this study aimed to look at the internal processes of a family and external influences. This dual approach was assisted by the use of both numerical and non-numerical evidence. Information which could be quantified would be helpful in discerning the systematic influences on family members' behaviour of social and environmental factors and personal characteristics. More qualitative or 'soft' data was essential to see how people explain and make sense of their own actions, the nature of children and social relationships. To seek both kinds of data can result in a loss of representativeness compared with surveys and a loss of richness compared with intensive studies. Hopefully, sufficient breadth and depth was achieved to produce a combination that may be more fruitful than just one or the other.

In small-scale research, there is a conflict between maximising the representativeness of the sample and minimising the number of significant variables. As it was hoped to understand a spectrum of practices and attitudes, it seemed desirable to investigate as far as possible a general section of the population rather than a sample selected for particular problems or usage of limited types of care. In order to simplify comparisons within the sample it was planned to restrict the study to two parent families, so that the relationship between internal and external sharing could be looked at. In addition, the ages of the children concerned were stan-

dardised. The age of three years was chosen as it was intermediate between infants and older pre-school children who
have received most research attention. On the basis of previous
research it was foreseen that some would have started at group
care and others not, so that comparisons could be made
between attenders and non-attenders. It had also been shown
that this is the age at which parental reports of problem behaviour reach a peak and there is the maximum discrepancy
between desire for group care and its availability (Bone, 1977;
Jenkins *et al.*, 1980). At an early stage, it was decided to meet
with parents, rather than carers or children. They would be
in a position to give an overview of their child's care history
to date and offer an integrated, albeit partial perspective on
that. Alternative methods such as observations of children or
discussions with carers would have been fine for a different
kind of study focusing on one specific care setting, but were
less well suited to the broad purposes of this research.

The investigation was carried out in the city of Edinburgh,
which forms part of Lothian region. This has the highest rate
of nursery school provision of all the local authorities in Scotland. Indeed the overall level of places in pre-school groups
(relative to the population of under-fives) is one of the highest
in Britain (McFadyen, 1977; van der Eycken *et al.*, 1979). The
policy of expansion continued larger than in many other places
and only came to a halt just after the present study took place
(Nursery Concerned, 1983–5; Wilson, 1981; Young, 1983).
Therefore Edinburgh presented the opportunity to examine
sharing care in an area which is comparatively rich in officially run pre-school facilities at a peak period of provision.

The ecological framework favoured a small area study. This
would also permit some familiarisation with the neighbourhood where the children lived and with the group care
provision available locally. It was decided to see families from
two areas rather than one to highlight contrasts in patterns
of shared care under different conditions. A two area approach
can also be a convenient way of obtaining a comparison by
social class. It was considered important to do this, because of
the known effects of socio-economic status on sharing care and
indeed numerous related aspects of family life (e.g. Newson
and Newson, 1963, 1970a). On the other hand, it must be

remembered that most of the class contrasts which have been identified involve differences in percentages which are sometimes quite small. The feature concerned may nevertheless become characterised as typically middle class or working class whereas it is simply rather more common in that class. After reviewing the relevant research, Littman *et al.* (1957) concluded that dissimilarities in child-rearing between members of different classes were neither general nor profound. Socialisation studies have often produced conflicting results or used inadequate methods to assess and measure child-bearing patterns (Johnsen and Leslie, 1965; Zigler and Child, 1973). For all these reasons it was essential to be cautious about generalising from any class distinctions which emerged in the study, especially as they would be derived only from two small areas. Furthermore it would be important to pay heed to similarities across social class.

It was decided to select two municipal wards roughly equidistant from the centre of Edinburgh. Demographic and social indicators for all the wards in the city were examined and ranked in order to choose one area of comparative advantage (Milburn) and one of considerable disadvantage (Whitlaw). Milburn is a residential area of traditional respectability and a high proportion of professional workers. Whitlaw is an industrial area, criss-crossed by rail, road and canal routes. It has poor housing and those people in work are mostly employed in manual or service occupations.

The ideal sampling frame would have been an up-to-date list of all families with children aged three. Attempts to gain access to such a list proved unsuccessful so instead names and addresses were extracted from centralised birth records. An important and unwished-for effect of approaching families of three-year-olds at the birth address was the exclusion of families who had moved in the meantime. Those who remained at their address after three years could be expected to have fewer problems, more local contacts and more opportunity to book a place for their child at a playgroup or nursery school than families who had moved.

From the original list of 264 names and addresses, eighty-five were still living at the same address three years later. This high rate of mobility probably reflects the general tendency of families with young children to move more than average (Ineichen, 1981; Rossi, 1955). Of those who remained, eighteen declined to participate, giving a refusal rate of 21 per cent. This is slightly higher than is normal for family research, but low in comparison with other studies requesting some commitment from *both* parents (La Rossa and La Rossa, 1981). Four couples were seen in a pilot study. This meant that the main sample interviewed consisted of sixty-three sets of respondents; thirty-six lived in Milburn and twenty-seven in Whitlaw. In addition, six families who had moved to other parts of Edinburgh were also visited. To ease identification in the text the initial letters in the names of children and parents will be used to indicate the nature of the families, as follows:

A–L Milburn resident e.g. Anthony Balfour
N–Z Whitlaw resident e.g. Stanley Tulloch*
P   *Pilot* study family e.g. Paul Preston*
M   Family who *moved* e.g. Mary Mitchell

Information from the last two types of family was used only in the qualitative analysis. The * sign after a name designates that the family is working class, according to a definition which will be explained in chapter 4. With two exceptions, all the couples had apparently remained together consistently since the child's birth. Over three quarters of the children were aged between thirty-six and forty months at the time of contact. The other nine were aged between forty and forty-six months.

From the outset it was decided to consider fathers' as well as mothers' viewpoints. Day care research has virtually ignored fathers. Whilst most care is done by mothers and they often arrange specific external sharing, fathers may affect broader decisions about their wives' work or their children's care arrangements (Gavron, 1966; Hunt, 1968). Their willingness and availability to act as carers themselves is crucial. It was thought preferable and more economical to speak to both part-ners together. A semi-structured joint interview was carried out with each couple, except in a few cases where the father attended only part or none of the interview. In order to obtain as much depth of material as possible in a single interview, the schedule was quite lengthy and most interviews lasted about three hours. A tape-recorder was used, so that a verbatim account was available. Qualitative analysis used these transcripts to identify and elaborate themes. Much of the data was also coded for computer analysis by means of the SCSS package (Nie *et al.*, 1980). The first part of the interview was devoted to a lengthy exploratory discussion of all occasions when the child had been looked after by anyone else, as far as the parents could recall. The circumstances and consequences of these occasions were followed up in a fairly free manner, prompted where necessary by appropriate questions. In the second half of the interview there was more orderly and standardised questioning about relevant aspects of the child's and parents' lives (see Appendix).

Some check on the validity of the information given was provided by multiple approaches to similar issues at different points in the interview and by having two respondents who could confirm or modify each other's accounts. Nevertheless, there are problems about relying too much on people's recall (Yarrow *et al.*, 1970). Therefore, interview material was supplemented by diary records. Parents were asked to fill in a standard form which gave information about their child's activities and carers over a two-week period. These diary sheets were divided into three sessions per day (morning, afternoon and evening). Records which were complete enough for quantitative analysis of all the sessions were returned in all but five cases.

Thus the following description of the main research findings makes use of numerical data, summarised comments and verbatim quotations. There is a danger that the incorporation of too many examples of these different kinds of evidence may render the text indigestible. In consequence, wherever possible only rough fractions and important figures are given. Percentages are used sparingly since they can give an impression of false precision and disguise low actual numbers, though they can be very useful for comparisons with other samples of different sizes. Space restrictions have enforced brevity in most quotations. Only a few could be included to illustrate each argument. There is a risk that examples were unwittingly selected to substantiate a preconceived idea. Somewhat different conclusions might have been reached from different excerpts. The ultimate value and validity of the material presented depends on the plausibility and consistency of the findings, and on critical appraisal and future testing by others (Popper, 1974; Ravetz, 1971; Spencer and Dale, 1979).

2 *Patterns of shared care*

It is the intention of this chapter to outline some of the basic features of shared care which were to be found amongst the families interviewed. Later on I hope to amplify and explain those patterns in various ways and to pinpoint some of their consequences.

First we shall examine the particular experiences of a small number of individual children. This will help to illustrate the diversity and complexity of care patterns and to identify some of their key elements. For example, who did children stay with, for how often and for what reasons? The second part of this chapter will then consider more systematically the range, variety and combinations of those elements for the whole sample. Although the families who were seen were not strictly representative of the population at large, there are also no strong reasons for seeing them as unusual, so that the picture which emerges should have relevance to parents and children more widely.

What follows are the brief details of seven children's experiences of shared care up to the time that their parents were interviewed. They were then all aged between three and three and a half. As a result of the way the sample was selected, all had been born into two parent families and their parents remained together three years later. In addition, all the fathers were in full-time work. Thus each had been brought up so far in what is often seen as the 'normal' family. That remains the pattern for the majority of young children, although illegitimacy, parental separations and high unemployment mean that increasing numbers of children grow up in other kinds of families (Gittins, 1985; Osborn *et al.*, 1984; Popay *et al.*, 1983; Segal, 1983).

Stephen and Mary

We begin by comparing two children in families where the mothers were not in paid employment. These were Stephen Powell who lived in Milburn and Mary Purdie* whose home was in Whitlaw. Stephen was the only child of his parents so far but Mrs Powell was expecting a new baby shortly. Mary was the middle child of three all aged under six. Her father was a well-paid lorry driver, whilst Stephen's had a stable professional job. Both families were therefore able to live in quite spacious accommodation with gardens, although the locality in which the Purdies* lived was, on their own admission, less attractive. House prices there were lower than in Stephen's neighbourhood.

Stephen's parents described him as a loving, serious boy. His father characterised him as 'not at all aggressive'. He was also mad about imaginary and toy cars at that time. Mary was said to be active, friendly and happy. She particularly loved dancing.

Like many others, both the mothers in these families had not wished to return to work after their children were born. They explained this with a mixture of reasons including a sense of duty, the anticipation of pleasure from staying home with the child and the assumption that this is what mothers characteristically do (in our society). Mrs Powell had been a nurse for ten years before Stephen was born but had not worked since. She was very committed to her career and was depressed for much of the first year of Stephen's life. She missed the company and daily structure which her work had provided. Yet she believed it was important for her to stay home to be with Stephen in his early years. By contrast, Mrs Purdie* admitted to no regrets about giving up work seven years previously. She said she had plenty of company close by and did not miss the extra money. Another important difference between the two families contributed to these contrasting reactions to giving up work. Mr and Mrs Purdie* had over a dozen close relatives living in Edinburgh, whereas all of Mr and Mrs Powell's few near relations lived over fifty miles away.

Stephen's parents knew very few people near their home when his mother stopped work to give birth and look after him. In any case they were reluctant for him to be cared for by a non-relative when he was a baby. Therefore, they recalled that he was hardly ever away from his mother in the first year. The only exception was that occasionally his grandma (Mrs Powell's mother) looked after him briefly during her periodic visits to stay with them for a week or so. By the time Stephen was a toddler Mrs Powell had come to know some other mothers with pre-school children living nearby. They had become acquainted through stopping to chat about each other's young ones as they passed in the street. Four mothers including Mrs Powell began to visit each other's home once or twice a week. When this happened the children played happily together and it seemed natural that now and then one of the mums left her own child and popped out to the shops or some other engagement: 'From 18 months, I started leaving him with friends along the street, but that was with difficulty. He was very reluctant to be left.' The initial reasons for doing this were so that Mrs Powell could go shopping alone and 'to give me a break'. At first Stephen resisted being left by his mother but by the time he was two he had accepted these arrangements and was no longer upset. Gradually he was left for longer periods with the two or three other mothers living close by. What began as one-off episodes developed into a more regular system. Eventually, the mothers took it in turns to look after all the children once each week: 'We swopped children to give each other freedom.' One of these women left the district and her place in the group was taken by someone else in the same street. The same set of families also established a small evening babysitting group for themselves. Mrs Powell explained how the women insisted that their husbands also take turns in going out to look after other children at night. Mr and Mrs Powell mainly made use of this babysitting group when they wanted to go out to a concert together.

During the later stages of her second pregnancy Mrs Powell also arranged for a teenage girl to take Stephen out from time to time in order to give herself some rest and to provide Stephen with some more energetic activity. This same girl liked to look after other children in the neighbourhood, for which she received payment. Usually she took Stephen to the park.

Mr and Mrs Powell were asked to explain why they chose the people they did to act as carers for Stephen. Mrs Powell said that they felt 'very strongly that we did not want anybody looking after our children that the child did not know quite well'. They would have preferred to use relatives but they lived too far away. Mr Powell added that the carers were 'friends whose reactions we could gauge and with whom we felt relaxed'.

Within the group of mothers that Mrs Powell had befriended it was the common expectation that their children would go to some kind of playgroup. They carefully discussed the pros and cons of different groups well before Stephen was old enough to attend one. Consequently Stephen was enrolled at a small private playgroup in the area. Mrs Powell was unsure if the playgroup supervisor was qualified but other mothers who had used it recommended it highly. The Powells said that they wanted him to go to the playgroup for 'socialisation'. They thought he would also have a wider range of activities than was possible at home. At its simplest, he would be able to do things there which he enjoyed. Mrs Powell did not want formal teaching for him since she felt able to do this herself at home. Stephen settled in readily at the playgroup and looked forward to going there, partly because he knew several playmates already through the 'swop care' group. However, he would probably go somewhere else when he was a year older. Mrs Powell explained that at 3–4 she wanted 'something to keep him happy and occupied, not too structured', whereas 'he will need something more structured for 4–5'. Mrs Powell did not participate in the playgroup at all, since it was run entirely by the supervisor and one helper.

Like the Powells, Mr and Mrs Purdie* also had strong views that children should not stay with people who were not already familiar to them. The Purdies* too believed that it was important for a young child to be mainly with the mother, yet later have opportunities to learn outside the home. This had led to a very different sequence of sharing care, however. Whereas for Stephen shared care had been carried out almost entirely by friends of his mother who lived within a few hundred yards of his home, Mary had apparently never been looked after by a non-relative before she was three. All her carers were kin who lived in other districts of Edinburgh about two miles away. The Purdies* saw several relatives two or three times per week. Much of Mrs Purdie's* daily tasks and social life involved the company of her sisters, parents and aunts. There had been no shortage of offers from them to have Mary stay. In fact, Mary's older brother Raymond had mostly gone to his maternal grandparents but their health had deteriorated considerably in the last couple of years. Therefore, it was normally Mrs Purdie's* married sister (Auntie Karen) who had looked after Mary besides her parents. Auntie Karen had older children of her own and was well used to looking after little ones. Moreover, Mary had always been happy to stay with her, which was less true with other relatives. Consequently, when Mrs Purdie* wanted to go to the shops unencumbered or had a dentist's appointment, it was usually Auntie Karen who took Mary and her two brothers. She was also the main person to come and babysit in the evenings when Mary's parents went out for a drink with friends on a Friday or Saturday night. As she grew older, Mary asked to go and stay at her aunt's home, since she enjoyed being there and playing with her cousins. She had spent two nights at Auntie Karen's home when she was just three. One other person who occasionally looked after Mary was her great aunt who liked to take her out for walks.

Mr and Mrs Purdie* were very aware that Karen looked after their children more often than they did hers. She seemed to enjoy this and had certainly never complained. Nonetheless, they felt there was an imbalance so they tried to make up for it in other ways. For instance they took her to places she wanted to get to in their car from time to time.

At the time of the interview Mary had just started at a local nursery school two weeks previously. Her older brother Raymond had gone to the same nursery. When the headmistress asked if his sister would be going too, Mrs Purdie* agreed to her name going on the waiting list. She had been wondering about using a nearby playgroup instead but eventually decided that 'they don't learn as much as with teachers'. It will be recalled that Stephen's parents expected him to change from his present group after a year, but Mr and Mrs

Purdie* took it for granted that Mary would remain at her nursery school until she was five.

The Purdies* explained the main reasons why they wanted Mary to go to nursery school. These were:

1 To have other children to play with.
2 To have more things to do – 'she was bored at home'.
3 To help prepare her for school – 'It breaks them in for school.'

It was early days but so far Mary had been very quiet at nursery school and did not play with the other children yet. Asked if it brought benefits for herself, Mrs Purdie* said it did not because it was time-consuming and complicated to take and collect Raymond and Mary at different times. Mary could stay at nursery school for a 'full' day (i.e. 9 o'clock to 2.15), but her mother wanted to take her for only a couple of hours in the morning. Mrs Purdie* explained – 'She's young – I feel as if she's a baby.' Mr Purdie* said that Mary going to nursery school would not affect him, except that occasionally when he was home during the day he was sorry that she was not there.

There were three nursery schools within walking distance of the family, compared with only one which was near to where Stephen Powell lived. Mrs Purdie* said that they had chosen this particular one because 'it had a good name for being educational'. Mrs Purdie* said that she would not want to be involved at all in running the class since she was too busy and felt she did not have enough patience, though her husband questioned this last point.

Already certain themes emerge from comparing these two children. There were some obvious differences which turned out to correspond with patterns which were typical of the two children's respective neighbourhoods, although they were by no means universal in either area. Thus, Stephen's shared care had been mainly by other local mothers, both individually and in an informal group. He had been looked after regularly and frequently by adults outside the nuclear family since he was two. Mary on the other hand had stayed only with relatives and on a less regular and less frequent basis. However, the periods of time spent with her carers had sometimes been quite long and unlike Stephen she had already stayed away from her parents overnight. Stephen's experience of shared care up to the age of three had involved much play with other children of his own age who were not related to him. Mary's had meant that she spent time with older cousins. Whilst Stephen had started at a playgroup where he already knew a number of the children, Mary was going to a nursery school where she started with no 'pals'.

Yet there were also similarities for the two children. Neither had been away from their mothers on a regular basis for long parts of the day before starting at playgroup or nursery. The people who had looked after them were all women, except for the occasional male babysitter in the evening for Stephen. Moreover, in the interviews it was mainly the mothers who talked about sharing care and the reasons for it.

The diaries kept by the two mothers for a fortnight strengthened the pictures which emerged from their descriptions during the interviews. Mary's diary was a brief one. In the two weeks she had spent all of the time with her mother (and sometimes both parents) except while she was at nursery school and also once when she went to Sunday school. The teacher at nursery school commented that Mary could now stay longer since she was settling better than had been the case a few weeks before. Mrs Purdie* noticed that Mary was 'talking more about nursery' too. The diary made no mention of any contact with neighbours, friends or other young children outside the nursery. Mary and her mother visited her Nanna and Auntie Karen, however. Her great aunt had called by to see them a couple of times too.

Mrs Powell kept a more full record of Stephen's activities. Besides his attendance at playgroup, there were three instances in the fortnight when he was away from home without his mother:

1 'Went to park with Doreen (sixteen-year-old girl who lives nearby and takes him out twice a week). He is very fond of her and looks forward to his outings.'
2 (Morning) 'Spent in neighbour's house in company of two girls aged three and twenty months. Part of the regular weekly exchange of children on a rotary system. He is very happy with three-year-olds but finds younger children's interference in play rather difficult to handle.'

3 (Afternoon) 'Spent with neighbour and her children due to pre-natal appointment of mother. The two three-year-olds dressed up and played mothers, organised dough and stuck shapes into it. Generally happy together, they were reluctant to part at the end of the afternoon.'

By the age of three, both Stephen and Mary had led quite active social lives. In their different ways they had interacted frequently with a range of other adults and children outside their nuclear families. Sometimes that interaction had resulted from or resulted in shared care. In contrast, a few children in the sample had spent their first few years in greater isolation and with comparatively few contacts outside the home. Ross Whigham* was one such child.

Ross

Mr and Mrs Whigham* lived in a tenement flat in the industrial part of Whitlaw. They had no relatives in Edinburgh apart from Mrs Whigham's* grandmother whom they saw every week. However, she was well into her eighties and seen as too old to look after a child on her own. Mrs Whigham's* widowed father came through from Glasgow to stay with them for a week or so now and then. They also visited Mr Whigham's* parents and his sister every week or two in a small town fifteen miles outside Edinburgh. Otherwise the family had very few social contacts. Mr Whigham* said he did not really have any friends. Mrs Whigham* did see a former colleague of hers from time to time. As for neighbours, they said that they hardly ever saw them because they were unfriendly or out at work most of the time.

The Whighams* had one child, Ross. From the portrait of him given by his parents he appeared less sociable and less adaptable than either Stephen or Mary. Though he was happy enough with his parents they depicted him as very shy with other people, often wilful and subject to 'strange' moods.

Mr Whigham* worked as a chef. His wife had been a nursery nurse for some years but had not worked since Ross was born. She felt strongly that she wanted to be home with her son.

Moreover Mr Whigham* pointed out that they did not need the money so what would be the point of her working?

According to his parents Ross had hardly ever been looked after by anyone else. The only occasion they could recall in his first year was when they left him briefly in a nursery at a holiday camp. He had been acutely distressed and difficult to console. Therefore they had resolved after that not to leave him with other people except in special circumstances. In any case, Mrs Whigham* remarked that since she had nobody close by to leave him with it had not really occurred to her that she might want or need to do so.

In the following two years, Mr Whigham's* sister and her boyfriend had taken Ross out on his own a couple of times during their visits to Edinburgh. Once they treated him to a trip to the zoo, for instance. Also, a few times Mrs Whigham* had popped out to the shops for about half an hour leaving Ross with her father during one of his stays with them. Mr and Mrs Whigham* said that they hardly ever went out in the evenings. Once or twice they had gone out for a meal to celebrate a birthday. They timed this to coincide with a visit by Mr Whigham's* sister or Mrs Whigham's* father so that one or other of them could babysit.

When the interview took place, Ross had been going to a church playgroup for a few weeks. The main reason for taking him there was 'companionship, because he had nobody else to play with'. In addition, Mrs Whigham* believed that 'he's got to learn to share and get on with other people'. She preferred him to go to a playgroup rather than nursery school because there 'they have them outside in all weathers'. Moreover the playgroup 'has very good equipment and the people in charge are very good'. Indeed Mrs Whigham* wanted Ross to stay there until he started school but the playgroup leaders were keen for children to move on to nursery school once the children were nearing four years. At the playgroup, mothers helped play with the children for a session at a time on a rota basis. Mrs Whigham* enjoyed taking her turn very much; she was then able to draw on skills from her earlier training and work.

Ross had not had a good start at playgroup: 'The first week I left he screamed every morning.' This slowly improved: 'Now he doesn't bother when I leave him' and 'he enjoys going', although he still mostly played alone or with an adult. Mrs Whigham* thought that starting at nursery school had affected him outside as well – 'It's made him a wee bit more clingy.' Mrs Whigham* herself was glad to have some time to do things on her own while Ross was at playgroup. Even so, 'the first two weeks he was left, I did miss him terribly. Going out to the shops, I kept putting my hand down for him and discovered he was not there.'

Thus, unlike Stephen and Mary, Ross had had hardly any experience of shared care before he went to group care at three years. His diary confirmed that he had not been apart from his mother at all in the two weeks, except for the playgroup. None of the few people whom he saw frequently (his aunt, his grandparents, his great grandmother) had any dependent children, so he had no playmates before starting at the playgroup. Indeed he had not yet made any new friends there, either. Ross apparently had no significant emotional or developmental problems but it is not hard to see that his life could have been richer than it was and that he had difficulties in dealing with the world outside his home. His parents themselves thought that he would have found it very hard to adjust when he came to start school were it not for the progress they expected him to make at playgroup.

None of the mothers of the three children who have been considered so far had worked at all since they were born, but evidently a crucial influence on children's patterns of shared care is whether their mother does work or not, for how long and with what kind of child care arrangement. Strictly speaking, shared care which occurs while mothers work is required to permit *both* parents to work at the same time but it is generally assumed that it is only the woman's work which gives rise to the alternative non-parental care. The people in this survey described it in that way too. We will now look at the circumstances of four children whose mothers had done paid work, with varying implications for the care of the children. These cases will also illustrate further how a pattern of shared care may develop over time or alter abruptly. We have already seen how Mary Purdie's* shared care arrangements remained much the same until she started at nursery school, whereas

Stephen Powell's had altered in the second year and then evolved further over the next eighteen months. It must not be forgotten that children with working mothers may also have the same kinds of shared care experience for other reasons as do children with non-working mothers.

In some respects the descriptions of the next two children (Aidan and Neil) fit quite well with the common image of 'working mothers' and their care arrangements. Both worked five days a week for several hours and the children were looked after by individual childminders from outside the family's existing social network. Closer examination reveals that the care histories of the children were more complex than this simple picture suggests. They also shared some features with children whose mothers did not work. Furthermore their situation is not as typical of working mother families as is often supposed, so afterwards we shall examine the very different care patterns of two other children, Emily and Derek.

Aidan

The Hunters had two children, Aidan aged three and his six-year-old sister, Jennifer. They described Aidan as an easy-going child who liked to be active and was fond of boisterous games. The family had no close relatives living near Edin-burgh at that time. However, for the first few months of his life Aidan's paternal grandmother had been living with the family. From time to time, Mrs Hunter left the baby with her mother-in-law during the daytime so that she could go out to do some shopping. When Aidan was six months old his grandmother went abroad to stay with her daughter.

Shortly afterwards, Mrs Hunter went back to work as a GP. She had done the same six months after Jennifer was born. This second time she had been more ambivalent about whether to start work again but she was worried about losing her place at the medical practice. Making up her mind was made much easier when the childminder who had looked after Jennifer offered to do the same for Aidan. The word childminder sounds rather impersonal but by now she had become very well known to the family who called her by her first name, Margaret. Although they were not friends in the sense of pursuing shared activities together, the two families were on very good terms. Sometimes the Hunters took out Margaret's children, who had become Jennifer's best friends. Therefore, although Mrs Hunter had not liked to ask Margaret directly, she was delighted that she was willing to care for Aidan while she and her husband were at work: 'I was really pleased because it kept it as a unit. Jennifer was quite close to her children.'

Therefore, ever since he was eight months old Aidan had been taken each weekday by his mother or father to stay with Margaret for about six hours. The diary showed that while he was at Margaret's Aidan sometimes played alone with cars or Lego but often played with her children or their friends. They also went to the shops and park together. Thus he was doing very much the kind of things a three-year-old might do at his own home.

Aidan's parents said that he had adapted very naturally to going to stay with Margaret. It had been part of his life since infancy and he had never shown signs of being upset at leaving his parents. Mrs Hunter believed her children had benefited from the arrangement: 'They are getting the affection of a mother. ( ) She does love them and she treats them very well.' She also thought that Margaret gave them more patience and attention than she was able to do herself. However, she and her husband recalled that at first they had not wanted to use a childminder but had been keen for Jenny to go to a day nursery. Mr Hunter said 'we would have preferred something run by the local authority – bona fide', but they did not qualify for a place. There were no relatives close enough to help and they did not like to ask friends. Mrs Hunter explained: 'I don't feel I could look after other people's kids, so I didn't think it was fair to ask one of my friends.' Also, 'our close friends are in the same position, as they are starting families'. Hence they had been happier to ask someone they did not know beforehand to look after the children rather than approach a friend.

Mr and Mrs Hunter said that nobody else had looked after Aidan apart from themselves during the daytime. Mr Hunter often came home early from work so it was usually possible to do things which might otherwise have led to shared care (e.g. shopping, appointments) either when Aidan was with Margaret or by internal sharing. However, the diary showed that Aidan was taken to Sunday school by the mother of a fellow pupil there.

When asked about what they did for evening babysitting, Mr Hunter's reply was 'We've not solved that one.' In other words, they did not have a consistent arrangement even though they went out together in the evening roughly once a month. Several different people had been used once or a few times each. They mentioned the teenage girl next door, two nurses on the stair, and two of Mrs Hunter's friends from her work. Once they had nobody to call on when they were invited to a function to do with Mr Hunter's work. Therefore they contacted a girl who had advertised at the local clinic and paid her to babysit. They had not been keen to do this but it had worked out all right. Mrs Hunter had learnt about a babysitting group in the area from people she had met at Sunday school. Mr Hunter was not keen to join for reasons that were not altogether clear. The main point he made was that they did not go out often so would be called out to babysit for others more often than they would need help themselves.

Just after his third birthday Aidan started at nursery school. He was taken there by Margaret, who also collected him, so his parents had little contact with it apart from special meetings. Aidan's diary indicated that he had begun to go and play at other children's homes after nursery school.

Neil

Neil Ogilvie* was an only child and his mother was not able to give birth to any more children. As in the families of Ross and Stephen, there was no older child in the family whose experience of shared care might act as something to follow, modify or avoid, depending on how it had worked out. This contrasts with Mary who had gone to the same nursery school as her older brother and with Aidan who was cared for by the childminder who had looked after his elder sister. By nature Neil was said to be lively, amusing and cheeky. His history of shared care exhibited both greater use of the family's kin network and also greater changeability than was the case for Aidan.

Mr and Mrs Ogilvie* did not remember sharing care much

in Neil's first year, except that from early babyhood he had gone to stay now and then overnight with his maternal grandparents. They also lived in Edinburgh but on the other side of town. Therefore, when Mr and Mrs Ogilvie* wanted a night out together, it suited the grandparents for him to come and stay, rather than for them to make a longish bus journey back and forth on the same evening. However, the arrangement was not purely practical in origin. Mrs Ogilvie's* parents very much enjoyed having Neil for a long period. It had also been a family tradition; Mrs Ogilvie* recalled that as a young child she had similarly gone to stay with her grannie. During the daytime, if Mrs Ogilvie* wanted to get on with doing something at home without Neil there, she took advantage of visits by her sixteen-year-old niece. She liked to take him out for walks.

Not long after Neil was born Mrs Ogilvie* decided she wanted to go back to work. She felt very confined in their small flat and missed the company she had in her former job. She began to work part-time in a shop. This did not necessitate external shared care because Mr Ogilvie* was at that time working short hours, mostly at night in a pub. Therefore he looked after Neil while his wife was at work. He enjoyed this and took responsibility for feeding and nappy changing. It amused him that he received strange looks when pushing the pram through the park.

After a year, by which time Neil was a toddler, Mrs Ogilvie* stopped work briefly and then started again in a different shop. This time the work was full-time and Mr Ogilvie* was now working in the daytime so he was no longer in a position to care for Neil. For a while he took Neil to Mrs Ogilvie's* sister. That could only be a temporary arrangement since she was expecting a baby and also lived some distance away. An old friend then helped out for a few weeks but clearly something more reliable was needed. Mr and Mrs Ogilvie* did not feel they could use Neil's grandparents because they did not live close enough and were all working themselves. Consequently, like the Hunters, they sought unsuccessfully to get a day nursery place. When Mrs Ogilvie* went to the one nearby she was told they were not a priority family and she was referred to a childminder, Mrs Marsh. Neil stayed with Mrs

Marsh until he was just over three, when unfortunately she fell ill. Then he transferred to another minder who was known to and recommended by Mrs Marsh.

Neil had been very happy with both childminders and indeed with the other people who had looked after him: 'He's never had any problems with going to anybody.' To be sure, when he first went to stay with a childminder, 'for the first week or so he was a bit gurney for ten minutes or so in the morning, but once we were out of sight he was all right, you know'. Mrs Ogilvie* thought that she had been 'right lucky because they've both been right motherly types'. Indeed 'he behaved better with Mrs Marsh than what he did with me. I think kids always play up their own mums.' One advantage of the arrangement was that he enjoyed playing with the other children there – it will be remembered that he had no brother or sister. There was more space for him, too: 'If the weather was good he was out in the garden all day which he really enjoyed, whereas with our flat . . . he's not so free.' (Neil and his parents lived in a small top-floor tenement flat with only a concrete shared back yard.)

Neil took the change of minder very well. Referring to this, Mrs Ogilvie* declared: 'He's just like one of the family. He goes everywhere with them.' The diary illustrated some of his activities there: he often played outside, usually with the minder's children; he met her husband and friends; one day the whole family went for an outing to the seaside with the minder's sister and nephew.

During all this time Neil continued to stay with his grandparents. Several other relatives (chiefly aunts, cousins and second cousins) took him out or babysat. At the time of the interview, the couple's main babysitter was Mrs Ogilvie's* young cousin. He was aged thirteen and stayed overnight with the family about once a month when Mr and Mrs Ogilvie* wished to go out. Occasionally, the lady downstairs babysat for them and they looked after her children in return. The eldest daughter in that family, who was eleven years old, also often took Neil down to her own home or to the back yard to play. Each week Neil accompanied her to Sunday school. Apparently he sat there quietly and liked to go.

Unlike the other children considered up to now, Neil was not attending a playgroup or nursery school. He had been booked in for some time at the nearest nursery school; his birthday was in March and his parents had hoped he could start at Easter just after he was three. There was no place at that time but Mrs Ogilvie* had been told by the Head that he would be able to go there with the new intake in August.

Neither Aidan's nor Neil's family networks were in a position to look after them for an extended period while both their parents worked. Let us now consider a family where that was possible.

Emily

Mr and Mrs Griffin were both teachers. They had two children, a boy aged five (Hugh) and a girl aged three (Emily). When interviewed, Mrs Griffin was expecting a third child in a few months. Emily was seen by her parents as a happy, sociable child who enjoyed active, outdoor games.

Very soon after she was born Emily developed feeding difficulties and her doctor also diagnosed heart trouble. She had to attend hospital frequently and was admitted for surgery at three months. Emily was away from home for a week. Partly as a result of anxiety about Emily's health, her parents were reluctant to leave her in anyone else's care during those early months.

Towards the end of Emily's first year, Mrs Griffin began doing some sessional teaching again. She asked her own mother to look after Emily. This was for two half days a week at first, but was later extended. Mrs Griffin's father brought her mother to the home in the car and stayed, 'pottering about', but Mrs Griffin's mother was clearly the one who was in charge of the children. This arrangement was still going on at the time of the interview.

In the second year of Emily's life, Mrs Griffin began a regular weekly swop with a 'friend' she had come to know who lived nearby and also had young children. The friend had social activities she wanted to get on with once a week whilst Mrs Griffin used the time to do extra teaching. Thus the arrangement grew up in a similar way to the swops described by Mrs Powell but for rather different purposes. It also involved a pair of mothers rather than several.

Some months later a second swop arrangement began with another mother in the street. She and Mrs Griffin had become acquainted through meeting at the playgroup which Hugh attended. Their swop occurred less often and less systematically than the first one. It happened more for the children to play together than for the adults' benefit, but Mrs Griffin recognised that it was useful to have the time free for housework, shopping or simply 'a break' for herself.

Throughout Emily's first three years, her maternal grandmother remained the person who looked after her the most besides her parents. Mrs Griffin stated the initial attractions of this: 'At the time, it seemed to me, if you were going to leave a baby, a small child, to go to work, a grandparent was ideal rather than finding a stranger who might be difficult to assess.'

There were also practical advantages. Her parents did not live far away, they had a car, they were retired, and her mother enjoyed doing it. The Griffins felt awkward about asking friends and would have felt obliged to pay them. As time went by, there turned out to be drawbacks and even some friction about grandma's care of Emily. According to Mrs Griffin, it was very tiring for her mother and Emily had been spoilt: 'She can't say "No" to them.' Mrs Griffin concluded: 'Now if I was going to leave the kids I would perhaps employ somebody else after very careful assessment of them.'

Lest it be thought that care by grandparents so that a mother could work was inherently problematic, it must be stressed that many other families had not found the same difficulties, though a few had. For instance, Ralph Quinn's* father worked during the day and his mother had worked five mornings a week since he was six months old. At first the main person to look after him had been his maternal grandmother but sometimes it was his paternal grandmother. Later on the latter's husband had retired and became actively involved with Ralph's care. He normally took him to nursery school by car. He collected Ralph later and took him to the park or brought him to stay with either of his grans. This had been successful for all concerned. Mrs Quinn* felt she had to work to avoid being very depressed and frustrated. Ralph very much enjoyed being with his grandparents: 'He's used to it. He used to say "Which gran is it today?". It was like part of his day. He's never bothered.'

Let us return again to Emily Griffin's situation. She had been mainly looked after by her grandmother and by two other local mothers that she knew well. Nonetheless, unlike Aidan and Neil, she had been very resistant to being left for a long time. Even with her grandmother she had initially been subdued when her mother left. When first taken to the friend round the corner for the weekly swop 'she would scream with rage for about 10–15 minutes, then settle down'. However, 'after a period of time she was quite happy to be left without any fuss'.

For evening care Emily's maternal grandparents were also used but the Griffins belonged to a babysitting circle too. This might seem unnecessary duplication but they were glad to have the choice. If Mrs Griffin's mother had been with Emily a lot during the week it seemed excessive to ask her to come out again on a Friday or Saturday night, so they preferred to ask a member of the babysitting group. On the other hand, sometimes nobody was free from the group or Mrs Griffin's parents offered to stay, so then the Griffins were happy to have them as sitters. The main reasons for needing a baby-sitter were an invitation to dinner with friends or the wish to go and see a film.

In contrast to the babysitting group which the Powells belonged to, this one did not involve the fathers in looking after other people's children. Mrs Griffin explained: 'If they've got a youngish child, I often feel that I ought to do it, because being female, you are supposed to be the one who is able to deal with a smallish child, which I feel in my case is not necessarily correct.' It transpired later that Mr Griffin was both more experienced and more comfortable than his wife with young children, at least before Hugh was born. She continued to find parenting problematic and lacked confidence in herself. Mrs Griffin normally arranged babysitting, as is clear from her additional explanation for expecting the wives to do all the babysitting – 'For some reason I feel that I shouldn't send them a strange daddy that they have never seen.'

Mrs Griffin had occasionally used a university creche for Emily when she went to a lecture. This was not very satisfactory since there were too many children of different ages for the two supervisors to cope with adequately. Emily had disliked going there but accepted it more as she grew older. When she was three Emily began going to a voluntary playgroup. Mrs Griffin would have preferred a nursery school but there was no place in the area. As a result of her work commitments, she did not often take part in running the group as some other mothers did. She had helped out occasionally, but 'I find it pretty boring and I think a lot of other mothers do too.'

Derek

Unlike the other children with working mothers, Derek had not been looked after by relatives, friends or childminders for this purpose. His parents had used a pattern which is increasingly common – the mother works at times when the father is at home.

Although she was a trained telephonist Mrs Baxter* had not returned to that job after Derek was born. She did not want to work full-time and there was no work available for the hours she was prepared to leave Derek and his older sister, Emma. Therefore, when Derek was nearly three years old, she had began working as a cleaner five evenings a week for three hours from 6 to 9 p.m. She would have liked to begin this before but Mr Baxter* had previously been running his own business and had frequently not come home until late at night. Recently he had changed his job so that he finished regularly between 5 and 5.30. Then it became possible for him to look after the children in the evenings so his wife could go out. Occasionally he returned late, in which case his mother or father came over briefly to cover the period between Mrs Baxter's* departure and his arrival. To the Baxters* the main advantages of this arrangement were that they did not have to share care for any substantial period and were not imposing on their relatives, who were the only people they would consider to look after the children. They were appalled at any idea that a 'stranger' might look after him so that both of them could work. However, their decision to rely on sharing care within the marriage in order that Mrs Baxter* could work had limited her choice of work and was not entirely satisfactory. She was very conscious of the low status and limited satisfaction of being a cleaner: 'Now I know I'm capable of a lot more than that, but the hours suit me at the moment with two young kids.' In fact she and her workmates were planning a night out together and 'We're not saying we're cleaners. We're going to say we're nurses.' Even so Mrs Baxter* was glad to be working, 'getting out and meeting the girls. I feel happier in myself, I do.' Her husband agreed that it was good for her to have a break from the home and the children. In the past, Mr Baxter had hardly been involved at all in the physical care of the children, which remained true for the times when Mrs Baxter* was home. He had never changed a nappy, for instance. When his wife started work, he became responsible for bathing Emma and Derek and putting them to bed. In addition, 'I do the kids' supper every night and Maureen (his wife) does my tea and dinner.'

The Baxters*, like several other couples in the sample, had managed care of the children between themselves so that both were able to work, the mother doing so part-time. Yet it would be wrong to conclude that they had not shared care outside the marital partnership. Since babyhood, Derek had stayed with several different relatives – both sets of grandparents, his father's sister, his father's brother and his mother's brother (aged sixteen). They all lived in Edinburgh, although not in the immediate district and Mrs Baxter's* family were the other side of town. Derek's aunt and uncles had chiefly babysat in the evenings so that his parents could go out for a meal together or go to a club with friends. In the daytime he had mostly been looked after by his 'old grannie' and his 'new grannie', as he called his paternal and maternal grandmothers respectively. The main person to look after him in the daytime was his father's mother who lived a mile away. Mr Baxter* described how she would call by and say 'Go away and get your messages, then, and I'll look after the bairns.' This prompting gave Mrs Baxter* a chance to do something on her own and also gave her mother-in-law time alone with her grandchildren. Sometimes Mrs Baxter* had a more specific reason herself for wanting to leave Derek, as when she had a hairdressing appointment. Then she was more inclined to contact her own mother first and, if she was free, take Derek over to her place.

Like Mary Purdie*, but unlike the other children we have looked at, Derek had apparently never been cared for by non-relatives before he was three. None of the family had any friendly relations with the neighbours. These were perceived as snobbish by the Baxters*, who were a working-class couple in predominantly middle-class Milburn. Mr Baxter* said, 'I never speak to anybody here, you know.' Mrs Baxter* said she had tried to engage people in conversation but they appeared stand-offish. As a result the family had not become involved at all in the kinds of weekly swops in which Stephen and Emily had got involved (independently from each other) a few streets away in different directions. Similarly, when they were asked what they thought about babysitting groups Mr and Mrs Baxter* expressed alarm about the idea. Mr Baxter could not imagine moving to a new area and 'meeting some neighbours . . . and letting a complete stranger into the house'. Mrs Baxter* added with incredulity, 'And letting them look after the children'. They argued that the only kind of person they would consider sharing care with would be 'the family or a very good friend'.

In fact, there was an exception to that rule since Emma had gone to nursery school, which of course was not run by a relative or very close friend. Evidently that kind of child care was not regarded in the same light as babysitting or sharing care for work. Derek himself had not yet started at nursery school but was booked to start at the end of the summer when he would be three and a half. In fact his parents had wanted him to start when he was two because he had appeared bored at home and was frustrated that he could not go into the nursery school with Emma. When he went up to the nursery with his mother to take and collect Emma, he would often rush around in the playground and play with some of the other children. Whereas Stephen and Emily's mothers had used playgroups since there was no nursery school place available,

Mr and Mrs Baxter* did not want to do that. It was important to them that children should learn things at a pre-school group and they did not think that would happen at a playgroup. Apart from the educational angle, the main reason for wanting the children to go to nursery school, according to Mrs Baxter*, was that 'It makes them that wee bit independent, which you don't really want anyway, but which they have to have. You don't really want to see them grow up and grow away from you, but that's what it's about, isn't it?' She believed that 'Once they are used to nursery they will adapt to anything, whereas the wee ones that's no been to nursery will maybe cry for their mums or no want to be left.'

General patterns of care

These brief summaries of the salient features of individual children's shared care histories have drawn attention to many of the themes which will be developed in the book. The variety of patterns is obvious, even within one smallish city amongst families who were all of Scottish or English backgrounds. Ross Whigham* had hardly been apart from his mother at all whereas Neil Ogilvie* was looked after by a childminder five days a week for eight hours each day. The frequency and extent of shared care for the other children ranged widely between those extremes. The kinds of people who had looked after the children included grandparents, aunts and uncles, a niece and a nephew, and a great aunt. Neighbours or friends living close by had also been important for some children. Nearly all of these had in fact been other mothers of young children. Most of the children had stayed with teachers or playgroup supervisors. Some had been with childminders, Sunday school teachers or people running a creche. In all cases, though, the primary responsibility for care of these children outside the nuclear family as well as within it had rested with women. There had been many different reasons for sharing care, such as shopping, appointments, both parents working or both parents doing social activities in the evenings. Shared care had also occurred for children to learn, play and make friends. It had sometimes happened at the behest of the carer rather than the parents.

All the parents had similar wishes for their children to go to a playgroup or nursery school but there were differing attitudes about what was best for the child and whether the mother should participate. These children's stories showed too that sharing care is usually a dynamic process which evolves and responds to changes in circumstances, parental perceptions and the family's social relations with other people. Each child's experience usually consisted of combinations of care by more than one individual or couple which developed or changed to make up a sequence of shared care. A longitudinal study would be the best way to find out how such care sequences evolve. Here it was necessary to rely on parents' recollections which may not always have been accurate. These naturally revealed some individual alterations in response to particular events or changes in the family or outside. It was also possible to detect certain more general trends. In only some cases had these sequences been consciously planned.

Some of the circumstances and events which lead to sharing care could be seen as idiosyncratic but it is also clear that there are important general similarities between some of the children which means that it is possible to discern crucial dimensions of care which may combine in regular ways. The later chapters set out to amplify and in part explain those distinctions and regularities. Understanding each child's situation requires detailed exploration of many aspects of the family and its environment, not all of which can be readily grasped in a single interview, however lengthy. The task of this report is somewhat different, namely to describe, classify and account for the more general or common features of sharing care, as illustrated by the seventy-three families who were seen. That involves to some extent disregarding some of the particularities of individual children's histories. Explanations of the care patterns will take two forms, although these will not always be kept separate. Firstly, the ways in which aspects of shared care appeared to be affected by certain 'objective' features of children's and families' social and physical environment will be outlined. Equally important, there will also be an examination of more 'subjective' influences as expressed by the parents themselves. These include their perceptions of children's needs and capacities, their views of parenthood and their attitudes to different kinds of people who might potentially look after children. Whilst it is hoped that the systematisation of the evidence will provide a useful framework to increase understanding of shared care, it is important not to lose sight of the detailed processes involved, nor assume an inevitability of outcomes. Sometimes, to be sure, parents described their actions in sharing care almost as if there was no alternative, but frequently there had been uncertainties about what to do, changes in attitude and arrangements, or careful weighing up of different possibilities. These complexities must remain in the forefront of any explanations of what happened.

Shared care outside organised groups

The starting point for understanding how sharing care arises and in turn affects children and their parents is a simple description of the key elements of care patterns which were to be found in the sample. First of all we shall consider care by individuals or couples (relatives, neighbours, minders etc.). This involved the care of just one or a few children at the same time. Such arrangements constituted the main form of shared care before the age of three for all the children in this sample. Larger officially recognised pre-school groups will be dealt with at the end of the chapter more briefly, for these have received most attention in the day care literature. Particular emphasis will be given to the relationship between these two types of care as this has hardly been examined in the past.

Frequency of care
How typical or unusual was the near-absence of shared care for Ross, the daily experience of non-parental care by Emily and Aidan or the more intermediate patterns of Stephen and Mary? For each of the three years since each child was born, approximate frequencies of normal care were established during the interview in order to show the broad evolution of care. For this purpose, brief atypical episodes were ignored. The predominance of parental care in our society is seen in the fact that about half of the families shared care only a few times in the first year, as far as they could remember. For

some children the pattern persisted. Fourteen children (just over one in five) were described as having been apart from both their parents during the day less than six times in the whole of the third year. Some parents struggled to recall the rare circumstances when their child had been left with someone else. A few had shared care so seldom that those occasions stood out sharply in their memories. Nevertheless, all of the children in the sample had been cared for by someone other than parents at some point in the three years.

Evidently it was by no means uncommon for children to be away from their mother or father hardly at all before they were three years old. However, some children had stayed with other people quite often as babies and most were experiencing quite frequent shared care by the time they were three. Sometimes the increase in frequency occurred gradually, but there were also more abrupt changes as when a mother started work or began a regular care arrangement with one or more friends. Thus by the time the children were aged between two and three the number of families who shared care at least once a week doubled to make up just over half of the sample. Then about one in six of the children were being looked after five days a week for part of the day while both parents worked. However, the majority of the children experienced shared care at intermediate frequencies ranging from about once a month to once or twice a week. In that sense, out of the children described earlier, Stephen, Mary and Derek were the most 'typical'.

For comparative purposes three kinds of shared care sequence were identified. These will be used in later chapters in order to see how children's overall care frequencies varied according to other features of their situation:

> **17 'low sharing' families** had shared care only a
> few times in each of two or three years.
> **25 'high sharing' families** had care frequencies
> of once a week or more in at least two of the years.
> **21 'medium sharing'** families made up the
> remainder of the sample.

The frequencies of care shown over the admittedly short period of the diaries confirmed that these categories represented significant differences between families reasonably accurately.

Both the interviews and diaries revealed that evening care occurred much less often than daytime care in most families. Only eight couples said they shared care in the evening as much as once a week or more. One third of the families used an evening carer only a few times a year. With a few exceptions, those families who shared care at least once a fortnight in the evenings also shared care at least weekly during the daytime. Similarly, most of the couples who were low sharers in the daytime also shared care rarely in the evenings (p < 0.001). This suggests an underlying dimension of parental readiness to leave the child which affected both parts of the day.

Types of carer

A second important dimension of shared care consists in the kinds of people who act as carers. How were they related to or known to the child? Were they men or women? Were the people who looked after the children parents themselves, single or childless? Did they look after them alone or with someone else? Do they have children or not? How far away do they live? The individual children described earlier illustrated that, with a few exceptions, there were three main types of carer:

1 **Relatives,** many of whom did not have young children themselves
2 **Local mothers with young children**
3 **Paid childcarers,** people such as a childminder or daily help who had no prior social relationship with the family and who received payment for looking after the child.

The comparative importance of these was brought out by the diaries. During the two week periods for which records were kept, 24 children were looked after by relatives (day and evening), 26 by friends and neighbours and just three by a paid childcarer. This may exaggerate the importance of non-kin, since relatives had been more important for many children when they were younger. In addition those children who were rarely away from their parents often had a relative as their main carer but had not stayed with them during the diary period. We shall now look at each of these principal types of carer a little more closely in turn.

All the children in the sample had been looked after by a relative at some point. In half the families the main (i.e. most frequent) daytime carer was a relative. There were eight children who had apparently never been cared for by anyone other than a relative, except for group care. There was a consistent ranking in the number of families using different kinds of relative as their main carer. These were (in order):

mothers' parents
fathers' parents
mothers' sister
other siblings of the parents
other relatives, usually maternal

Thus there were two strong biases in favour of the mother's side of the family more than the father's side and of grandparents more than other relatives. For the sample as a whole this hierarchy of main daytime carers was quite clear cut and was also repeated for most other aspects of care and contact, but it must be emphasised that for many individual children the order of importance of each type of relative differed from this pattern. Moreover, as a result of the large variations in the frequency with which families shared care, some children had several people they stayed with more often than another child's main carer. For example, Emily Griffin was looked after by each one of her three principal carers (her grandmother and two local friends of her mother) much more often than Ross Whigham* had been by anyone.

By and large parents tended to choose relative carers from amongst the members of their own original nuclear families, i.e. the child's grandparents, aunts or uncles. To be sure, some children were cared for by other relatives, like Neil Ogilvie's* cousin and Mary Purdie's* great aunt, but that was not very common. Grandparents accounted for one third of all the main carers and nearly as many of the children's second most frequent carers. Moreover, 90 per cent of the children had been looked after at some time by maternal grandparents and two thirds by their paternal grandparents, so that it was extremely rare for a child never to have been looked after by grandparents despite the distance at which a fair number of them lived. Considerably fewer children (eight) had kin other than grandparents as their main carer, but the child's aunts and uncles were quite often the second or third most important carers.

In a small number of families, the children had a brother or sister who was old enough to look after them on their own, but in only one instance was an older sister the main carer. During the diary period three children were looked after by older sisters (aged nineteen, eighteen and nine) without their parents being there. It would seem that parents in Britain are much less willing to hand over full supervision of a young child to an older one than in non-industrial societies (Weisner and Gallimore, 1977).

Most of the children's carers who were relatives did not live in the local district, although about one in three did live that close. Some grandparents, aunts and uncles who lived up to fifty miles away were regular or even main carers. Rather than ask non-relatives to act as carers, nearly one fifth of the families (more in the first year) preferred to ask a relative to come into Edinburgh to babysit or arranged to go out only during a visit to or by relatives. In this respect Ross Whigham* was by no means unusual, therefore.

Table 2.1 *Kinds of people used as main and second carers*

| | Number of families who use each kind of carer (N = 63) | | | |
	Kin	*Friends neighbours or circle*	*Paid child-carer*	*Nobody*
Main Daytime Carer	31	23	8	1
Second Daytime Carer	33	26	0	4
Main Evening Babysitter	33	23	6	1
Second Evening Babysitter	34	23	1	5

Whilst relatives were the most frequent carers in slightly more than one half of the families, it is also clear from Table 2.1 that for many children unrelated people were equally or more important. In over one third of families the main carer was someone other than a relative who lived within a short walk of the child's home. Most of these were other mothers of pre-school children. They lived in the same street or an adjacent one and had to a greater or lesser extent become a friend of the child's mother. In addition some children were looked after by their immediate neighbours. Some younger children simply wandered in next door to see someone they knew very well. In other instances it was deliberately planned by the adults. Although a few of these next-door neighbours happened also to have young children, they were just as likely to be middle aged or elderly. Parents' friends living outside the surrounding few streets had been used for daytime care in only a few cases and then not very often. About one third of couples had used people who worked or used to work with or for one of them – colleagues or occasionally secretaries. This had virtually always been on an occasional basis, unless they also happened to have young children and live nearby.

The third important type of carer, and the one perhaps uppermost in people's minds when they think of children being away from their parents, is the paid childcarer. In fact, relatively few families (less than a third) had used any carers other than people in their social network before their child went to some form of group care. Four families had used a paid childcarer outside the home (i.e. a childminder) and nine had used a paid childcarer in the child's home (i.e. au pair, daily or agency help). Daily helps were mostly used for babies and for care of short duration, whereas other paid childcarers were mostly used for older children and for longer. Three out of the four families who used a childminder began to do so only after the child was two. All but one of the families who had used a childminder or au pair for any length of time had had a change of person in that position. Whereas most new carers from amongst relatives, neighbours or friends were already familiar to the child in some way, these discontinuities of paid childcarers nearly always meant that the new carer was previously unknown to the child.

As with daytime care, just over half of the main evening carers were relatives. Maternal grandparents were again most often the first choice as carers. Their prominence was particularly apparent from an examination of the diaries. Including both daytime and evening care, twenty children had been cared for by their maternal grandparents in two weeks but only four by paternal grandparents who were the next most common kind of relative. The rest of the evening carers were for the most part again local parents but unlike daytime carers some of these were not well known to the parents and a few were men. This is because fourteen families used a babysitting circle. Babysitting circles may be distinguished from other care arrangements in that they are formalised associations of local parents whose agreed function is to organise sharing care. In theory though not always in practice any member may be called on to babysit for any other. The detailed functioning of circles will be discussed in chapter 3.

Most families did not have exactly the same set of people for daytime and evening care, but nearly always there was some degree of overlap. Many had the same kind of people for both daytime and evening care even though they turned to different individuals. Thus, grandparents might be more used in the daytime and an aunt in the evening. Several children went to a few local mothers in the daytime, but a wider number of circle members came to babysit in the evening. Only ten families combined a non-relative as their main daytime carer and a relative as their main evening carer, or vice versa. Although most children had been cared for by both relatives and non-relatives at some time, few had been looked after frequently by both. In the evenings, about half the families relied almost entirely on a combination of relatives for care. A quarter of the whole sample rarely used anybody but grandparents. On the other hand only about half of the couples who belonged to a babysitting circle relied exclusively on that when they were going out in the evenings. Three families used both their circle and one or more relatives quite often, as did Mr and Mrs Griffin. A further four normally called on circle members for babysitting but had grandparents as a back-up arrangement. Evidently circles are not simply organisations for those without relatives on hand, as some respondents thought.

Most of the families who shared care only a few times a year had a relative as their main carer. It seems that parents who were loath to share care often were also reluctant to do so beyond the extended family. Those families who shared care at medium frequencies usually had either kin or local people as main carers. Daily care was normally by a childminder, au pair or relative. Members of babysitting circles were significantly more likely than others to share care frequently in the evenings. One half of circle members did so at least once per fortnight, compared with one quarter of the rest of the sample.

The diaries recorded by the parents in this study also shed some light on the frequency with which they had acted as carers themselves. They showed the presence of other children in the home but did not note occasions when the parents went out to babysit. The number of families who shared care in their own home *for* other parents was roughly the same as the number who shared care *of* their own children in the fortnight. Interestingly, none of the people interviewed (who by definition were parents of young children) had looked after a child who was related to them during the diary two weeks. We shall see later that there was a general tendency not to ask relatives with young children to act as carers. The children who had stayed with the sample families were described as either friends of the children in the family or else as children of friends or neighbours. The majority of the children's friends who came to play or stay without their parents were of the same sex as the child the diary was about. Most were aged between three and four. The tendency to mix with children of the same age and sex is a common feature of even pre-school children's friendships (Rubin, 1980).

Characteristics of carers
The vast majority of carers were women. That was true of relatives and non-relatives, of daytime and evening care. To have discovered otherwise would have been most surprising given what we know of traditional expectations about the care of young children. Ninety per cent of the main daytime carers (fifty-four) were women who looked after the child on their

own. The few men who did contribute to daytime shared care, either jointly with their wives or occasionally on their own, were virtually always grandfathers or uncles who were retired or had jobs which sometimes freed them during the day. Theoretically men and women were more equally available for evening care but most evening carers were women too. Nevertheless, more men were involved with evening than daytime care. The most important male carers were grandfathers, who usually but not invariably looked after the child jointly with their wives. Single uncles and teenage boys were also not uncommon as evening carers. It was rare for adult men who were unrelated to the child to be involved with care. The main partial exception to this was that in most babysitting circles some of the men went out to look after other people's children. Even so, usually the women acted as carers more frequently. In two of the circles no men babysat. Of the fourteen couples in the sample who were circle members only four said that they both went out to babysit equally often. In the other cases the husband either babysat for others less than his wife (four) or did not do so at all (six). Some fathers regarded themselves as in a back-up position, going out to babysit only when their wives were unable to do so for some reason. In effect, many mothers were doing most of the return for a service which benefited both partners.

That these young children were not entirely unfamiliar with care by a man other than their father, however, is shown by the fact that this had happened at least once for two thirds of the children. Yet it had occurred frequently for only six children. Therefore most would be growing up with the experience and perhaps the expectation that child care outside the nuclear family as well as within it is primarily a female task.

Nearly all the daytime carers were married with young or grown up children of their own. A higher proportion of evening carers were single or did not have young children, although these were still very much in the minority. This resulted from the greater prominence of teenagers, single female friends and unmarried uncles, who were less free to act as carers during the day when at work or school.

Stephen, Neil and Derek had all been looked after quite often by teenagers and this turned out to be a fairly common practice. In the whole sample, thirty children were said to have been looked after at some time by a total of forty-four carers who were still in their teens. Three quarters were non-relatives. About half of these teenage carers were aged seventeen or under. Eight were strictly below the legal minimum age (16) for being in charge of a child and the youngest was aged eleven. Only about one fifth of the teenager carers were boys but they had all looked after the children a fair amount, whereas a number of the girls had been used only once or twice. A few teenagers had taken children out after school or at week-ends but for the most part families used teenage carers in the evenings. Some of these had looked after the children only once or a few times when regular carers were not available. However, a teenager was the main evening carer for nine of the sixty-three children.

Combinations and changes of carer

Quite a few relatives looked after children in a pair. This usually involved grandmother and grandfather or aunt and uncle but now and then another combination like aunt and cousin or two aunts. Care by non-related couples together was less common but, as we have seen, sharing by two or more women in a 'swop' was by no means unusual.

The diaries showed that over a third of the children had been looked after by more than one carer on separate occasions in the two weeks but only six had stayed with three or more. Over a longer period most of the children had several carers. All the people who look after a particular child during a period of a few months may be regarded as making up that child's carer set. Just under half the families had a carer set of seven or more people. The upper limit of 'active' carers was about a dozen, though some children whose parents were in a babysitting circle with thirty to forty members potentially had more people who might come and look after them. Families with mainly non-relatives as carers tended to have larger carer sets than those who mostly used kin carers. A larger carer set did not necessarily mean it was easier to share care frequently or on demand because a few families had several carers whom they used only occasionally, whilst one or two main carers like grandparents or a childminder could be very readily available

for frequent care. A large carer set was especially characteristic of those children who stayed with several relatives or
several street friends once or twice a week. Both those children
who were rarely away from their parents and those who were
away daily for work reasons stayed mainly with one person or
couple.

The seven children considered at the beginning of the
chapter illustrated how carer sets often do not remain the
same. Aidan Hunter's grandmother emigrated. Neil Ogilvie*
moved from one childminder to another. As babies Stephen
Powell and Emily Griffin were looked after apart from their
parents only by their grandmothers, but then began staying
with street friends when they were toddlers. Thus, an existing
carer may stop looking after the child and may be replaced.
New people can join an existing carer set. Just as important
is that the comparative importance of carers may change.

For most of the children, not only did shared care become
more frequent as they grew older but the number of different
people looking after them became larger too. Sixteen children
did have roughly the same carer set over the three years, but
for three quarters of the sample the number of carers
increased. This entailed a substantial expansion of the
daytime carer set by more than three carers in half of the
cases. In the first year over 50 per cent of the families used
only one or two carers but in the third year this proportion
had fallen to under 20 per cent. By and large the differences
between the sizes of carer set of individual children were maintained even though most grew bigger. Those children who
began with just one or two carers as babies usually still had
less than six carers by the time they were three years old.

Most of the 'new' carers were local mothers or paid childcarers since relatives who looked after the child more than
occasionally usually did so from an early age. Of course, some
alterations of the carer set were caused by individual events,
such as a grandparent's stroke or a street friend leaving the
district. By far the most common factor was that many families
came to know better and/or trust more other mothers who
lived nearby. Therefore a typical progression showed a shift
towards greater use of people living within close walking
distance in addition to or partly instead of kin who were

further away. This took two main forms. Firstly, there might be an addition of one or two local mothers to a carer set which remained chiefly made up of kin. Secondly, in some families, relatives were the main carers early on but were later over-taken in care frequency by street friends. This did not necess-arily mean that the relatives were used less often than before (although that did happen sometimes) but simply that non-relative care had increased in comparative importance.

The number of families with maternal grandparents as main carers declined from twenty-six in the first year to only sixteen in the third year. There was a similar fall in the number of families with paternal grandparents as main carer but the number of families with other relatives as main carer remained fairly constant. The place of grandparents as main or second carers was normally taken by street friends and to a lesser extent by paid childcarers. It is evident, then, that the use of local people as carers by many families did not mean that they had no kin available because often relatives had been important carers for those families during babyhood and mostly remained so later on. They had simply become less prominent as sharing care amongst local friends became more frequent. Only rarely was there a change in the opposite direc-tion, with a non-relative as main carer in babyhood and a relative later. There were also a few parents who had non-local 'old friends' or ex-neighbours as carers for older brothers and sisters or when the child was younger, but who increas-ingly turned to local people as time went by.

Expansion of the number of carers was equally likely to occur in the second or third year depending on whether a family began to share care with several mothers round about either earlier or later. About one quarter of the children had quite a sharp increase in their carer sets over a short space of time. This generally occurred when the mother joined or helped create some form of multiple exchange sharing care network in the street or adjacent streets similar to the one described by Mrs Powell.

Although it was apparent that for many families proximity became more important than long-established relationships as the child grew older, this shift in favour of localised sharing of care with non-kin should not be exaggerated. Over one in three of the families retained the same predominantly kin carer set throughout the three years. In the third year there were still six families who had relatives living outside Edinburgh as their main or second carers.

To sum up, the sequences of main carer amongst the sixty-three sample families may be described as follows:

20 Grandparents for all three years
 8 Other sequences of kin only
10 Switch from grandparent to local mother
 8 Local mother all three years
 9 Local mother or paid childcarer all three years
 4 Switch from local mother or immediate neighbour to relative
 4 Other sequence

The location of shared care

Where shared care takes place affects the context of that experience for the child and so may have social or emotional consequences. If the carer comes to the child's home, then the familiarity of place, belongings and playthings make this less of a change and perhaps less of a threat than if the child goes to the carer's home. On the other hand, as Mrs Ogilvie* observed, someone else's home and garden may be more interesting and exciting. It may involve play with other children and experience of different activities and rules from those at home. We have also seen that some shared care involved being taken out to places of interest, like the park, the zoo or the seaside. That was mostly done by relatives or, in the case of walks and visits to the park, teenagers. Nearly all the children had been looked after at some point both at home and away from home. Evening care normally took place in the child's home (three quarters of the sessions recorded in the diary). Parents' statements showed that during babyhood not only had their children been left with fewer people less often than happened later, but also shared care had then occurred mainly at home. Often this consisted of mothers popping out during visits by relatives. By the third year, most shared care for most children took place at the carer's home. This applied particularly when children stayed with local mothers. Only a small number of children were still being looked after mainly in their own home by carers once they were three years old. These were usually in families where sharing care remained infrequent and almost exclusively by close relatives. This meant thàt the experience of shared care by about one in six of the children was restricted in frequency, range of carers and location. The few exceptions to the association between infrequent sharing and home care were those children who were left fairly often at home with an au pair or daily help.

In many countries children live in much larger households than is generally the case in Britain, so that parents may share care with kinfolk or more rarely servants (Minturn and Lambert, 1964). In this study, just eight children had someone in the same household as themselves besides their parents, brothers or sisters. In five cases, the person concerned was an important carer for the child; these consisted of an au pair (two), a grandparent (two) and a student lodger.

Overnight care
Of the sixty-three children in the main sample, thirty-eight had been apart from both of their parents for one or more nights in their first three years. Only five children had stayed in hospital overnight without a parent present. The same number of children had been admitted to hospital overnight accompanied by their mothers. This illustrates how a much lower proportion of children go into hospital alone nowadays than was the case a generation ago (Douglas, 1975). It would seem that nowadays the greater willingness by hospitals to let a parent stay with a child overnight has significantly reduced the amount of total separation from familiar people in the potentially alarming circumstances of a hospital. In part, this is a beneficial consequence of the work of Bowlby and the Robertsons (1970), which has been much criticised in other respects.

However, the vast majority of overnight stays had been with relatives or friends. Excluding hospitalisations, just over half of the children (thirty-five) had spent one or more nights away from their parents. Relatives were even more predominant as overnight carers than they were for day and evening care. One half of children had stayed overnight with a relative; this was over twice as many as had been looked after by a non-relative overnight (thirteen). On the other hand the bias to maternal relatives was less marked than for other care: one third of children had stayed with maternal grandparents overnight. Slightly smaller and roughly equal proportions had stayed with each of paternal grandparents, aunts and uncles, friends and neighbours. Three children had been looked after overnight by an au pair or daily help but none by a childminder. Of all the children who had ever been apart from their parents overnight, four fifths (twenty-six) had been cared for by grandparents either solely or as well as others.

The mean number of nights a child had been apart from parents overnight before their third birthday was twelve, i.e. about four per year. This average has little real meaning for there was a very wide range from none to one hundred. Nearly all the stays with non-relatives had been for one or two nights only per child and virtually all the long periods of overnight care or repeated brief overnight stays were with relatives. This contrasts with daytime patterns. It suggests an unwillingness to use friends and neighbours for more extended forms of shared care.

Only twelve children had been cared for in their own home overnight (for an average of three to four nights per child concerned), compared with thirty-four children away from home (for an average of twenty nights per child). With respect to location, then, overnight care resembled daytime care more than evening care. Sometimes it appeared to represent the equivalent and extension of away-from-home evening care. If the child went to a carer's home to stay for the evening, then usually he or she would stay overnight too in order to minimise disruption for both carer and child.

Half the children who had been cared for overnight had stayed with more than one person. This usually involved a combination of relatives. For five of the seven children who had stayed with both sets of grandparents there had been an approximately equal number of nights with each set of grandparents. In other words, a balance had been maintained with both sides of the family. When children had spent nights with a friend or neighbour, the children had nearly always also had overnight care from kin too. Thus the use of non-kin for overnight care was mostly by those generally predisposed to overnight care with relatives.

Some differences in the timing of overnight care were noticeable over the three years. A few children had just one extended period of overnight care, as a result of their own or their mother's illness or hospitalisation. The remainder of the children who had experienced overnight care were divided fairly evenly into two types. The first group were like Mary Purdie*. They had spent just one or a few occasional nights with a relative or non-relative. The second group included Neil Ogilvie*. They had been looked after on a more regular and frequent basis for one or two nights on each occasion, usually at week-ends. Such recurrent overnight care had always been by either grandparents or (less commonly) married aunts and uncles. The main increase in the number of children staying overnight with relatives occurred between the age of one and two. In contrast, there was a sudden increase in the number of children who were looked after by non-kin only after the age of two, when parents felt the child was old enough to cope and understand. Although the frequency of overnight care did not usually vary much once started, the growing numbers of children who began overnight care each year resulted in an increase of the mean number of nights each year from 2.3 in year one to 4.8 in year three.

Group care

Our attention now moves outside the children's social networks in order to consider their experience of organised groups. The two main forms of group care used by parents in this sample were playgroups and nursery school. These are indeed the only two types of group care available to two parent families in normal circumstances, as the Hunters and the Ogilvies* discovered when they were seeking full day care for their children. None of the children in the main sample had been to a day nursery. Three major themes emerged in the study with regard to group care. Firstly, despite some important differences, both playgroups and nursery schools seemed to be serving broadly similar functions for families and children, as will be seen more clearly in the next chapter.

Secondly, it was apparent that usage of group care had become almost universal shortly after the age of three. Thirdly, group care varied considerably in the extent to which it represented a sharp break or a more familiar transition from the child's previous experience.

Of the sixty-three children whose parents were interviewed, over three quarters (forty-nine) were already attending group care at the time of interview. This was surprising as it represents a much higher rate of attendance for this age group than has been found in other studies, not only nationally but in nearby areas (Bone, 1977; Haystead *et al.*, 1980; Watt, 1976). This results in part from the high level of pre-school provision in Edinburgh. The nature of the sample was also important, since this omitted single parent families (who receive priority for a day nursery place if they request one) and newcomers to the area (who may be less willing or able to obtain a group care place).

The near unanimity about group care usage was further emphasised by the fact that the fourteen children not currently attending did not form a distinctive group of non-users, as had been expected. Like Neil and Derek, all were booked into a group and were due to commence shortly. The only significant way in which they differed from the others was in their birth month. They all had their third birthdays towards the end of the school year, mostly between April and July. This meant that they had been too young to start at the main intake times of pre-school groups in August and January, but were expected to start within a few months of the interviews at the beginning of the next school year. This delay was frustrating for some of the parents but the main reason for emphasising this point is that it demonstrates the quasi-universality of starting group care by just over three among this sample of families. All but a few of the study children's older siblings had attended a pre-school group too. This supports a double argument that will be further substantiated in later chapters. Firstly, in many ways both playgroups and nursery schools are a response to common needs in children as perceived by adults. They perform similar although not identical functions even if they are organised and sponsored in different ways. They may also cater for somewhat different age ranges. By three and a half virtually all the children in this sample would be in one or the other. Secondly, if the high level of provision in Edinburgh were extended nationally, then it seems probable that usage elsewhere might also become quasi-universal.

Of the children attending group care, just over half (twenty-seven) were at a local authority nursery school, with whom was included one child at a university nursery school for the purposes of analysis. Nursery school hours varied a great deal. Some places were part-time (two to three hours) whilst full-time places ranged from four to six hours. The remainder of the children attended playgroups or private nursery schools (Table 2.2). Usually the hours attended were similar to those for a part-time nursery school place. All nursery schools and some playgroups only admit children after their third birthday and this obviously had great impact on the age at which children started group care. Only one quarter of the sample had started at group care before they were three – usually just a few months earlier.

Table 2.2 *Types of group care attended or planned*

1 *Attenders = 49 Actual Attendance*	
Local Authority Nursery School	27
Voluntary Playgroup	12
Private Playgroup	7
Private School	2
University Nursery School	1
2 *Non-attenders = 14 Planned Attendance*	
Local Authority School	10
Playgroup	4

Except for a few children with working mothers, group care frequency was greater than frequency of non-group sharing care. The hours children attended group care ranged from two days a week for two hours to five six-hour days. A comparison could be made from the diaries of the amount of time the children spent in group and non-group care at the age of three. Children spent *on average* about one quarter of all forty-two sessions in the diary fortnight away from their mothers. Just under two thirds of these sessions were spent at group care. It must be remembered that most of the children had only started group care within the previous few months, so that before then non-group care was paramount. Going to a nursery school or playgroup did not appear to attenuate the frequency of non-group care for most children. Attenders had only a slightly lower mean number of sessions with individual carers than the non-attenders.

Occasionally, group care replaced entirely an earlier arrangement for sharing care. For instance, when Mrs Villiers* first went back to work part-time her mother had looked after Simon. This arrangement was discontinued once he started at nursery school because she was able to get to work and back during the nursery hours. Much more often the pre-existing arrangement carried on, although sometimes in a modified form. Several grandparents and paid childcarers who had been caring for the child while both parents worked continued to help with taking, collecting and probably some additional period of care once the child was at playgroup or nursery school. That applied to Ralph Quinn* and Aidan Hunter, for instance, whose grandfather and childminder respectively did this. In fact, all the children with childminders went to group care, just like other children. Some parents who had a regular swop care arrangement with local friends every week or fortnight changed to a less frequent, more ad hoc arrangement once the child started at group care. The arrangement was not needed so much because the child spent less time at home and the mother now had free time when the child was at group care.

Both nursery schools and playgroups included children with a wide range of shared care experience. However, all the children from low sharing families attended a playgroup (or private school), compared with only half of those from medium sharing families and one quarter of those from high sharing families ($p < 0.05$). Thus, parents who did not share care much within their social networks were more likely to send their children to groups which were of shorter hours and so also minimised separations from mothers.

Contrary to conventional assumptions about the novelty for children of starting to go to playgroup or nursery school, a majority in this sample (thirty-nine out of sixty-three) had already had some experience in a largish, organised and continuing group previously. Just under half the children (twenty-seven) had been to a mother and toddler group. Strictly, these do not constitute shared care as defined in this study since the mothers did not leave their children, although sometimes they played in a separate room. The phrase 'mother and toddler group' might suggest that they would be most attractive to mothers who are less ready than others to be apart from their children. On the contrary, most of the families who had used such groups were medium or high sharers with large carer sets. They saw mother and toddler groups as part of a gradually expanding sequence of social experience for their children. For instance, Mrs Urquhart* wanted to 'break him in . . . sort of . . . for nursery, you know. Get him used to being away from me just once a week.' Those working mothers who shared care with highest frequency from an early age were not generally available to attend with their children. Low sharers were perhaps disinclined to encourage their children to mix early in a group setting.

More surprisingly, just over one third of the families (twenty-two) reported that their children had been in various other forms of group without their parents (Table 2.3). These will be referred to as 'miscellaneous groups'. They have been ignored in the literature but had considerable positive or negative implications for a fair number of the children in this sample. The most important were church creches and Sunday schools. The former look after very young children while parents are in church whereas the latter provide introductory religious instruction for children over three. Some had been going continuously to a church creche since an early age, but others had only just started at Sunday school. At least one fifth of the children had been to one or both of these, usually on a weekly basis. Another kind of miscellaneous group is a sports creche where children are looked after so that their mothers can do keep-fit or play a game such as badminton. A few children had been in a sports creche weekly and a couple more occasionally. Some children had not settled well at a sports or church creche so then the arrangement had been stopped. Sometimes an individual carer then looked after the

Table 2.3 *Attendance at miscellaneous groups*

1 *Interview information – number of children said to have attended in the 3 years*

Church Creche or Sunday School	11
Sports Creche	5
Ballet Class	3
Other	6
Total who attended any kind = 22 (3 attended more than one)	

2 *Diary information – number of children who attended during the diary fortnight*

Sunday School	12
Ballet Class	4
Ballet Class and Sunday School	1
Sports Creche	1
Other	2
Total who attended any kind	20

Note that two other children went to a mother and toddler group during the diary fortnight

child for the same purpose. A fair number of children had taken part in a weekly ballet or dancing class, but this had not been happening for long since the starting age is normally three. There were several other types of group which had been attended by one child each, such as a group for gifted children and an adult learning project creche.

Not only did children begin attending playgroup or nursery school with widely differing histories of shared care but their parents had varying plans for them thereafter. Transfers from one group to another are not uncommon even though there are usually only about two years until children start school. Nine children had already changed group by the time of interview. In addition twelve couples said that they possibly or definitely would change group when the child was four years old. The most common changes involved a shift from playgroup to nursery school at the age of three or four. There were also a few instances of changes from one kind of playgroup to another. Two families planned a triple group sequence; this entailed an initial playgroup from two and a half to three, a second more 'formal' playgroup from three to four, and finally nursery school from four to five. If parental projections were accurate, about three quarters of the children would be attending nursery school between four and five. There were no examples of a child transferring *from* a nursery school to another establishment, but in all somewhat over half of playgroup users (seventeen out of twenty-nine) had either already made a change of group or planned to do so at the age of four. In many cases the playgroup performed a preparatory function for nursery school. Notwithstanding, a sizeable proportion of playgroup users did see it as a self-sufficient pre-school experience right up to the age of five.

For the sake of clarity this exposition of care patterns has not incorporated the circumstances and reasons which gave rise to them. Yet to make sense of the varying instances of shared care it is of course essential to understand why and how they came about. Therefore, the next chapter will add colour to the present monochrome picture by sketching in the details of the processes of shared care.

3 Processes of sharing care

Parents' motivations for sharing care

In this chapter we shall consider the immediate situations and factors which led parents to share care and also some of the consequences of care arrangements for the adults and children concerned. As a first step in understanding how care patterns came about it is useful to describe systematically the reasons parents themselves gave for sharing care and for choosing their particular types of care arrangements. To many parents their reasons for sharing care seemed obvious and normal. Indeed there was a fairly small range of situations which couples invoked to explain why they had shared care. Yet it also became clear from comparing the actions of different families that parents exercised considerable discretion about whether to share care or not. In similar situations some families had regularly shared care whereas others had done so either occasionally or not at all. None of the reasons given for sharing care were expressed by every couple. It was also evident that the same family were prompted to share care for a particular reason on one or more occasions but had not done so in very similar circumstances at other times.

A record was made during and after the interviews of all the reasons given for non-group daytime care arrangements recalled by all families for each of the three years (Table 3.1). These were largely but by no means exclusively a reflection of certain aspects of the mothers' day to day tasks which may be carried out more easily without children being there. The most frequently mentioned of these were shopping and appointments with doctors, dentists, hairdressers, etc. Mothers' leisure and social activities were less prominent as reasons for sharing care. Each year, about one in five mothers had shared care in the daytime in order to take part in specific

Table 3.1 *The most common reasons for non-group daytime care*

Reason given for care	Number of families who gave this reason for any one year		
	Year 1	Year 2	Year 3
A *Mother-based reason*			
Shopping	47***	47***	49***
Appointments[1]	23**	24**	25**
Social activity/Sport[2]	11*	11*	12*
A break[2]	12*	11*	19*
Work[3]	10*	17*	17*
Mother's stay in hospital	3	4	5
B *Child-based reason*			
Intrinsic pleasure of child and/or carer	15*	28**	40***
C *Other reasons*			
Parents' joint activity[4]	10*	10*	11*
Support father care[5]	0	1	3
Sibling-based reason[6]	6	8	9
Other	3	1	1

Key * Mentioned by 10 or more families; ** by 20–30 families; *** by 40+ families.
Notes
1 Appointment at doctor, dentist, hairdresser, hospital.
2 Specific activities are distinguished from a more generalised desire for a break.
3 Mother's work is meant here. It is normally implied in all the reasons that father is at work or otherwise not caring.
4 Normally a weekend reason for care, such as a wedding, funeral, weekend away or holiday.
5 When father normally cares while mother works.
6 Includes parents' contacts with siblings' school or pre-school group, and parents' desire to spend time alone with a sibling.

social activities like playing squash or attending a meeting. In addition an increasing number each year said they shared care partly or fully in order to give themselves a more generalised 'break' from the home and child care. Even so, only one third of all the mothers indicated that they had ever shared care in order to have such a break.

Family ceremonies (weddings, anniversaries, funerals)

constituted a prominent occasional reason for sharing care, even for parents who otherwise seldom shared care. Only a few children had needed an alternative caregiver because their mothers had gone into hospital but this did account for the most extended periods of continuous shared care.

Interestingly, even though we are only considering shared care by individuals and not official groups at present, a desire to provide play and social activities for the child was an important factor which led mothers to share care. In fact there were two overlapping varieties of what may be called 'child-oriented' care. In the first type, relatives were eager to have the child come and stay with them simply for the pleasure of the child's company. In the second type, local mothers with young children arranged for their children to play together. For the sample as a whole sharing care for 'child-oriented' reasons occurred more often and for more children as they grew older. This contrasted strikingly with the pattern of other reasons for sharing care which Table 3.1 shows to have been fairly constant over three years. One factor in the increase of 'child-oriented' sharing was a belief that carers found older children more enjoyable or easier to manage. Just as important was that some children themselves began to ask for one or both of these types of care to be arranged once they were of an age to express their wishes. Over half the parents reported that their children had asked to stay with another person sometimes or often. On the other hand thirteen children had apparently never taken the initiative in this way.

In the day care literature non-group shared care has largely been identified with 'work care', i.e. arrangements to enable a mother to work. Without denying that there are major implications for shared care when both parents work, this is a considerable oversimplification. For two out of three of the families in this study the mother's work had played no part at all in their patterns of external shared care. Although thirty-eight of the sixty-three mothers had worked at some time since the child's birth, only twenty-one of these had needed to share care outside the marital partnership in order to do so.

Some dimensions of care varied according to the reasons for sharing care. Naturally, children with working mothers tended to include those with the highest frequencies of non-parental care ($p < 0.001$) but their carer sets showed the same range in size as children with non-working mothers. Sharing care for social or child-oriented reasons generally went together with both large carer sets and care frequencies of at least once a week. Low sharing families had usually eschewed making care arrangements for either child-oriented reasons or for the mother's benefit (work, a break or social activity). For them, shared care was only legitimate in exceptional circumstances, such as family ceremonies or appointments.

In fact not only low-sharing parents but many others had some sense that sharing care should occur only when it was seen as essential in some way. This idea was compatible with contrasting frequencies of care because there were differing interpretations of when it was 'necessary' for children to be included or excluded in certain adult activities. As Mrs Edwards explained: 'That's what I mean by "You have to". Obviously, you don't have to – it's just to make life easier.'

Most people recognised that sometimes it was justifiably more convenient to do something like popping out to the shops 'without the children under your feet' (Mrs Griffin). Some mothers felt more strongly that there were times when 'you have *got* to leave them' or 'you *need* a break'. By contrast, a few parents like Mrs Whigham* perceived virtually no daytime circumstances in which they would feel any need to leave the child with someone else. Several mothers seemed to need to keep their children close for their own emotional reasons, especially if the organisation of family life left them isolated or lacking external outlets for personal satisfaction. Thus, Mr Laurie had two jobs and his wife commented that 'that is why I depend on the children so much – you know, for company. That's one of the reasons I never go anywhere without them.' Perceptions of when there was a need to share care could also be affected by the availability of trusted carers. For example, Mr and Mrs Kinnear had gone out a fair amount while Mr Kinnear's father looked after their first son. By the time they had their young twins the grandfather was considered too old to be a carer and they said they did not need to go out.

The interviews and diaries provided clear evidence that children sometimes accompanied parents for the same kinds of activity as led to shared care at other times. Shopping was both the most common reason given for shared care and the most widespread activity of mothers and children together outside the home in the diary fortnight. Mothers had differing opinions about when it was desirable to take a child along or ask someone else to share care. Appointments with doctors or dentists were seen by some parents as boring or alarming for children whilst others liked to include their children in order to extend their knowledge or allay potential fears. Decisions whether to share care or not also depended on the circumstances, the child's age and the availability of alternative carers including the father. Some children were taken to local shops but were left with a carer when their mother went into town so they did not have to cope with the large crowds. Difficult weather might tip the scales in favour of leaving a child with someone else while the mother went out shopping or took an older child to school. The length of time for which care would be needed could be important in assessing the child's reactions to being taken along somewhere or staying with someone else. A long period might be seen as too much to ask of a carer. Alternatively, for a short period, 'it wouldn't be worth asking anybody to look after him – it would be just as quick to take him' (Mrs Reynolds*).

Mothers also held contrasting ideas about how their decisions to share care or take children with them were affected by a child's age and the number of children in the family. Babies were often seen as easier to take along than toddlers, because they were lighter and unable to wander off. Some parents were disinclined to bring slightly older children with them for fear they might stray or get bored, but others thought it was easier to take them since they were more able to understand and cope. To take more than one child could be a handful when going shopping so that some mothers preferred to share care. On the other hand, 'the more there are the more you feel you couldn't possibly impose on somebody so that you just have to take them with you' (Mrs Henderson).

Unlike daytime care, evening care was rarely arranged for practical reasons but mostly for parents' social outings. Normally the couple went out together but occasionally they were engaged in separate work or social activities on the same evening. A few liked to take children with them in the evenings and would only accept invitations for visits on this understanding. The vast majority of people took it for granted that children needed to be in bed and should not have their sleep unsettled.

Overnight care had sometimes resulted from the admission of the child or mother to hospital. More often it was occasioned by parents' late evening social activities, when it served as a form of prolonged evening babysitting. Regular overnight care was also sometimes arranged for child-oriented reasons. These two main factors in overnight care often combined. If a relative asked for the child to come and stay, this was used by the parents as an opportunity to go out. Alternatively they might simply welcome the chance to have uninterrupted sleep or a quiet week-end to themselves. For some children there had been a few nights of overnight care when their parents went to family ceremonies or spent a week-end away. These two explanations accounted for most of the overnight care by non-relatives. For seven children, an extended period of overnight care had resulted from their parents' holiday away together.

Parents' reasons for sending a child to a playgroup or nursery school were usually not the same as their explanations for sharing care with individual carers, but there was some overlap with the 'child-oriented' care which had become increasingly important after toddlerhood. Several writers have stressed that most families are motivated to use group care for the child's social benefit rather than for educational reasons (Haystead et al., 1980; Watt, 1976). This was largely confirmed in this study but it was also apparent that for most parents there are multiple considerations which favour the use of group care. Over three quarters of the families gave at least three different reasons for their child going to playgroup or nursery school. The comparatively good level of pre-school provision in Edinburgh meant that group care had achieved a widespread legitimacy. As a result parents often simply assumed their children would attend without seriously questioning this. Mrs Boyd expressed a common feeling – 'I didn't give it a lot of thought. It seemed the obvious thing to do.' There were just a few who were reluctant to adhere to this norm; they said they only sent their child because otherwise he or she would lack friends or be different when entering school.

Table 3.2 *The most common reasons for wanting a place in group care*

Reasons mentioned	Number of families (N = 63)	
For child to mix	55	C
Play opportunities	31	C
Preparation for school	26	C
Independence for child	20	C
For child to learn	18	C
Child was bored	11	C
A break for mother	8	M
Social norm	7	O
Follow older sibling	7	O
External authority for child	6	C
Pressure on parents	6	P
To help child share	5	C
To help with child's behaviour	4	C
To widen horizons for child	4	C
To assist mother's work/study	3	M
For child to have fun	4	C
Child wishes to accompany or do same as sibling	3	C

Key
C = Child-based reason   P = Parents-based reason
M = Mother-based reason   O = Other reason
Notes
1 For the 13 families whose child had not yet started group care, reasons relate to planned arrangements rather than previously made arrangements.
2 Most families mentioned several reasons, so there is much double recording.

Nearly all the families included social benefits for the child amongst the reasons they gave for arranging the place at group care (Table 3.2). This factor was mentioned first by most of them. They explained that they wanted their children to go to playgroup or nursery school so that they could 'mix with other children', 'make friends' or 'socialise'. Some kind of opportunity to play was the next most common reason given. In many cases this meant that parents thought their child was ready for and interested in playing with others or with the wide range of play materials. In a few families the parents wanted a shy child to develop affiliative and play skills. The other main reasons given for the use of group care were (in order) preparation for the routines and practices of school, independence for the child, and learning elementary skills. Evidently, early education and help in adjustment to later education were important though secondary considerations for most families at this stage. For some low sharing parents this reason tipped the balance in favour of using group care, about which they otherwise had some reservations.

Therefore, unlike much shared care before three, group care was mainly regarded as a means of helping the child to start adapting to a wider social world than the immediate family and its realm of contacts. A few parents explicitly stated that it was a bridge from the comfort of the family to the tough outside world. While group care was primarily valued for its immediate, intrinsic merits for the child there was also often a future orientation in that families saw it as a form of gradual introduction to school. The kind of preparation which was wanted was usually depicted largely in social/emotional terms. This included growing accustomed to being in a large group away from home and learning the routines of school life. Fewer parents emphasised a wish for their children to gain specific knowledge or cognitive skills at this stage. With the exception of the few reluctant users, parents saw group care as providing things for the child which they could not do themselves. It was complementary to family care, not a substitute for it.

Overtly, there were few practical reasons given for the use of group care when compared with individual care arrangements. Fifteen families gave mother-oriented reasons for group care, but always in association with a child-oriented reason. Only three mothers openly stated that they hoped that group care would help them to start work. More commonly, mothers looked forward to a break from the child or a relief from the pressures of constant caring. This was the case for both families with twins.

Given the wide variation in non-group care sequences,

especially with regard to frequency, it might have been anticipated that these would affect motivations for group care. This
was not the case. Low, medium and high sharing families had
similar reasons for wanting group care. Families who had
hardly shared care at all did *not* feel they should also shelter
their children from group care. Nor did those parents whose
children had a range of carers and contacts regard group care
as superfluous. On the whole, the kinds of motivation for group
care also did not differ among nursery schools, private and
voluntary playgroups. This helps justify the practice here of
linking them together for most purposes as offering substantially similar services.

Choice of individual carers

Frequently, a decision to share care was inextricably linked
with the choice of a particular care arrangement but analyti-
cally it is useful to distinguish these two processes. Many
people did not actively set out to 'choose' carers. To some
it appeared self-evident that certain people would naturally
become carers. Thus Mrs McDonald did not consider anybody
apart from her mother to look after Martin. She said 'I've got
no-one else. I trust my Mum.' For others their own awareness
of alternatives or offers by potential carers made the decision
more conscious and sometimes more problematic. By and large
there seemed to be two major elements in the selection process.
In the first place only certain categories of people were
considered. Then there might be further selectivity within
those categories according to individuals' characters. Within
the relevant types of people, parents normally selected only a
few as carers, according to practical considerations or personal
qualities. For example, being good with children or more
willing to put oneself out explained why some friends, aunts,
uncles or grandparents were used as carers rather than
someone else with the same kind of relationship.

The negotiation of the carer role is a two way process, in
which both parents and carer need to be agreeable to arrangements. Usually, parents chose from people who had indicated
a willingness to care or from whom a readiness was anticipated
through prior close relationships. In other cases, incentives

could be offered to carers in the form of material reward or exchange services. Often willingness was taken for granted on both sides but some parents were loath to ask a potential carer until an offer was made. As we saw in the last chapter, Mrs Hunter had been uncertain whether to return to work after Aidan was born but resolution of her doubts was assisted when his older sister's minder said she would look after him. Several relatives were acceptable as carers for Robert Ormiston* when his mother was at work on a Saturday morning but it was her aunt who took the initiative and so he stayed with her. Some relatives were like Derek Baxter's* paternal grandmother in that they were not merely enthusiastic about looking after the child but virtually insisted on it. Simon Villiers'* sixteen-year-old cousin was possessive about her role as his main carer and indicated to his parents that she would be hurt if someone else was asked to stay with him when his parents went out.

All parents were asked why their main carer was that particular person. As far as possible explanations were sought for the selection of other carers too. These did not reveal all the factors affecting choice. It was very rare for parents to specify that carers should be women, have had experience of young children of their own, be grandparents, or come from the mothers' rather than fathers' family. Yet, as we saw, these attributes were very prominent in carer sets. Perhaps parents were not consciously aware of the significance of these factors or maybe they saw them as too obvious to be worth stating. It was also important to ask why significant or willing network members had not become carers, for the composition of a carer set depended not just on positive selection but also on the non-use of others. Over half the families reported at least one person who had shown willingness to care for the children but had not actually done so. For instance, some parents were not happy to have as evening carers people who they thought might panic if their child woke up.

Most of those interviewed provided practical reasons for the choice of their main carer, such as nearness, availability and willingness. This disguised the fact that pragmatic considerations were used within taken-for-granted categories of people. Only a few of those living near at hand became carers, some available people were not asked and the offers of willing people were sometimes not taken up. In discussion, many parents indicated that only certain kinds of people were acceptable for care. This is illustrated by Mr Vallance's* comment at the end of an interview: 'You've made us think about a few things. Our circle is not as big as we thought. You think you have a lot of friends, but it's surprising how few we'd leave our kids with. It makes you realise what constricts you.' Mrs Vallance* had in fact begun the interview by saying that they used her mother for care 'because she was the only one that was available'. She later admitted that there were other non-practical factors. She declared 'I wouldn't trust anybody else' and 'we've got the same ideas about things, you know'. Several other couples explained their choice of main carer by stating why they used one relative rather than another, thereby implying that only kinfolk entered into consideration. The main non-practical factors affecting selection of carers may be described as:

relational   the carer is a relative or friend of the child's parents

personal   the carer knows the child well or the child trusts the carer

evaluative   the parents trust the competence or skills of the carer

Some parents explained their choice of carers by saying simply 'family'. Preferences within the kin set depended on such factors as distance, health, age, work or other commitments, and having children or not. For evening care, grandparents might be preferred to younger relatives as they often had fewer social commitments of their own. In a few families, parents' siblings or cousins were favoured in comparison with grandparents because they were more mobile or more flexible about staying late. Interestingly, families whose main carers were relatives were just as likely to give nearness or convenience as a major reason for choosing them as others, even though far fewer of those relatives lived nearby. It appeared that for non-relatives nearness generally meant within walking distance, whereas for kin it referred to any practicable distance which might well be a different part of Edinburgh. Although there was a widespread view that kin should be the first choice as carers unless that was impractical, there were a minority of families who positively preferred non-relatives as carers. For instance, some thought that care by other local parents helped integrate the child more readily with everyday contacts in the street. Non-kin care could also avoid some of the emotional complications which some respondents thought arose when grandparents were carers.

Evaluation of the carer's competence was mentioned much less than might be expected. Selection of carers from among local friends or neighbours were sometimes attributed to particular skills (e.g. nursing) or similar values and ways of treating the child to those of the parents. This was rarely of conscious importance in the selection of relative carers. Presumably the ability to meet the child's needs in ways which parents approved of was ascribed to kin more automatically.

For one quarter of the families, opportunity to reciprocate care was important in choice of main carer. This chiefly referred to arrangements with other local parents and only once to a relative. Mrs Clark noted that 'there are some (neighbours) you would use rather than others, because you could repay them in kind'. Reciprocity is discussed in more detail later in this chapter.

Most parents stressed that carers should be well known to themselves or the child. Many asserted strongly that they would not countenance care of their child by a stranger or outsider. In social policy writings, analysis of the concept of stranger has mostly dealt with anonymous, distance service givers (e.g. Titmuss, 1970; Watson, 1980). In urban areas like Milburn and Whitlaw people are surrounded by many people who are strangers in the sense of being unfamiliar to themselves or their children. These strangers living nearby are potentially relevant for social contacts or sharing care. However, families meant different things when they referred to strangers. To some it meant any non-relative, whilst to others it meant people not well known to themselves or the child.

Three main kinds of attitudes to strangers were detected in this study, mainly in relation to evening care. These may be designated:

1 aversion
2 conversion
3 acceptance

Well over half the parents strongly objected to stranger care. Nearly all low sharing families and those with kin as main daytime carers felt aversion to any possibility of a stranger looking after their children. Apparently, restrictiveness or expansiveness both in the frequency of shared care and in the boundaries of persons trusted to care tend to go together. The main reasons for concern about stranger care were that the child would be anxious or frightened, that the carer could not cope if the child needed something, or that the carer might be a threat to the safety of the child or home. Aversion to stranger care was a major factor in unwillingness to belong to baby-sitting circles. A few members of circles were themselves opposed to strangers coming to babysit but felt that their particular circle was small enough for all the carers to be familiar.

Some couples were prepared to consider care by a person they or the child did not know well, but with important qualifi-cations (e.g. only when the child was asleep). Others thought it was all right provided that there was opportunity to 'convert' the stranger into a familiar person by inviting the person round for tea or coffee beforehand. In relation to evening care, only thirteen families indicated that they felt no qualms about having a babysitter they did not know well. All of those who had accepting attitudes to strangers had non-kin as their main daytime and evening carers. They were either high or medium frequency sharers. They were apparently unconcerned about their child's reactions to unfamiliar people as such, although they might well want to be assured of the carer's competence. Against the prevailing current of opinion, there were a few parents who expressed a definite preference to pay a stranger in some circumstances. Advantages cited included the precise format nature of the arrangement which obviated feelings of imposition and the fact that paid childcarers might more readily be brought to the child's home. In short, payment to strangers increased parental control over the situation. Mrs Miller's parents and other relatives lived in Edinburgh but, when asked what they would do if she was in hospital for a period, she replied 'I think we would prefer to employ some-body rather than a more casual arrangement, so it was more watertight.' Mrs Henderson had paid a friend's au pair to look after Douglas while she studied at the library, because his grandmother's timing had been too unreliable.

The fact that most carers were women went largely unquestioned, but this was more of an issue in babysitting groups. Some recipients of care felt it made no difference whether the circle carer would be a man or woman. Others wanted a woman because they assumed she would be more able to cope than a man, especially with the practicalities of baby care. Female carers were also usually more familiar to the child from daytime contacts. As it happens, some of the fathers were quite confident about their ability to look after other people's children. Others did feel inexperienced or simply assumed that this was primarily a woman's role.

Like gender, age was not a prominent positive factor in the choice of carers but did play a part in ruling out certain individuals or kinds of people. Some parents felt it was valuable for their child to spend time alone with an adolescent but many said they would not use teenagers as carers because of doubts about their competence or trustworthiness. Many offers of care by elderly relatives or neighbours were not taken up. Parents were concerned that they might be too tired or stressed, or would not provide adequate supervision and stimulation. Health could be more important than absolute age for there were some important carers in their seventies whereas some younger people were ruled out because of frailty, disability or vulnerability to stress.

Parent-carer relationships

A few children had carers who were known almost exclusively for that function, as in the case of a childminder, teenage babysitter or circle member. Much more typically sharing care was only a part, and often a small part, of the total relationship between the family and the carer as relative, friend or neighbour. Therefore, expectations and rules about the carer's role could vary greatly depending on the nature and quality of the non-care relationship with that person. Frequently, care arrangements built up gradually and with only partial deliberateness, as when a grandmother's care became regularised on a weekly basis or ad hoc swops developed into multiple, systematic exchanges. When agreement is reached to share care there is inevitably some kind of unwritten 'contract' between parents and carer about the terms of the arrangement, even if this is often vague and largely implicit. On the whole people seemed to make explicit their expectations about the practical side of things, like the time and place for sharing care. Parents were much less likely to spell out or even consider very carefully how the carer should amuse or handle the child more generally. Carers normally had a fair amount of discretion to do what they wanted, in the way they wanted. This is not to say that there were no rules of expected behaviour, but these were largely implicit and only became apparent when they were breached. Thus some parents complained about certain actions or inaction by carers such as panicking with a crying child, failing to tolerate exuberant behaviour or spoiling the child. All these judgments were made from the parents' perspective of course and doubtless the carers would have expressed a different viewpoint.

Comments about ill-treatment of the children by a carer were very rare although Mr and Mrs Nichols* did change Winnie's childminder because they thought she was learning aggression and bad language. In contrast, overindulgence was deprecated by quite a few parents especially if the child was more difficult to control at home later. Problems to do with spoiling arose mainly though not invariably with relatives. Mrs Laurie stopped arranging for her own grandparents to have her son and daughter to stay because she believed they indulged the children excessively. That had resulted in conflict because the children wanted to carry on doing just as they pleased when back with their parents. Mr Tulloch* likewise had become unhappy about using his brother-in-law as a baby-sitter. He explained that whilst he himself was trying to teach Stanley right from wrong, his wife's brother let him do what he liked so that 'the bairn's in two minds'. Mrs Urquhart* was loath to ask her sister to look after Thomas, because 'anything he wants he gets, you know, and it's not fair when they come home. And I've tried to explain it to her, but I don't want to hurt her feelings, you know.' This illustrates the particular difficulty of clarifying care 'contracts' with relatives in that it might disturb the wider relationship.

Paid childcarers and circles were seen by some as avoiding such pitfalls. It was thought that more clear cut stipulations could be made. Nonetheless a few parents complained of what they regarded as breaches of unwritten rules. Mrs Miller complained that her daily help had not looked after the children as she wanted. Two parents criticised other circle members for not adhering to what they regarded as shared expectations about the obligations of a babysitter from the group. In one case the carer had called parents back home instead of coping with a crying child. In the second example the family were dismayed that the babysitter was not prepared to stay after midnight.

Generally, decisions about where care should take place depended on the time of day and the convenience of the carer. In the daytime, it was generally assumed that friends and neighbours preferred being in their own home. It might also be seen as advantageous to the child, perhaps because there was a garden or novel playthings. In the case of some grandparents and older friends or neighbours it was preferred that the carer come to the child's home, where the environment was more oriented to the child's amusement or safety and to the protection of precious possessions. Such carers did not have children of their own and so were also more free to come to the child's home. The concern to fit in with the convenience of the carer, which was prominent in the daytime, was overridden in the evenings by a general wish not to disturb a sleeping child. It was also seen as more important for sleepy or sleeping children to be in their most familiar environment in case they woke up. If it was most convenient for a relative carer to have the child at their home, then the child would normally stay on overnight.

Reasons for changes in the relative importance of carers

Changes of carer could involve ceasing to use a carer, starting to use new people or altering the relative frequencies of existing carers. On the whole, arrangements with relatives were less liable to fluctuate than those with friends or neighbours but there were exceptions to this. A few grandparents became less frequent carers because of their age and declining fitness, especially if additional children in the family made looking after them a greater strain. In a few instances this paralleled the increased maturity of a teenage relative, who then became preferred as a carer. A grandparent's death had deprived five families of a major carer. Strokes and heart attacks had incapacitated several others as carers. In a few families, a grandmother starting work or one of parents' sisters having a baby had reduced their availability for care.

Alterations in care patterns with non-kin resulted more often from moving in and out of the local area, the differential development of friendships and changing perceptions of the advisability of non-kin care. A few ex-neighbours were still prominent carers but normally residential mobility of non-kin put an end to sharing care. Those with a considerable street network of carers had alternative and additional people to make good the reduction in care resources caused by someone moving away. On the other hand a few families had relied almost exclusively on a close neighbour and when that person moved they were loath to use less favoured carers. As in the case of those reliant on care by a grandparent who died, frequency of sharing fell sharply after the loss. The changes which occurred for all but one of the families who had used a childminder resulted from changes in care needs or the emergence of a more favoured carer. Only in the case of Winnie Nichols* noted above was dissatisfaction with the quality of care responsible for the move. Discontinuity of placements is a well-known feature of minding (Bryant *et al.*, 1980; Mayall and Petrie, 1977).

Differentiation within carer sets

As virtually every family had more than one person in its carer set, there needed to be some basis for selection on particular occasions. Differentiation amongst combinations of carers took three main forms – non-preferential, hierarchical and specialised. Sometimes, several major carers were seen as more or less equally acceptable so that choice depended on who was contactable and available. This was true of some street networks, circles and multiple kin carer sets. In contrast to these intersubstitutable carer sets many combinations exhibited a hierarchy. One or two carers were definitely preferred whilst other people would only be used when the first choice carers were not free. For instance, Mrs Urquhart* listed her order of preferences: first came either set of grandparents, then her sister or sister-in-law, then a friend downstairs and finally a friend down the street. In hierarchical carer sets, the person(s) who looked after the child most frequently and recently were the ones who would usually be asked first next time. By contrast, in non-preferential carer sets there was often an attempt to spread the 'burden' of care by choosing someone different each time. This also helped to sustain care relationships with several people who might otherwise drop out of swop arrangements if not called on for a long time.

Specialisation took three main forms according to the time of day, reasons for sharing care and location. Different carers could be used or the same carers used with differing frequencies according to whether the timing of care was day or evening, weekday or week-end, early or late finish in the evenings. Care of Robert Ormiston* was provided by one aunt during weekdays, his great aunt at week-ends and another of his mother's sisters in the evenings. The length of a care session might affect choice. Mrs Taylor* said, 'I couldna ask my Mum if it's got to be a late finish.' When Mrs Cairns wanted brief care she asked street friends or her husband but for a more infrequent but longer period she turned to her mother-in-law. There was sometimes a difference between carers who could be asked at short notice and those who required advance warning because of distance, commitments or personality. Stewart Raeburn's paternal grandmother was mostly a carer for planned occasions because she lived twelve miles away. Examples of functional specialisation included use of paid childcarer or grandparents while mother worked, but street friends at other times. This occurred to give the child a chance to play with friends or to minimise the mother's sense of indebtedness and imposition with respect to the work carer. A few parents gave instances of locational specialisation so that the child would stay with the carer who lived nearest to the place where the parent (normally the mother) was going, such as shops, dentist or hospital. A different kind of locational specialisation occurred when care sessions were organised around visits to or by a more distant carer. Some children were looked after by relatives during a holiday or week-end stay, while the parents went out.

Choice of overnight and crisis carers

Major care commitments place a greater imposition on the carer and require more adjustment by the child. In consequence, it was to be expected that somewhat different criteria might apply. This was indeed the case. All the people interviewed were asked to say who would be their first choice as carer for an overnight stay, whether they had actually shared care overnight or not. Three quarters of the respondents nominated a relative – a considerably higher proportion than was the case for more routine daytime care. Some parents who shared care frequently with non-relatives nearby in the daytime or evening had gone to considerable trouble to arrange overnight care with a relative some distance away, because 'you can't ask friends to look after children overnight' (Mrs Johnstone). Mrs Traynor* described their fifteen mile round trips to take and collect the children for week-end stays with her sister's family:

> It can be an awful upheaval. You have to pack your case, and when Sheila was a baby, it was taking the cot, the pram and everything. But I would rather do that knowing they were going to be happy with the person, rather than running upstairs (for someone) to watch them.

Non-routine needs for care may also lead families to look outside their normal carer set. Besides mothers' work which is dealt with in chapter 6, this had taken three main forms as follows (with the numbers of families concerned in parentheses):
Brief emergency (8)
Major crisis (16)
Birth of younger sibling (18)
By brief emergency is meant an accident or sudden illness to a family member. In most cases such situations had led to

sharing care with stair or street neighbours because of the immediacy of the need for assistance.

A major crisis consisted of a more prolonged and unexpected illness or hospitalisation of the mother for periods ranging from a few nights to two months. During such a crisis it was mainly grandparents and fathers who had looked after the children, often in combination. Some stressed the importance of keeping care within the nuclear family, despite the financial loss. Mr Laurie said, 'We'd rather put ourselves out than other people, you know.' Major crises sometimes altered well-established ideas about carer choice and frequency. The Irvines had always felt strongly that only parents should look after children. Unexpectedly, Mrs Irvine had to spend two months in hospital so they arranged for their daughter to stay all the time with Mr Irvine's parents. She came through the experience happily and they concluded that they had previously been too circumspect about sharing care.

Birth of a younger sibling is distinguished here from other major illnesses or hospital stays by mothers because this normally involves more predictability and opportunity to plan for care. Mothers' admissions to hospital for both childbirth and illness have been important reasons why children are admitted to local authority care (Packman, 1973; Statistics, 1984). Therefore, it is important to understand how ordinary families cope with this from their own resources. In this sample, all the families who had had to deal with such a critical disruption of maternal care had managed without resort to residential care. The arrangements made resembled closely those described by Bell et al. (1983). In six instances the father had taken time off work to care for the child, usually with the help of grandparents or a neighbour. In the other twelve cases grandparents or the mother's sister had looked after the child, either completely or more commonly until the father got home from work. Four of the children had gone to stay overnight with their grandparents. Grandmothers sometimes provided services like cooking and washing for the father as well as the child and in two cases both went to stay with the grandparents. Victor Shaw* was given an early place in a playgroup to make it easier for his maternal grandmother to cope. This was the sole example of the use of official services in a crisis.

Whether they had experienced a care crisis or not all the parents were asked how they thought they would deal with a stay in hospital by mother for a few nights and for some weeks. For short term absences of mother, nearly all of the parents thought they would rely on the father or the extended family. Several families nominated relatives who lived at a distance in preference to local friends who were the main everyday carers. In the case of a prolonged absence of the mothers, fifty out of sixty-three families envisaged that grandparents or parents' sisters would be the main carers. Distance was not necessarily seen as a problem. Mrs Kerr said 'My first choice would be my mother, though that is rather difficult as she is at the other end of the country. I think at this age it would have to be a grannie.' Fathers' work commitments meant that they were chiefly seen as a back up to others after work, especially for long periods. It was generally felt that friends or neighbours could or should not be called on to help for lengthy continuous periods. In fact more families said they would prefer to pay a stranger for crisis care than said they would use a friend.

Most families seemed to have a fairly clear choice of 'crisis' carer and some had a range of relatives they thought they could call on but several parents did hesitate about whom they would choose. These were families who had no close relatives in Edinburgh or perhaps only ones who were very elderly or unfit. The general feeling that care in a major crisis should come from relatives meant that even some parents who had a large local carer set felt anxious about how they would cope because they had no kin living nearby. Even after consideration four couples said they had nobody they felt able to ask for help in such a predicament.

Choice of group care

In a number of cases the group a child attended was chosen because an older sibling attended (twenty) or occasionally because a parent had attended (three). Otherwise, using the classification devised for individual carers, the main influences on group care choice were practical and evaluative rather than relational or personal. Nearly all the families considered only two or three facilities in their local area. Direct assessments of group care before booking a place were often superficial because parents usually had only brief contact before accepting a place or indeed before the child started, unless an older sibling had attended the same group. Therefore, the advice of acquaintances and friends in the neighbourhood was often critical in determining which establishment was chosen.

Well over half the parents said they had first learnt of the group from a neighbour or friend. Often they had been given a specific recommendation about one particular group. Sometimes evaluation of different groups was the product of comparative discussions in pairs or groups of mothers and it was simply a shared assumption that it would be a good idea to follow what friends or neighbours had done. A few families took very different views of the same establishment but in general there was a considerable degree of consensus about which were good ones and about the few which merited criticism. Given that most parents hardly knew the group beforehand, it is not surprising that they said they were most influenced in their choice of group by such factors as the amount of open space and equipment rather than the personal qualities of the staff. The decisions of only one out of every four families appeared to have been affected by whether the group was a playgroup or nursery school.

With a few exceptions official sources of information and evaluation of group care were much less significant than informal contacts (Table 3.3). Less than one third of respondents said that they had received any kind of advice from a professional person about sharing care. This was sometimes a reminder about group care in general and sometimes a recommendation about a particular group. Just four families had first learnt of the group they used (or planned to use) from an official source. By far the most important professionals were health visitors who gave some kind of advice to nearly one quarter of the families. This represents an interesting prolongation of the influence of health provision on pre-schooling, despite the statutory transfer of direct responsibili-

Table 3.3 *Sources of information and advice about group care*

1 *How family first learnt of facility used for child or for which child is booked in*	
Source of information	*Number of families* (N = 63)
Friends or neighbours	38
Father's contacts	6
Mother sought out information	5
Health visitor or social worker	4
Mother went as child	3
Relatives or relative's friends	3
Mother passed by facility	2
Advert	2

2 *Advice from officials about care*	
Source of advice	*Number of families who had received any advice at all about group care* (N = 63)
None	44
Health visitor only	11
Social work department only	3
Health visitor and SWD	1
Hospital social worker	1
GP	1
Clinic doctor	1
GP and health visitor	1

ties for providing and regulating pre-school groups to education and social work departments. Occasionally, the health visitor had suggested that a group care placement would help relieve family stresses, such as a relationship difficulty with the child or a difficult pregnancy. In three cases this idea was very much welcomed but two mothers had resented the idea that separation of the child was proposed as a solution. Despite the importance of health visitors compared with other officials, three quarters of parents had had no advice from one about group care. It seemed that, unless the child had a problem, advice depended on the chance factor of the particular knowledge and interest of the individual health visitor. No family had apparently received any information from the education department which runs all nursery schools. In spite of the paucity of official communication most parents claimed that they had been able to get all the information they needed, usually from people in their social networks. Just a few parents wanted more direct imparting of knowledge by those actually managing or running the facilities.

Parents and group care

Considerably more mothers (over three quarters) felt that they benefited from group care than had acknowledged any personal gain as a reason for using group care in the first place (one quarter). As we shall see later, this fits with a more general norm that mothers should avoid arranging care for overtly selfish reasons but may take advantages of care which is fixed up for the child's benefit. The most important gains mentioned were opportunities to do things like shopping or attend appointments without children present. In other words, it was possible to use group care *incidentally* for the same kind of reasons that shared care was *deliberately* arranged before. Some mothers also welcomed the fact that they had more time to devote to their own interests or look for work. Ten mothers said their overall relationship with the key child was helped by the separation because this reduced tension from constant interaction or led to mutual pleasure at reunion. Mothers' morale could be much improved. Mrs Traynor* described how she 'was getting a bit depressed, fed up from trying to keep Sheila happy, run the home. I feel freer since she went to nursery.' Group care mostly gives time resources to mothers, but thirteen mothers drew attention to the disadvantage that time was taken up in accompanying and staying with the child. Relatively few expressed a sense of missing the child but three mothers did experience a considerable feeling of loss with their child away.

Nearly all the fathers felt that group care made little impact on their lives. The main exceptions concerned shiftworkers, who either missed seeing the child when home during the day or were glad to have more peaceful sleep. Eight fathers accompanied their child to or from group care frequently. At the other extreme, one quarter (seventeen) had never been there at all,

In this sample, most of the mothers had so far had no participation apart from taking/collecting the child or social/fundraising activities. Some might well have become more involved later when their children had been attending longer. About one quarter sometimes took part in running a playgroup on a rota basis. Only three mothers in all had any management role as committee members. This degree of involvement is much less than many commentators would think satisfactory but in fact many women in the sample did not agree with the policy assumption that mothers should participate a lot. Overall the mothers were fairly evenly divided into those who saw involvement as a good thing and those who were not keen or not free (Table 3.4). There was some mis-matching, in that there were mothers in favour of involvement who had no opportunity for it and several who did assist with care who would have preferred not to. Those who were very positive about involvement were glad of the opportunity to see how their children were getting on, to meet other mothers or to satisfy a general liking for being with young children. There was little evidence that a transfer of educational ideas was either desired or actually happened although this has been seen as a major purpose of participation (Bronfenbrenner and Mahoney, 1975). Reluctance to participate did not necessarily signify lack of interest in the children. Some mothers thought that their prolonged presence would contradict a prime purpose of group care by inhibiting the child from making friends, gaining independence or learning. For example Mrs Balfour said 'If I were to stay there, he wouldn't do anything of any value.' Mrs Sim* believed that 'If mothers were there, I think the children would be more intent to come up to them all the time.'

Most nursery staff are not keen for children to start group care before the age of three (Morsbach et al., 1981). In this sample, roughly half of the families said they would have liked this. Not many seemed to feel strongly about it, however, and there was very little support for group care before two. Previous research has also shown a substantial number of

Table 3.4 *Mothers' views about participation at group care*

	Prefer involvement	Mixed feelings/ not mind	Prefer non- involvement
Middle Class (N = 33)	11	7	15
Working Class (N = 30)	10	5	14
Total (N = 63)	21	12	29

parents wanting a younger start for their children. This finding has been juxtaposed with knowledge of the increase in mother's work to imply a causal connection between the two (Bone, 1977; Hughes *et al.*, 1980). However, in this study, the main reasons for wanting an earlier entry to group care were to give the child more company, friends, enjoyment or stimulation at a younger age than entry requirements currently permit.

A much smaller proportion of low sharers than medium or high sharers wanted an early start to group care (p < 0.1). This suggests an underlying dimension in families related to (un)willingness to share care extensively or early. Therefore, families who were low sharers and were against an early start to group care were classified as 'protective'. By this definition, there were twelve protective families. This grouping was felt to have face validity as it corresponded more or less to impressions gained during the interview about which families were very concerned that all but minimal sharing was wrong or upsetting to the child. It must be emphasised that this grouping of families is not to be seen as in any way pathological like those on which Levy (1947) based his study of overprotectiveness. Nonetheless some of them did express in *much milder form* some of the features he recognised, particularly inhibition of the child's social maturity. Most protective families relied almost entirely on one or two relatives as carers. None had accepting attitudes towards care by strangers (p < 0.01).

Opinions were obtained about the difference between play-groups and nursery schools. Some researchers have seen the contrasts between the two general kinds of group as of less significance than the differences between individual establishments (Bruner, 1980). This was true for a good many parents too, but some did have strong feelings that one type was better than another. Virtually all the mothers but only half of the fathers seemed clear what the differences are. When asked which they preferred, far more respondents said nursery schools. Nearly half the mothers currently using a playgroup said they would have preferred a nursery school place if one had been available. There were no examples of the reverse.

Nursery school preference most often derived from beliefs that it offered better trained or more professional staff and/or rather more structured activity and formal teaching. Therefore, although most parents wanted group care for their children mainly for social reasons, this was often wanted within a setting which encourages learning and development. Those who preferred playgroups mostly did so on the grounds of the informality, smaller size of group and/or shorter hours. These included a high proportion of low sharers, but also some medium and high sharers. The question of mother participation seemed to have little influence on preferences. In some ways it seems that parents tended to see playgroups more in terms of their original intentions, i.e. as a substitute for nursery school in a more intimate setting, rather than the later purpose of community involvement.

The couples interviewed were invited to comment on the fact that most children (in Edinburgh) now go to some form of group care, whereas most of their parents did not. Nearly all were unreservedly positive about this major change in the social experience of early childhood. Many were of the view that it helped children prepare for school and avoid the upset of sudden entry to school at the age of five. Several parents volunteered the word trauma to describe this. These responses also illustrate that different kinds of question related to the same topic can elicit different sorts of answer, since avoidance of school-entry trauma was hardly mentioned at all amongst reasons for wanting a place at group care or benefits to the child from actual attendance. A frequent observation was that group care is now more necessary than in the past because of the greater restrictions of urban life, particularly caused by motor traffic. Just five mothers expressed some doubts about the expansion of group care. This arose either from resentment at what they felt as normative pressures that all children should be taken to group care or from a belief that children can prosper just as well at home.

Milburn and Whitlaw are particularly well provided for by national standards so not surprisingly there were high levels of satisfaction with the level of local pre-school provision. Comments about group care staff were almost all favourable too, even though these were initially strangers to the child and parents. The main exception to this positive appraisal of local facilities was that one in five of all families (thirteen) wanted a nursery school place nearer to their home. As most families did in fact have ready access to a nursery school, this does mean that a large proportion of the rest would have liked one close by.

Reciprocity

In certain respects shared care may be regarded as a service. It either gives parents freedom to do things unencumbered by direct child care responsibilities or provides something which the parents believe is of benefit to their children. Consequently it is helpful to consider how far it is characterised by the same kind of principles which have been observed from social and economic exchange in other contexts and cultures (Ekeh, 1974; McCormack, 1976; Mauss, 1954).

Sometimes the care service was given free of charge. The pleasure of the child's company and the 'psychological rewards' of altruism or giving aid within the extended family was felt by both parties to be an adequate recompense (Wispe, 1978). More usually parents felt that providing such inner rewards to others was insufficient. The idea of receiving something for nothing made most people uncomfortable. Therefore, some kind of payment in cash, time or kind was felt to be desirable or obligatory. It seemed that there was a general incompatibility between social and cash relationships as far as adults are concerned. It was rare for relatives or friends to be paid for care and typically there was a lack of interpersonal closeness maintained with paid childcarers. The principal exceptions to this were teenagers, who were often both paid for care and socially close to the family. The difference in age and status meant that cash payment was seen as more acceptable. With adult relatives it was often the case that no form of return for a care service was seen as necessary but parents mostly did feel that some kind of non-monetary 'repayment' was required for non-kin adults. These distinctions will now be elaborated.

A few parents felt that no return was necessary for sharing care because the carers enjoyed looking after the children or would be offended at the implication that they needed any incentive to care for the children. Repayment for care was also sometimes actively evaded or discouraged by carers. Even though Emily Griffin's parents insisted on paying her grandmother to look after her while they both worked, she reasserted the exchange imbalance and hence her altruism by spending the money on clothes for Emily. Mrs Ogilvie* remarked that 'I once offered my Mum something in fact. She told me more or less to get lost, sort of thing, that she didn't want paying to watch her own grandson. ( ) So after that, it was just a case of taking a box of chocolates.' These remarks exemplify a typical dilemma in that receiving money for shared care would often be felt as an affront by a close relative and even some non-relatives, yet parents wanted to show appreciation and reduce their feelings of indebtedness. This was illustrated by the fact that a question phrased 'Do you pay back in any way?' met with a frosty reception in the pilot interviews. Once this was reformulated in the main sample as 'Do you do anything in return?', respondents were much more forthcoming. They revealed that they resolved the problem of reciprocity by means of some kind of symbolic action or counter-gift which did not threaten the carer's sense of altruism. These included giving occasional presents (like Mrs Ogilvie's* chocolates), providing meals for the carer or performing some other service. Often there was deliberately no immediacy or exact comparability of return. For example, some parents gave extras at Christmas or on a birthday, when presents were already legitimate. Preparedness to help kin carers in future was seen by some as sufficient to reduce the feeling that help went in one direction only. For instance one or two fathers said they would do odd repairs for the child's grandparents. Other couples indicated they would or did give help with things that ageing relatives could no longer do for themselves. By disguising or separating the 'repayment' for sharing care, the parents as recipients of the service were able to fulfil their sense of obligation to reciprocate, without thereby threatening the carer's sense that they were acting altruistically.

At the time of interview, only six of the sixty-three families were making cash payments to individual carers for daytime non-group care. This entailed a weekly cost substantially above that of other forms of care and always resulted from both parents working. Evening care was more likely to involve payment largely because of the wider use of teenagers. About one third of families had used a paid babysitter at some time and ten families did so regularly. There was a wide range in the size of payment from a nominal amount to two pounds an hour (1981 prices). A few parents were spending several pounds a week on a private nursery school or playgroup but for the vast majority the costs of group care were nil or small (apart from lunches) as a result of public subsidy.

In relation to child care time is as much a resource to be exchanged as money. Many people preferred reciprocal sharing to cost-free care, because it removed feelings of indebtedness or imposition. It was easier to approach a carer for help not as a favour but as a part of ongoing exchange. Mr and Mrs Finlayson described how they used to ask his (childless) brother and sister-in-law to babysit frequently. This gradually tapered off 'because we're not reciprocating'. At the same time they made greater use of street friends who had been making care requests to them more than vice versa. The imbalance in both directions was thus reduced.

Frequent daytime sharing care for other than work reasons with non-relatives usually involved some kind of return care. The arrangements had varying degrees of formalisation, exemplified by those involving Stephen Powell and Emily Griffin which were described in the last chapter. Thirteen mothers engaged in some kind of regular weekly swop and a further twenty had a less systematic kind of reciprocal arrangement.

About half of the swop arrangements involved a network of more than two mothers whilst the rest were swops between pairs of mothers. Some of the former had developed into 'mini-groups' in which three to five mothers took it in turns to look after all their children at once while the others had a break. These mostly arose when children were first aged one and a half to two. Some had conscious purposes of preparation for group care, as well as giving opportunities for the children to play and for the mothers to meet socially. Although the mini-groups operated in similar ways the descriptions given by several individuals suggested that their particular one had developed spontaneously rather than from imitation of one already in existence. For instance:

Mrs Finlayson   'I suppose we all instigated it. It just emerged. . . .'

Mr Finlayson   'I suppose they were all doing the odd swop and it became apparent that there was a better way of doing it.'

Mrs Finlayson   'We did it to give the children a chance to play together. To give ourselves a morning off. ( ) We met a lot anyway, so it seemed sensible to have a regular arrangement.'

Swops were almost entirely confined to street friends with children of similar age so that care needs and demands were readily matched. Reciprocal care had the advantage of being constantly renewable. Care of children acted not just as a repayment but also as a downpayment against which it was easier to draw care services for oneself in future.

This norm of reciprocity (Gouldner, 1960) was seen not just in the preference for swop arrangements but also in the discomfort felt about non-equivalent exchange in relation to non-kin care. Several parents were reluctant to 'take advantage' of people without young children as there would be difficulty in finding a suitable return. Mrs Hunter declined her neighbours' offers of care because they felt 'like a favour'. She and others also wished to retain offers from those without children for emergencies so that a stock of goodwill was not used up. Sometimes the demand for care was too large to fit with the norm of approximately balanced exchange with friends who had children. Mrs Allan explained that when they went ski-ing, they took their son seventy miles to stay with relatives rather than leave him with friends in the same street, because 'then you've got to repay it in some way ( ) – I mean by looking after their children some time. ( ) The difficulty is not everyone wants to go away for a week-end, you know.'

Babysitting circles and reciprocity

Throughout the country babysitting groups have grown up in many areas, but there are also plenty of districts where they are absent. Little is known about their history, forms and functions. Yet this form of mutual aid merits special attention as an example of a successful neighbourhood self-help group dealing with the care of dependants by non-kin. The concept and practice of babysitting circles has developed and operated autonomously without professional encouragement. Since this study took place in only two small areas it cannot yield a comprehensive picture of circles but can illustrate some of their key features in a way which extends beyond individuals' experiences. It was clear from the interviews that knowledge about circles was highly variable and attitudes to them differed markedly from one person to another. The information about how circles work came only from accounts of individual members and not direct observation so the following picture is partial and tentative.

All the circles described by respondents had a limited terri- torial basis usually of a few adjacent streets. A few were confined to a single street but the largest ranged over a few square miles. The care service was limited to one dependent group (children) so that all members were at the same life- cycle stage (early parenthood). The basic mechanism was that parents provided care for other families in return for care of their own child at other times. There was no need for immediacy or equivalence of return care between any one pair of families. The exchange requirement was that each member's giving and receiving should be in approximate equilibrium over a period, so that there was no imbalance with the group as a whole. In this way circles provide an example of a general-ised exchange system (Befu, 1977; Fox, 1975). Indeed the very word *circle* evokes memories of the famous Kula *Ring* of Melanesian traders described by Malinowski (1922) and others. By spreading care arrangements in an organised way amongst a number of families, circles helped remove some of the emotional constraints to sharing care which result from fears of imposing on others and doubts about others' willing-ness to care. Circles had general rules which specified how the exchange arrangements were to be made. Sometimes these were written down and circulated with membership lists. There might also be subsidiary regulations, such as a require-ment that female carers be walked home late at night.

The reciprocal care service offered by circles involves ex-change of time as a commodity. Free time was given up by the carer and gained by the parents receiving the care service. The tasks of the circle organisation were to evaluate time costs, provide a means of matching supply and demand, and achieve a fair balance of input and output for each family. There have been only a few attempts by economists to analyse choices about the allocation of time as a scarce resource in similar ways to choices concerning money or material goods (Sharp, 1980). There has been a tendency to describe time allocation decisions in terms of financial equivalents, particu-larly using the concept of earnings foregone in using time for non-work purposes (Becker, 1965). This is undoubtedly important, but it is probable that in addition individuals are affected by distinct non-monetary considerations when they determine how they use their non-work time.

Economic and accounting analogies were apparent to several members. They used terms like credit and debit, being in the red or black, or even being bankrupt. In addition, the ways in which some respondents explained their decisions about circles were comprehensible in terms of economic concepts. Some couples chose not to join circles because the opportunity costs from spending their time in return babysitting were considered too great. This would mean giving up 'two nights for one', as Mrs Davies put it. Non-work time was a highly valued resource which they wished to retain for preferred leisure or domestic activities. A few parents had left a circle or decided not to join because they saw their care demands as too low or inelastic, so they would always be in credit to the circle. Usually such decisions to terminate inequitable exchange were linked to the availability of alternative carer resources like kin or a paid childcarer (Burgess and Nielsen, 1974). Several parents were conscious of the substitutablity of time and money. Circles could be attractive for saving money to those whose main alternative form of care was seen as paying teenagers or an agency. On the other hand, Mr Elliott argued that it was silly to waste his wife's time out babysitting when they could easily afford to pay people.

The babysitting groups in this sample had two formal methods of balancing supply and demand. One was based on book-keeping principles and the other relied on the exchange of some kind of object which acted as a time measure. Three families belonged to a circle with a book system and ten families belonged to an exchange medium circle. In addition Mr and Mrs Carlisle belonged to two groups, one of each type. The book-keeping model involved keeping a record of the time units or points for each care occasion and maintaining a balance sheet of giving and receiving care. This was a centralised system in which one family or mother at a time kept the record book in rotation. The person holding the book was responsible for matching demands for care with carers' balance sheet at the time. The book-keeping system meant that the links between a consumer and provider of a care service on any particular occasion were determined by the book person and not the participants. This had the effect of extending care connections fairly evenly throughout the membership. Informal communication might modify this theoretical impartiality to take some account of personal preferences, especially if there was a 'good reason' such as wanting a more familiar person for a baby. This system had the advantage of good information flow about families' credit balance. It made possible quick adjustments to prevent large imbalances occurring. The main drawbacks seemed to be that making arrangements could be very burdensome for the book holder and other members had restricted choice about who would babysit for them. (Other more flexible variants of this are known to the author from outside this study. For example, a monthly list of members' credit and debit balances may be issued to guide people about which person to approach first to babysit, namely those who have a deficit of giving shared care compared with receiving it. Although one person compiles the list, specific care arrangements are fixed up between the members concerned.)

Exchange medium circles used beans or some kind of artificial tokens. These had values equivalent to time periods and were paid to carers at each care session. In one circle, the standard time unit of exchange was the whole session, which Mr and Mrs Carlisle saw as unfair, because they had to go out and babysit longer and later than they required a carer to do themselves. In all the others, finer gradations of time were measured. They attempted somewhat crudely to take account of both variations in the length of care session and differences in the subjective valuation of identical periods of time. Normally, there was a basic rate for evening hours or half hours. Periods considered to be more inconvenient such as before six or after midnight were then weighted by rates of pay higher by 50 or 100 per cent. Both the standard and weighted time equivalents varied from group to group. A few respondents thought that the weighting had become so elaborate that it was dysfunctional because the calculations became offputting.

Use of tokens and beans opened up the possibility of forgery. A few sceptical parents thought there were dangers of this taking place but none had experience of it. This highlights the degree of trust with respect to honesty as well as access to one's child and home which circle membership was normally assumed to guarantee.

The exchange medium system was more decentralised than the book-keeping system since arrangements were made directly between the pair of families concerned. There was no formal means of communication about which families were in credit or debit, but usually those families who had spent a lot of their tokens passed the word around that they would welcome requests to go and babysit so they might replenish their supply of tokens.

The beans and tokens served some of the functions that characterise money (Newlyn, 1962):

1 Permitting a separation in time of giving and return. This is essential in relation to shared care, where both sets of parents are enabled to go out and care for two sets of children by doing so on different occasions
2 Acting as a store of value
3 Providing a unit of account

It is interesting that money itself was not used. The main practical implication of this was that tokens were highly specific in their convertibility, namely for care services only. This meant that the supply could be controlled by a limited initial allocation and there was little incentive for wealth accumulation. Use of cash would have made control of the overall supply much harder and so have removed one of the limiting factors on excesses of giving and receiving. Perhaps just as important would be the fact that cash payment could introduce commercial and power overtones, which most circle members were keen to avoid (Baldwin, 1978; Blau, 1964).

When asked how their particular group had been established, most respondents replied that two or three neighbouring mothers had developed the idea and organisation, usually with the more passive involvement of at least a few others. Several had grown up within the recent experience of the family being interviewed but others had been established much longer. The resulting circles range considerably in size. All the book circles had remained fairly small with fewer than twenty members. Most exchange medium circles had grown to a membership of twenty-five to fifty. Functional necessity probably kept book systems from expanding too much as this would result in an excessive workload for the book holder. Those circles in which only women babysat were small ones. Some circles deliberately restricted the size of membership to ensure that everyone was well known to each other and to minimise travel. Where such constraints did not operate it appeared that there was a natural tendency for circles to grow, as friends of members and friends of friends were introduced. More formality and greater involvement of men in babysitting was characteristic of the large, longer established circles. This suggests that they might be the end-products of typical sequences of development. Bigger groups were liked for the greater certainty of carer availability and a wider range of social contacts. Moreover, circles with a wide geographical spread meant that those living in streets with few young children could become linked to families further away. On the other hand, there were indications of fissiparous tendencies in very large circles. One small book circle comprised members who had come together out of disaffection with the unfairness and complications of a large bean group. Another circle had considered dividing into smaller district groups.

Entry to circles was easier in some cases than others. Some small circles limited eligibility to the same street or to people well known to each other. Larger circles had more open membership. Several respondents asserted that only trustworthy people would be admitted and that there were adequate vetting procedures, such as the need for nomination by an existing member or ratification at a circle meeting. Nevertheless, several remarks by members indicated that any newcomer to the area with young children was invited to join. One or two gave inadvertent examples of encouraging people they hardly knew to belong. It was widely accepted that trust of one's home and child could be automatically given to an unknown member. This seemed related to an assumption that only similar people would want to join or be invited to join. Mrs Miller and Mrs Balfour both stated explicitly that trust derived from having members of the same 'social type'. There was also perhaps an underlying presumption that only similar and suitable people would be likely to live in the same area.

Quite often some or all of the mothers from a circle would also share care for each other during the day. Normally this was regarded as separate, so that it did not involve the tokens or recording associated with evening care. The arrangement was an individual matter for the pair of families concerned. It was explained that daytime care required less inconvenience or disruption of planned activities for the carer, partly because she would be in her own home with her own children anyway. Occasionally a circle member did provide daytime care as part of the circle system, with an appropriate weighting for daytime hours. This happened, for instance, when a single mother needed to build up credit for evening sessions or if a child was cared for at a week-end and so might be a greater imposition than usual.

It was evident from parents' descriptions that circles had important social as well as practical functions. Most had been started by sets of street friends. Once established they assisted in the initiation and development of friendships. Sometimes an individual's social motivation was overt. Mrs Booth said 'I joined the sitting circle to get to know people.' Most of the circles held meetings to discuss organisational matters but often these associations led to the development of non-business aspects too. They could become opportunities for lavish spreads to be provided, for children to play and for social conversations. Some circles had specifically arranged recreational activities for the group, such as dinner parties or outings together. Conversely, social relationships also gave rise to babysitting groups, since several had grown out of mothers' morning coffee gatherings.

Some circles had a specific organiser or secretary, although there was usually a new occupant of that position from time to time. Members of the other groups asserted that they did not have leaders as such. Mrs Finlayson claimed, 'It doesn't really have an organiser, it runs itself.' Mrs Kerr described her circle as being leaderless and 'a mutually organised group'. Without direct observations it is difficult to test such perceptions, but it seemed that there was a concern to avoid giving individuals permanent positions of power within circles. A loose structure was possible because usually circles included subsets of mothers who were in frequent everyday interaction. This could give rise to clique formation. Mrs Gunn remarked, 'I think we're all like that, circles within circles.' Exchange medium groups were more conducive to this because they permitted more individual choice of carer. This was reinforced by the tendency to prefer known people as carers, so that a subset in a token group might arrange care largely internally, using the wider circle only as a back up arrangement. Subset formation could be based on locality, membership length or age of children.

Usually, men were only marginally involved in the organisation of circles, even if they participated a fair amount in care itself. In small circles the involvement of men seemed to depend a lot on the attitude of the mothers. Mrs Gunn's circle had not even considered the possibility of men being involved.

In contrast, the small group being set up by Mrs Powell and her street friends insisted on maximising the participation of fathers. A minority of the fathers in the sample babysat fairly often, usually in the larger circles. Some regarded this as the easy option, because there was more likely to be quiet and an opportunity to read or work than at home. A few men were reluctant to babysit because 'it's women's work' (Mr Gunn) or 'it's organised by women' (Mr Finlayson). Others felt they could not cope with young children. Some mothers accepted it as their role, but at least two mothers expressed some resentment at 'chauvinism' and having to 'pay for every night out' by giving up more of their time which their husbands did not.

Besides true circles, there were small care networks some of which may well have been embryonic circles, for this was how some of the big ones had originated. In these networks, a few families practised generalised exchange on an ad hoc basis with no formal attempts to maintain exact equivalence. Rough balancing was achieved by individuals' sense of indebtedness. Such networks offered a wider care resource base than pair swopping without the full obligations of circle membership. Progressive formalisation may not be inevitable as some mothers were determined to retain simplicity and intimacy.

Children's reactions to care

This chapter has been concerned mainly with the viewpoints of the adult participants in shared care. No observations were made of the children nor were any tests used, so that information about their involvement and responses is second-hand. Parents were asked to describe how their children had responded to their experiences of shared care and what changes had been noticed. This provides a subjective picture of children's reactions, but one which is based on the perceptions of those best informed about them.

Many of the parents revealed that they had had considerable anxiety about how their children would cope with being looked after by someone else. Often they expressed reluctance to risk separation from their child. Some evinced great relief when the child had fared much better with the carer than had been foreseen. Of course some children responded differently to different carers or care situations, and their reactions also changed as they grew older. Besides, high sharing families provided more occasions of non-parental care for the child and therefore more opportunities for varied responses than low sharing families did. Nevertheless, most of the children were depicted as having a general propensity either to happy or to unhappy reactions. Other research has produced mixed evidence as to the constancy or changeability of children's modes of reaction to separations and new experiences (Danziger, 1970; Waldrop and Halverson, 1975). This means that the patterns of distress which occurred in this study do not necessarily have any long-term implications – children can and do show considerable change and resilience as they grow up (Clarke and Clarke, 1976).

Over half the parents (thirty-nine) thought their children had always stayed quite happily with their daytime carers. For example, Adam Christie had stayed weekly from babyhood, first with relatives and later in a swop with street friends. His father remarked that 'He's always been very happy' (when left with the carer). A few children were reticent with most people but quite content to stay with a very familiar person such as a grandparent or neighbour. Nicola Sadler* was described by her parents as a shy girl, but she was always pleased to be looked after by her mother's parents because 'she's just been brought up with them and she's not strange with them in any way'. It was a common observation that children might cry briefly when the parent first left, but then settle happily as they accepted the situation and the carer responded appropriately. Eleanor Buchan had screamed when she first stayed with a street neighbour to play with her children. According to her mother, before long she was 'very happy there, feels very much at home, very mothered and appreciated, and has blossomed I think'. Evidently, the effects of care by familiar people in everyday circumstances bears little relation to the findings of distress from either institutional care or laboratory situations. The children who had shown considerable upset at being left and/or unwillingness to be left exhibited this chiefly before two years of age. Developmental studies have also found the period from about seven to twenty-four months to be the time when children are more likely to be distressed at separation from their mothers (Schaffer, 1977). On the other hand, many of the children had happily begun to stay more often with an expanding carer set of familiar people in the second year, just at that time when sensitivity to care by strangers is at its height. Reactions to daytime care did not seem closely related to differences in most care dimensions, except that a somewhat higher proportion of children with low frequency of sharing in the first two years was more likely to be upset when left (p < 0.1).

Usually, children had had fewer experiences of upset in the evenings. Many slept soundly and were unaware of parental absence. Some did wake but had not been bothered to find their parents not there. Eight children, i.e. about one eighth of the sample, had been persistently difficult to leave both day and night through the three years.

Several of the children who had stayed overnight in hospital had very negative reactions. They were disturbed not only by the unfamiliar settings but also the stresses of illness and treatment (see also Rutter, 1980a). For instance, Malcolm Miller had been a secure baby who slept 'beautifully', but he became clingy and disturbed at nights after a stay in hospital. In contrast to hospital stays, overnight care in the child's or carer's home had resulted in upset for only three children. For two of these the reason for the overnight stay was that their mother was in hospital. The vast majority had apparently enjoyed and benefited from overnight care, even though many of the overnight stays occurred during that critical period when any prolonged separation from mother has been seen as harmful by attachment theorists (Bowlby, 1973). A typical conclusion was that of Mrs Davies: 'I think they've done her good. I think they add to a child's confidence.' The generally favourable outcomes contradict a fairly common view that overnight separations from parents are undesirable for children aged under three. The fact that a lower proportion of children had apparently been distressed by overnight care compared with daytime care suggests that parents were particularly careful in choosing carers and contexts for overnight care which minimised the risk of upset. Some parents were worried about negative effects and were surprised that the child responded to the positive relationship with the carer:

| Mrs Forbes | We were concerned about how she would react to us disappearing off, (but) we had told her she was going to Grannie and she was delighted in fact. |
| Mrs Laurie | She loved it (but) I think because I'm used to being with her, I go into her room and her not being there. . . . I can't bear to leave them. |

Half of the children who attended mother and toddler or miscellaneous groups had some kind of negative reaction. This proportion was much higher than for other forms of care. A particularly high proportion of children attending church or sports creches had been unhappy or even acutely distressed. Fraser Booth 'cried and cried' at a church creche and his parents believed this had long-term effects on him. Mrs Booth said 'He stayed with no-one for the next year. It did him tremendous harm.' Although irregular or early attendance may have contributed to the distress in some cases, there were also a number of complaints about limited accommodation, inadequate means of amusing the children and changes of supervisors. Mrs Laurie described their church creche as having 'too many babies there for too few people. They just sort of put them in a room for the hour that you are in church.' Mrs Powell described how a toddler group she attended had been poorly run because the mothers were so exhausted they 'just wanted to sit and put their feet up for ten minutes'. However, four children had enjoyed going to creches regularly since babyhood. Descriptions of ballet classes and Sunday schools were nearly all favourable which reflects the fact that attendance only began after the children were three.

Most children in this sample had only been attending nursery school or playgroup for a few weeks or months. Therefore it was only possible to ascertain how they were getting on initially rather than assess their longer term adjustment. Other research has shown that most children have some difficulty at first but are usually well integrated by two to three months (Caldwell, 1973; Denzin, 1977). Nonetheless, many parents in the present study had been worried about how their child would 'settle' in this first introduction to long term daily group experience. In the event most of their children did adjust rapidly and well to group care. There were far fewer troubled reactions than was the case for miscellaneous or toddler groups. This was doubtless helped by the careful attention given to the introductory period by both staff and parents, as well as the children's greater age and experience. There were just a few who seemed to have been completely unhappy about the whole experience. Such was the value placed on attendance at playgroups and nursery schools that the parents chose to weather such a period of unhappy resistance by the child, which was occasionally quite prolonged. This included a few couples who had expressed strong disapproval of leaving an upset child in other contexts.

Half of the children attending playgroups were upset when starting, compared with only one quarter at nursery school. As can be seen later, this should not be taken to mean that playgroups provided a more upsetting experience, but rather that children who were vulnerable to separation anxiety were more likely to attend playgroups. There was suggestive statistical evidence that poor initial reactions to group care were associated with a history of less frequent shared care in a small carer set ($p < 0.1$). Half the children in low sharing families and two thirds of those in protective families reacted poorly to group care, compared with only one in four children in high sharing families. It could be that previous experience of being apart from parents helped children adapt to group care. Nevertheless, a number of children with minimal exposure to shared care did settle well in group care. Attendance at mother and toddlers groups which is often seen as preparation for playgroup or nursery school did not lead to any better or worse settling in group care.

It might be expected that any one child would tend to respond in similar ways to all of the different kinds of sharing care and that children with a history of resistance to separation from parents would not adapt well to group care. This was borne out to a considerable degree here. Over 80 per cent of children who had reacted well to care by friends and relatives also adapted well to group care, whereas most of those children who had previously been reluctant to be left with individual carers also had difficulty in settling at group care (p < 0.01). Even so a few previously adaptable children were unhappy when starting group care and over one third of the children who had earlier reacted poorly to individual shared care did fit in well. The majority of the children who had reacted negatively to mother and toddler or miscellaneous groups did not repeat this at group care.

The partial correspondence in reactions permitted the children to be classified as to whether their overall experience of shared care was mainly good (twenty-five), mainly bad (sixteen) or mixed (twenty-two). Those children who had had mostly negative reactions came chiefly from low or medium sharing families (p < 0.05). Nearly all the children had found at least one of the forms of care upsetting at some stage. Thus it could be unwise for adults to generalise too much from a child's response to just one kind of non-parental care.

Parents were asked how their child got on with other children at group care and how their behaviour had changed since starting. About one quarter of children attending group care were described as playing quietly or not mixing well. Again such children were found more often in playgroups (p < 0.05) and in low sharing families. Nine children had made new friends from group care. This low figure reflects the fact that in most cases they had only recently started. In the main, reported behaviour changes were positive. The one most frequently reported was that the child sang songs a lot more as a result of starting group care. This may seem trivial but there is evidence that the kind of rhythmic and repetitive songs learnt in playgroups and nursery schools form a valuable means of verbal and cognitive development (Hayes et al., 1982). Some children had also developed reading and play techniques which gave parents ideas about what to do at home too. Ten children were thought to have learnt positive things from other children, such as more effective communication or a specific play skill. About one quarter of children attending group care were said to have learnt things parents mildly disapproved of, like swearing or cheekiness.

So far we have discussed in the main either individual children or the sample as a whole. Now it is time to look at variations which reflected the social and material circumstances of different types of family.

4 *Social class, area of residence and sharing care*

The meaning and assessment of social class membership

The general properties of shared care have been delineated in the last two chapters. The remainder of the book discusses how these fitted in with important aspects of children's and parents' daily lives. First of all differences and similarities associated with families' social class and area of residence will be looked at, since these formed a fundamental part of the sampling frame for reasons discussed in chapter 1.

Part of the intention behind using a two-area sample was to produce a clear class comparison. Families still had to be differentiated individually by social class, however, because inevitably the correspondence between class and area of residence is not total. With a fairly small sample it was not possible to take account of very detailed variations in socio-economic status and mobility as is necessary for specialist investigations of social class (Goldthorpe *et al.*, 1980; Richardson, 1977). For more general purposes it is usually assumed that all members of a family are in the same class, which is indicated by the father's job. The most common means of classifying jobs is to use the Registrar General's groupings of occupations (OPCS, 1980). This is often simplified into a twofold division by which those with manual jobs are called working class and those with non-manual jobs are called middle class (e.g. Young and Willmott, 1957:171). For several reasons this approach was not felt to be fully adequate for the present study. There were some jobs which appeared to be wrongly classified and it did not seem right to alter these on an arbitrary basis as did the Newsons (1963). Refinements of the Registrar General's classification (such as that of Goldthorpe and Hope, 1974) produce far too many categories for a small scale study. Another problem about using men's jobs as the sole basis for judging socio-economic status is that it discounts the independent class status of women (Stanworth, 1984). This seemed to be particularly unfortunate for a child care topic in which women play such a prominent part. Finally, important non-occupational factors in class are left out when people's jobs are used as the only criterion.

To help overcome these difficulties it was decided to use an index which tried to treat men and women equally, took account of various factors over the life-cycle besides current occupation and also incorporated some element of self-description. Otto (1975) has criticised the use of such composite indices in family research because the individual items are conceptually distinct and coincide only partially in practice. This seems to miss the point. It is precisely because single indicators are sometimes mis-matched with other criteria that an assemblage of indicators is needed for more accurate allocation and also to reveal intermediate and mixed class categories. Previous attempts to compile a suitable index of social class were examined (Blau and Duncan, 1975; Goldthorpe *et al.*, 1969; Osborn and Morris, 1979; Townsend, 1979). It was not possible to adapt any of these for present purposes in their entirety. Either they did not avoid all the defects noted above or else they required data which was not available. Consequently a new index was developed for the present study which included the more relevant characteristics from these writings.

It was necessary for the index to yield a simple reduction to a middle-class/working-class dichotomy as subtler distinctions would rarely reach statistical significance with a small sample. Yet it would be useful to retain a capacity for finer divisions. Several indicators of social class were transformed into variables with two values of either a broadly working-class (Score 1) or middle-class nature (Score 2). Both parents were allocated a score of 1 or 2 for their parents' occupations, their own educational qualifications, whether they attended private school or not, their current occupations and their own ideas of what class they belonged to. Mothers' occupational status was judged according to their job before having children because a number had not worked since or had taken jobs of lower status subsequently. It is not intended to suggest that either families or society can be neatly divided up into only two groupings in one or all of these criteria. However, the area basis of sampling had achieved a sample with relatively few border-line families.

A family class index was calculated for each family by adding the sum for each parent on all the individual indicators together with a score for net family income. Table 4.1 shows in detail how this was done. The resulting index had a maximum score of 22 and a minimum of 11. It was occasionally used as a continuous variable expressing the degree of 'middle-classness' or 'working-classness' of a family for correlation with other variables, but was most useful as the basis for a twofold division of the sample. Families with a final score of 15 or below were deemed working class and those with a score of 16 or over were regarded as middle class. This was the major classification used in the study and the one to which future references apply. In the text working-class families are distinguished by appending an asterisk to their surnames. The distribution of families produced by the index fitted well with the subjective assessments made of families during the interviews. For some purposes a threefold classification was used to separate out a category of fifteen 'intermediate class' families. For instance, there were couples where one or both partners had been upwardly mobile and others in which the husband and wife had different class backgrounds. Finally, a fourfold division distinguished between 'solid' and 'intermediate' middle-class and 'solid' and 'intermediate' working-class families.

The final classification was compared with the Registrar General's grouping of occupations (Table 4.2). The study index produced one middle-class family with a father doing a manual job and seven working-class families whose father held a non-manual job. Mothers' jobs revealed more anomalies, partly because the Registrar General's classification is ill-suited to many of the occupations typically performed by women (Llewellyn, 1981). There were five working-class families living in Milburn and two middle-class families in Whitlaw. These were not mis-classifications, but families who on most criteria were different from the prevailing kind of family in their area. In spite of these exceptions, the correspondence between area and class according to the index was strong (p < 0.001). In consequence, area and class comparisons gave very similar results for most purposes.

That this class basis of comparison was not a fiction of the

Table 4.1 *Formation of the class index used in the study*

1 *Class Indicator Used*
Each family was allocated to a score of 1 or 2 on each class indicator. If information was not available (only a few instances) the average of other indicators was used. The final class index score was the sum for each family of the score on every indicator.

	Meaning of the score	
Indicator	*Score 1*	*Score 2*
1 Father's Father's Occupation	Registrar General's Classification IIIM, IV or V	Registrar General's Classification I, II or IIIN
2 Mother's Father's Occupation	– ditto –	– ditto –
3 Father's Present Occupation	– ditto –	– ditto –
4 Mother's Occupation before Pregnancy	– ditto –	– ditto –
5 Father's Schooling	Local Authority/ Religious	Private, Fee-paying
6 Mother's Schooling	– ditto –	– ditto –
7 Father's Qualifications	Only School or Minor Post-School Qualifications	Nursing, Diploma or Degree Qualifications
8 Mother's Qualifications	– ditto –	– ditto –
9 Father's Self-Description	Working-Class or Ordinary	Middle-Class or Professional
10 Mother's Self-Description	– ditto –	– ditto –
11 Family Income (net of Tax, National Insurance)	Under £140 per week	£140 and over per week

2 *Total Class Index Used*

The class index for each family was the sum of its scores on each of the 11 indicators above, thus giving a maximum possible score of 22 and a minimum of 11.

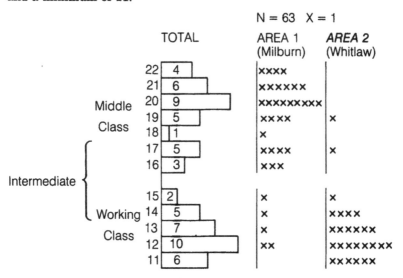

N = 63   X = 1

	TOTAL	AREA 1 (Milburn)	AREA 2 (Whitlaw)
Middle Class	22 | 4	xxxx	
	21 | 6	xxxxxx	
	20 | 9	xxxxxxxxx	
	19 | 5	xxxx	x
	18 | 1	x	
	17 | 5	xxxx	x
	16 | 3	xxx	
Working Class	15 | 2	x	x
	14 | 5	x	xxxx
	13 | 7	x	xxxxxx
	12 | 10	xx	xxxxxxxx
	11 | 6		xxxxxx

Intermediate { (brace spanning 17 to 14)

3 *Summary Class Indexes*

The above index was subdivided with three degrees of distinction.

(1) Twofold	This is the main class index used.		
	Label	*Total Class Index Score*	*Number of families*
	Middle Class	(16–22)	33
	Working Class	(11–15)	30
(2) Threefold			
	Solid Middle Class	(18–22)	25
	Intermediate	(14–17)	15
	Solid Working Class	(11–15)	23
(3) Fourfold			
	Solid Middle Class	(18–22)	25
	Intermediate Middle Class	(16–17)	8
	Intermediate Working Class	(14–15)	7
	Solid Working Class	(11–13)	23

Table 4.2 *Registrar General's rankings of parents' jobs*

	Father at time of interview	*Mother before pregnancy*	*Mother at time of interview*
Class I	12	2	2
Class II	21	26	8
Class III Non-manual	7	26	6
Class III Manual	20	3	2
Class IV	3	4	1
Class V	–	2	5
	63	63	24

Notes
1 The two unemployed fathers were ranked according to the previous job.
2 Those who had been University students before pregnancy were included in Class II.

Summary			
Class I–III NM	63.5%	86%	66.5%
Class III M–V	36.5%	14%	33.5%

outside observer was shown by parents' replies when asked what class they thought they belonged to and what other classes exist. This study's overall twofold grouping of families, as well as the criteria for judging class membership and the particular allocation of the families, were all broadly consistent with the views of most parents themselves. Over two thirds of respondents saw society as divided into some form of hierarchy. This took the form of either a simple middle-class/working-class dichotomy or a fourfold classification with upper and lower gradations of both middle and working classes. Mostly, people's own perceptions of the class they belonged to agreed with the class allocation from the study index. Some exceptions did occur as was to be expected (Gouder, 1975; Krausz, 1969). A few people denied the existence of classes.

Class and patterns of care

Some working-class parents thought that middle-class parents leave their children more readily. They cited the use of nannies and private boarding schools as evidence for this belief.

Conversely, some middle-class parents considered that working-class parents shared care more, because they were thought to belong to close-knit communities, experience greater economic pressures for mothers to work or make greater use of nurseries. In actuality the influence of social class was rather more complex.

Comparisons tend to emphasise contrasts, so it is important to stress at the outset that there were important universalities which applied across class. This was especially true with respect to reasons for sharing care and the evaluations of group care. Nevertheless it is hoped to demonstrate that there were large dissimilarities too, which were connected to important differences in the social experience of children and parents. In particular, most middle-class families shared care more often and among a wider range of carers outside the family's kin network than most working-class families. Whilst the latter usually selected carers from within their existing social networks of relatives and old-established friends, middle-class parents appeared to be more adept at recruiting new members both to their social networks and to their carer sets by developing acquaintanceships with families at a similar life-cycle stage living nearby. This meant that middle-class carers were usually concentrated in nearby streets whilst working-class carers often lived further afield. There was evidence that this class difference occurred even when such factors as availability of relatives and area of residence are allowed for. For working-class parents there seemed to be a less marked distinction made between daytime, evening and overnight care, because often the same relatives would be used for all these temporal dimensions of care. Overnight care by kin was often seen as an alternative to evening care, whereas nearly all middle-class parents only contemplated overnight care in special circumstances.

These striking differences will now be illustrated in more detail. It was not so much the absolute usage of relatives which distinguished families of different class as the comparative importance of kin vis-à-vis other kinds of carers. For over three quarters of the working-class families the main daytime carer was a relative, whereas for over three quarters of middle-class families the main carer was a non-relative. This marked contrast should not hide the fact that many middle-class families did make significant use of kin for care. It was just that often they were less prominent because of the families' high use of non-kin too. The minority of middle-class families who did have relatives as their main or second carers mostly shared care less often than other middle-class respondents (p < 0.1). In both classes the most common relative main carers were maternal grandparents, but use of relatives other than grandparents, aunts or uncles as carers was virtually a working-class preserve. Interestingly, in the diary fortnight slightly *more* middle-class than working-class families shared care with relatives (fourteen, as opposed to ten). This resulted from the fact that a number of the working-class families whose principal carers were relatives did not share care at all in the diary fortnight, whereas nearly all of the middle-class families who used relatives regularly did so during that period. The diaries also showed that middle-class care by the child's relations occurred mostly at home, whilst care of working-class children by relatives was more often away from home. Working-class mothers often dropped children off at their mum's or sister's home before going to the shops or doing something else, whereas middle-class mothers mostly took advantage of a visit by a grandmother to go out.

Even more significant than the dissimilarities with respect to kin care were the marked differences in the extent of shared care with non-kin. During the diary fortnight three quarters of the middle-class children stayed with friends or neighbours without their parents being there. This was the case for only four of the working-class children. Likewise twenty-six of the thirty-three middle-class families had a friend or neighbour as main carer either in the daytime or in the evening. In only one case was this the next door neighbour. Just four working-class parents said their main daytime or evening carer was a friend or neighbour. Two of these were immediate neighbours. A fair number of working-class families had used street friends for care at some point, but usually in a subsidiary capacity to relatives. Whilst they might be happy for their child to spend time during the day with a friend along the street, they were reluctant to take that person away from their family commitments or consider having non-family in the home during the evening.

Analysis of the overall make up of carer sets revealed that nearly all the working-class children were looked after mainly by their relations and perhaps one or two neighbours or parents' friends at most. On the other hand, many middle-class carer sets comprised several street or other local mothers and close relatives, as well as babysitting circle members in some cases. Most working-class families restricted both day and evening care to the same kind of people. In many cases the same individuals were used for both types of care. By contrast, eight middle-class children had a relative as main day or evening carer combined with a street friend or circle for the opposite time of day. This was true for just one working-class child. In these families it was clearly not distance of kin which resulted in the use of non-kin as a main carer by the family.

All the nine families who had used a daily help, agency help or au pair at any time in the three years (i.e. a paid childcarer in the child's home) were middle class. This represented nearly one third of middle-class families. However, there was no simple relationship between class or income and the amount of money spent on sharing care. Childminders (i.e. paid child-carers outside the home) had been used in both classes. Some well off middle-class families spent more than most on babysitting or private group care, but many did not. A few low earning families paid a fair amount each week for a playgroup, whilst some high earning families paid nothing for group care because their child went to a nursery school and did not stay to lunch. Nevertheless, it was clear that the larger monetary and accommodation resources of most middle-class families gave them a wider range of shared care options.

The proportion of children who had been looked after by teenagers during the day or evening was the same in both classes. However, twelve working-class children had been looked after by a teenage relative (excluding siblings) and no middle-class children. Conversely, twice as many middle-class as working-class children had been cared for by a non-relative teenager. A small number of middle-class families had used teenage 'strangers', recruited through advertisements or church groups. Families in both classes had teenagers as their main evening babysitters, but for more of the middle-class families teenagers had been an occasional back up to their regular arrangement. Only three middle-class children were reported to have been taken out regularly by teenagers in the daytime, compared with ten working-class children.

Similar proportions of children in both classes had been looked after at least once by a man alone (apart from their own fathers) but this disguises a big difference in detail. Nearly all cases of middle-class children being looked after by males occurred in the evenings and that chiefly involved men from a babysitting group. In a few cases it meant an uncle or non-related teenage boy. Half of the working-class children had been looked after by males in the daytime. Care by uncles and grandfathers alone was much more common in working-class families. To sum up, more working-class children were quite used to shared care by a man when they were awake but fewer were accustomed to care by men who were unrelated to them at any time.

Sequences of shared care indicated that the class difference in the kinds of carers used had been much less pronounced in the first year compared with later (Table 4.3). Nearly as many middle-class families reported having had grandparents as main carers in the first year as working-class families. At this age some of the largest carer sets were to be found amongst working-class families because several relatives had looked after the baby. Quite a few middle-class families who would later share extensively with street networks had relied mainly on grandparents and one or two close friends in the first year. In all, the number of middle-class families with a relative as main carer fell from sixteen in the first year to six in the third year, whilst the number of working-class families in that position remained steady at twenty-four. There was a definite shift towards greater usage of street and local friends in the second and third years by most middle-class families. Those few middle-class families who did not incorporate several 'local people' in their carer set were low sharers. This demonstrates further that it was not simply differential availability of kin and non-kin which accounted for the class contrasts in care patterns.

Table 4.3 *Sequences of main carer*

	Working Class	Middle Class	Total
1 Grandparents for all 3 years	15	5	(20)
2 Other all kin sequences	6	2	(8)
3 Switch from kin to local person	2	8	(10)
4 Local people or paid person for all 3 years	3	14	(17)
5 Switch from locals to kin	3	1	(4)
6 Other sequence	1	3	(4)

Besides being more stable in composition, most working-class carer sets were smaller and expanded more slowly than those of most middle-class children. This was largely a consequence of many middle-class families incorporating several new local carers into their carer sets from the second year onwards. The smaller number of working-class couples who shared care with local people usually did so less often and with one or two individuals only. A significantly higher proportion of middle-class children had a larger carer set of more than five individuals (p < 0.05). The difference was even more pronounced for evening care. However, the families who had fewer than three carers in each year (low static sequence) were equally distributed between the classes. Here is evidence that besides the class contrasts there is a dimension of limited sharing care which occurred equally in both classes.

The evening care arrangments of middle-class families also altered more over the years than those of working-class families. These changes were mostly from grandparents to circles or friends, although four families did use mainly grandparents all through. Half of the working-class children had the same kin evening babysitters throughout the three years. The changes that did occur were mostly from grandparents to other relatives who were preferred on the grounds of age, health or convenience.

If class differences in care by kin and non-kin were fairly predictable from sociological studies, it was less easy to foretell what might be the case with care frequency. According to parents' recollections the frequency of sharing care during the first year had been fairly similar in both classes. Thereafter, it appeared that many more middle-class families shared care at least once a week in the daytime and at least monthly in the evening ($p < 0.001$). A strong class contrast in the number of sessions of shared care was confirmed by the diaries ($p = 0.001$). Half of the working-class children experienced no sharing care in the two weeks compared with only three middle-class children. 'Protective' families, however, were evenly divided between the two classes. It was in fact intermediate class families that contained the largest proportion of people who were low sharing. These families were neither part of a close kin network nor integrated with many street friends. Low frequency care was rare among middle-class families, but when it did occur it affected both day and evening care. Diary and interview data indicated that the small minority of middle-class families who shared care rarely did so mainly with kin. Similarly, there was also a minority of working-class families with high frequency non-kin or mixed care, who had stepped beyond the general boundaries of restricted care amongst kin and one or two close friends.

Since middle-class parents shared care much more with other parents of young children living nearby it was to be expected that they would in turn look after other people's children more often. In the diary fortnight, over three quarters of middle-class parents had children from outside the family stay with them. Many of these were under five. Only one third of working-class families had looked after other children and most of these were over five. It was noteworthy that the middle-class children's older brothers and sisters also had more of their friends to stay, even allowing for the number of siblings concerned. From this it may be inferred that middle-class children tended to have more friends who come to stay with them at home not only at the age of three but also when they are older.

Whereas sharing care in the daytime and evenings tended to occur more often for middle-class children, regular overnight stays were mostly a working-class phenomenon. Nearly as many middle-class children as working-class children had had at least one overnight stay apart from their parents by the age of three but in most cases this comprised one or two nights only in the second or third year. By contrast, the working-class children who had overnight stays at all had usually been away for several nights each year from infancy or the toddler stage onwards. Families from both classes mainly used grandparents and occasionally a close friend, but overnight stays with aunts and uncles were largely confined to the working-class children. A few working-class parents had arranged a single night of shared care by non-kin, but this was virtually always with long-established friends on an occasion when kin carers were going to the same family ceremony as the parents. Within the working-class families, those who arranged overnight stays tended to be high frequency sharers in the daytime ($p < 0.01$).

These class differences conform with a common middle-class belief that overnight care even with close relatives should not occur until the child is thought to be old enough to understand and cope with the changes involved. Thus, even high sharing middle-class families were usually reluctant to share care overnight. Only one middle-class family had arranged regular overnight stays with grandparents for babysitting, and then only after the child was two. On the other hand, high or medium sharing working-class families commonly arranged overnight care with relatives from an early age and took it for granted that the child would be happy to stay. The routine acceptance of overnight care by all concerned rendered changes in the child's cognitive or emotional capacities irrelevant. Some delayed until after babyhood out of concern not to impose too much or because of the practicalities of arranging feeds, nappies and travel.

In Milburn there were only two nursery schools but several playgroups whilst in Whitlaw that position was reversed. Usage of the two types of group care naturally reflected this difference in provision. A large majority of the working-class children went to a local authority nursery school and the rest attended community playgroups. Middle-class children were more evenly distributed between nursery schools and playgroups, some of which were private. There were some indications that distinctive kinds of families in both areas sought out the facilities which were under-represented in that area.

Among middle-class families those parents who made most use of 'local people' for sharing care were more likely to start group care early and to use a local authority nursery school ($p < 0.05$). Conversely, among working-class families, usage of playgroups was strongly associated with low sharing ($p < 0.001$). There was no class difference in attendance at church creches and Sunday schools, but more of the children who had been to ballet classes and toddler groups were middle class. So were all of those who had stayed at a sports creche.

Of families who had made or planned a change of group, few were working class. These mostly preferred a short period for their children in a playgroup before a transfer to nursery school when they were aged three or three and a half. Middle-class families who wanted a change were more numerous and mostly expected to make the shift from playgroup to nursery school later, when the child was about four. This corresponds with the fact that many middle-class parents liked to arrange care experiences for their children in graduated steps of increasing size and formality, i.e. pair swops: mini-group: play-group: nursery school: school.

Class and processes of non-group care

The basic routine reasons for care, such as shopping and appointments, were common to all types of family. There were also no class differences in the proportions of families who shared care in order that the mother might work or for parents' social activities. However, in two important respects there were significant differences in reasons for non-group care. Firstly, sharing care for child-oriented reasons tended to begin in the first and second years in working-class families but occurred later for most middle-class children. In fact this represented two distinct kinds of care process. Many working-class children were cared for from babyhood by relatives who wished to do so because they enjoyed the child's company. This was sometimes a tradition continued from previous generations or an expected pattern following similar arrangements for older siblings or cousins. These served to strengthen particular kin ties, especially with grandparents or maternal aunts. For middle-class children the child-oriented care mostly involved women who lived close to each other wanting their children to play together. For instance Mrs Allan joined a weekly swop 'so that he would get to know other children'. Mrs Balfour said she sometimes shared care with local friends 'for his having fun – it's not always that I want to do something'. Many of the middle-class children actively asked to play with friends or were invited to lunch or tea. It was also mainly middle-class parents who said they arranged care partly to help the child prepare for group care through swops and mini-groups. Only a few working-class families arranged care specifically for the children to play together.

The second major class difference was that far more middle-class mothers (eighteen) than working-class mothers (seven) stated that they had shared care at some time for a general 'break'. Eight of the nine mothers who had shared care in order to take part in a sport were middle class too. Perhaps working-class parents obtained breaks 'naturally' from the child-oriented care by kin, so there was less need to arrange care specifically for that purpose. It is also possible that they felt less need of breaks or entitlement to them. Boulton (1983) noted that more working-class mothers gained greater intrinsic pleasure from child care and were less frustrated by it.

Thus, daytime reasons for care reflected common practical needs but also contrasting attitudes to children's and mothers' 'needs' for independent activities. Reasons for evening care similarly reflected differences in life-styles. Most commonly, working-class couples said they arranged evening care in order to go to some public place of entertainment. Just a few shared care while they attended private gatherings, which generally consisted of parties for birthdays, anniversaries or New Year. Many more middle-class families shared care for small scale domestic occasions, i.e. to visit friends and attend dinner parties. There were also unsurprising class differences in the kinds of public entertainments which parents attended together in the evenings. Two thirds of working-class respondents mentioned going to a dance, compared with only four middle-class families. Far more working-class families mentioned having a meal out, going to a club or attending a wedding celebration. On the other hand, only for middle-class families were concerts, theatre, ballet, opera or social functions at work important. Most working-class parents said that overnight care was multi-functional in giving the carer and child pleasure at the same time as freeing the parents for a quiet week-end or a late night out. It often acted as an extended form of evening babysitting. It was also arranged on a less regular basis for weddings, funerals or family celebrations. By contrast, middle-class children mostly experienced overnight care as an occasional or one-off stay whilst their parents went away for a week-end for a special social or leisure activity.

Reasons given for choice of carers showed considerable class overlap. However, there were differences corresponding to the relative importance of kin and of reciprocal care by trusted local people. Far more working-class parents said they chose their main carer for relational reasons, because they were 'family' (p < 0.001). Some working-class parents said they had never considered asking anybody but relatives to look after their children. A common phrase was that only 'family or very close friends' would be considered for sharing care. The majority of middle-class parents did have a preference for care by relatives too, especially for a young child, but they were generally much more content with care by non-relatives. Some thought it made no difference, like Mr Edwards: 'I wouldn't have said we feel that family has some special qualities that we prefer to our friends.' A minority saw disadvantages to kin care, such as spoiling the children or being 'a bit oppressive' for the parents themselves (Mr Balfour). Significantly more middle-class couples referred to a person's competence or manner in dealing with children when they described how they decided who was acceptable as a carer and who was not (p < 0.01). This does not mean that working-class parents were unconcerned about a potential or actual carer's ability or skill but they simply took it for granted among the close relatives who were considered relevant. Middle-class parents were more often choosing from among a number of local people those they had most trust in.

All but one of the families who mentioned opportunity to reciprocate as a factor in selection of carers were middle class (p = 0.001). This was associated with important differences in how other families with young children were perceived. Middle-class parents tended to view others at the same life-cycle stage as ideal carers. Not only did they have the desired recent experience in handling young children but there would also be opportunities for peer interaction and swop care. Working-class parents seemed much more likely to perceive the presence of other young children as a reason for *not* sharing with another family, especially in the evening. Comments indicated a reluctance to draw other mothers away from their commitments to their own children or to their husbands. The possibility of the man babysitting was barely considered. Moreover, the idea of a couple dividing up in order to babysit for someone else seemed to be much less familiar amongst working-class families. It was therefore thought that friends or even the child's aunts could not come out to share care, as they needed to stay at home with their children. Hence many of the friends used for evening care had not (yet) started a family of their own.

Parents' attitudes about openness to care by strangers appeared to be strongly connected to class, although this was modified by the influence of protectiveness. Working-class families were almost always hostile to the idea of stranger care, whereas middle-class families divided fairly evenly into those who did not mind and those who were against ($p < 0.01$). Most intermediate class families exhibited aversion or conversion attitudes to care by strangers, so that high readiness to accept stranger care was mainly confined to solid middle-class families ($p < 0.01$). Fisher (1981) has stated that people in large urban centres need to make a distinction amongst people they encounter between a private world of 'intimates' and a public world of 'outsiders'. In these terms it would seem that more middle-class families readily extended the boundaries of their private worlds. Those middle-class parents who preferred to convert strangers mostly thought that a single meeting would suffice so the child knew who the person was. The few working-class parents who could even contemplate stranger care envisaged conversion as a lengthy process of becoming well-acquainted. However, all the 'protective' families were against stranger care, regardless of class.

Middle-class objections to stranger care were nearly always related to concern about possible anxiety by the child. Mr Griffin said: 'I wouldn't like really the kids to wake up and

... you know, unnecessarily ... and be frightened.' There could be identification with the child's viewpoint. For example Mrs Clark said 'If I was in their situation, I wouldn't like to be left with someone I didn't know.' A few parents were more worried that the child(ren) might be difficult for the stranger to cope with, whereas a relative or friend would be more understanding and tolerant. Those who were willing to use strangers for evening care either were confident the child would not wake or else thought that waking to find a strange person would not be alarming. Mrs Jackson remarked with equanimity 'It's just pot luck how a child reacts'. Some people felt it made no difference to the children whether they knew a babysitter or not. This could be assisted by the children's awareness of the concept of the 'babysitter' role, so that they learned to have confidence in the person in that position, even if the individual concerned was initially unknown to them. Several middle-class parents thought that a carer's ability to deal with an awake or upset child in a reassuring manner was more important than familiarity. Unlike most working-class parents, they did not feel that there was a necessary identification between competence and familiarity. Talking of circle members, Mrs Boyd said 'Even if I didn't know them, I didn't particularly sort of worry. I mean some of them brought their own babies along, so obviously they were right into the problem of feeding or whatever. You could confidently leave them.' Some parents like the Jacksons and Arnots had been anxious about the idea of stranger care at first but had become gradually desensitised when care by non-relatives and then strangers did not give rise to the anticipated difficulties. This could be helped by the belief that strangers were convertible into familiar carers. Mrs Henderson had thought 'it's rotten for the children to have people coming and they don't know them. But they get to know them, if you keep inviting the same people.' Even so, doubts might persist. Mrs Miller belonged to a circle but admitted that 'we can't go out with the same ease of mind as if grandparents come here'.

Concern about children being upset on waking to a strange face or simply refusing to stay with a stranger was also found with working-class families. In addition there were more general fears about allowing a stranger access to the house or about the stranger's competence to care for the child. Fathers in particular felt protective of their home and child:

> **Mr Purdie*** You're leaving them with your children, so it must be somebody that you can trust in every way. You're leaving them with your house, too ( ) and if they are looking around, they don't give attention to what they are there for.
>
> **Mr Preston*** There's no way I'd leave my kids with strangers. I wouldna feel safe having a stranger walking through my house.
>
> **Mr Weir*** Even having strangers in the house, I wouldna take the responsibility. What would they do when they were in, sort of thing?

It was also mainly working-class parents who expressed worries about the danger of physical harm to the child. Mrs Sadler* spoke of the possibility of cruelty and Mr Wallace* noted darkly that 'it's not everybody that likes children'.

There were also differences in setting the boundary between strangers and other people. For most middle-class couples, the main criterion was whether the child knew the person or not. Many working-class parents defined strangers much more narrowly, sometimes simply by contrasting them with close relatives. For example:

> **Mr Robertson*** I wouldna have any sort of stranger watching them, only a relative that I know very well.
>
> **Mr Ferguson*** I feel happier with family. I think the children would feel happier, too. I don't know how the children would take to a stranger.

Consequently, even people who were quite well known socially might be classed as strangers in this context. When Mr Purdie* was asked to explain who he meant by strangers he replied 'People we know, nice enough – friends'. Several parents, when questioned about the possible use of neighbours or friends for care, would introduce the word stranger or outsider and indicate that only kin could be trusted with the children. The following exchange demonstrates how talk of friends was sometimes linked by respondents to general fears about non-kin:

Mr Tulloch*   It would be just immediate family.
I don't think I trust anybody else
(to look after Stanley).
Interviewer   Not even close friends?
Mr Tulloch*   No. Look at the things you read.
These people get a babysitter they
ken for 15 years and the next thing
you know the bairn is burnt.

Some middle-class parents from a working-class background retained a wide definition of and aversion to stranger care. Mrs Laurie declared 'No way would a stranger come to look after them. ( ) I've got a couple of friends – well, I class as fairly good friends – but I would never ask them to look after the children.' Others adopted a more pragmatic approach like Mrs Allan who had joined a large circle because 'we would never go out otherwise'.

These different attitudes to stranger care help explain the more restricted carer sets and care frequencies of most working-class families, especially in the evenings. Even those working-class parents who did leave their children at a friend's or neighbour's home during the day were reluctant to have non-kin *alone* in the home at night. The more extended and extendable boundaries of trusted carers set by most middle-class parents also meant that they were more free to go out often *together* than most working-class parents.

Selection of crisis carers did not show the same class divergences. The middle-class families who normally shared care with many 'locals' felt that it was right to turn to relatives for major continuous care needs. Working-class families who usually did not include neighbours in their carer sets might consider them for a brief emergency. When mothers went into hospital for a confinement or illness, middle-class parents relied mostly on fathers and grandmothers for child care, just like the working-class families. In response to a more hypothetical question about what they would do in the event of a short-term hospitalisation of the mother, the couples who nominated the father as chief carer mainly held professional jobs ($p < 0.01$). This may correspond to differences in values, but it was also harder for manual workers to arrange time off without loss of earnings. However, for a longer term absence of mother the vast majority of families in both classes opted for relatives other than father as the prime carer. One in five middle-class families said they would use a paid childcarer, which was not suggested by any working-class parents. This perhaps helps explain why it is mostly children from working-class families who are received into local authority care when their mothers are in hospital and the family's network cannot or does not look after the child (Packman, 1968). Middle-class parents who also need to look outside their social networks at times of crisis may often be in a position to pay for someone to come into the home. Working-class attitudes to strangers in the home might preclude such an option, even if finance and accommodation permitted it.

Class and group care processes

In spite of the class contrasts evident in non-group sharing and in the types of group used, there were no significant class differences in the primary reasons given for placing the child in group care. However, it was notable that about one third of working-class families had hoped that group care would perform some kind of training function for the child, such as making the child's eating patterns more acceptable or teaching hygiene and self-care. This was not mentioned by any middle-class family. There were also no major contrasts in the factors affecting the choice of group care facility or in perceived benefits from group care for the children. The main exception to this was that somewhat more middle-class parents preferred short hours of attendance and a higher proportion of working-class mothers wanted group care for their child before the age of three.

Approximately three quarters of the working-class parents in the sample (nineteen) admitted to worries about how the child would get on at group care compared with only just over one third of the middle-class parents (twelve). Although in general children's reactions to all types of shared care did not differ markedly between the two major class groupings, a higher proportion of solid working-class children did have adjustment difficulties at group care. This may be related to the fact that fewer working-class children had had much previous experience of shared care involving peers, whether informally or in toddler and miscellaneous groups. The class differences with regard to local child-oriented sharing also meant that middle-class children were significantly more likely to know other children at the same group when they started. Over half the working-class children (sixteen) had had no prior acquaintanceship with any of the children at their group but this was the case for only five middle-class children. The particular importance of group care in providing peer contacts for working-class children was further emphasised by the fact that nearly half of them had no close friends locally of their own age when starting group care, compared with merely two middle-class children.

Parental participation in group care has been seen as a largely middle-class attribute (van der Eycken, 1977). With regard to actual participation, this was borne out by this study as in others. Given their readier access to playgroups, it follows that more middle-class mothers participated in rota duties ($p < 0.05$). Nevertheless, very similar percentages of mothers in both classes said they were against or in favour of involvement in running the group (Table 3.4). It would seem that the difference in actual involvement resulted from the larger number of playgroups sited near to middle-class families and not from big differences in attitude to parent involvement. Quite a few working-class mothers were keen to give time, ideas and interest. It is probable that the low extent of interest found in some studies may reflect lack of opportunity for the families concerned or samples which included only those living in the most difficult circumstances. This study also showed that some middle-class mothers took part in group rotas reluctantly. In both social classes those who shared care least often were those most likely to be keen on mother involvement in group care. Possibly readiness to participate in pre-school groups is in part linked to a specially strong desire to maintain the closeness of the mother-child relationship and this attitude is unrelated to class.

It was seen earlier that far more of the middle-class children went to playgroups. Yet when they were asked about their ideal preferences between playgroups and nursery schools, parents from the two classes had similar proportions supporting one or the other. Again it appears that availability of different kinds of facility leads to class differences in practice which mask uniformities in preference. The gap between actual and desired provision was most apparent in Milburn. One third of the Milburn families saw a deficiency of local authority nursery school places as the main need in the area for improving pre-school services. Several used nursery schools outside the area because they could not obtain places locally.

Class and reciprocity

Working-class parents were markedly less likely to swop care with other parents and hardly any belonged to any kind of formalised shared care network. Some working-class mothers did have ad hoc reciprocal arrangements with a street friend or a sister. These were virtually all confined to a pair of mothers and the swops were usually occasional. They nearly always happened only in the daytime, which may be linked to the reluctance noted above about having strangers in the home alone. By contrast, about half of the middle-class mothers were involved with several others in multiple or mini-group swop arrangements in the daytime. The care exchange usually took place regularly every week or once a fortnight. Most of the remaining middle-class families had regular exchanges with one or more other mothers on a pair basis. In the evenings, very few working-class families engaged in any kind of reciprocal sharing but the majority of middle-class families did so, either by means of circles or through less formalised street friend networks.

The kinds of repayment made to different types of carer (teenagers, relatives or other parents) were broadly similar in both classes. It follows that working-class families were much more likely to 'repay' carers by means of gifts, services or nothing specific rather than cash or return care, because their main carers were usually kin. Hence it was not the case that reciprocity was less important in working-class families, merely that it took different forms. In a number of working-class families there occurred what might be termed 'intergenerational reciprocity'. Sometimes the mother had been looked after as a child by her own older sister. She later looked after her sister's children and now that sister or one of her children was looking after the key child. Alternatively, a single or childless married aunt had sometimes looked after the child and there was an expectation that the mother would offer return care when that aunt had her own children. In a few families, the mother had looked after her younger sister, who was now old enough to care for the key child.

In these two areas, babysitting circles turned out to be not just primarily but totally middle-class organisations. All the families who had ever belonged to a circle (eighteen) or were considering that they might join a circle (four) were middle class. The remaining middle-class families were very familiar with the concept of a circle whereas about half the working-class mothers and even more of the fathers were unfamiliar with the idea. When they were told what circles were a high percentage of working-class parents expressed strong hostility to them. This chiefly resulted from concern about stranger care but also involved doubts about wives going out alone or being able to cope with someone else's child. Circles require a degree of confidence in permitting unattended access to one's own home and of being alone in someone else's home. Most working-class couples lacked this sense of trust except with respect to relatives. Not only were fewer middle-class respondents opposed to circles but they usually gave different kinds of reason for their opposition. Most often they thought that circles would take up too much of their time or else fathers' evening commitments meant their availability to babysit would be restricted or unreliable. A few were also put off by the formality or 'tweeness' they perceived in circles.

Parents' geographical origins and mobility

Social distinctions and movements often coincide or overlap with geographical ones. In particular, more people with middle-class occupations tend to move further from their original kin networks and live in more favourable environments. Hence it is necessary to examine how far the class differences which were observed might be explicable in terms of mobility and physical environment. In a limited study like this a definitive answer could not be expected but some clues were elucidated.

Geographical mobility has implications for a family's network, reference groups and hence its practices and values with respect to sharing care. It is sometimes conjoined with social mobility and sometimes not (Bell, 1968; Goldthorpe and Llewellyn, 1977), but the present sample was too small to produce helpful comparisons of the different combinations. The most important distinction in origins appeared to be whether the parent had been brought up in the Edinburgh area (loosely defined as within about twenty-five miles of the city) or came from further afield. To describe these two types of people we may borrow terms from Mrs Boyd, who said 'The main difference I find in this area is that between the natives and the incomers.' As expected, far more of the 'incomers' lived in Milburn and were middle class.

It might be thought that the class differences in social and care patterns could be explicable by differences in geographical mobility and the (usually) consequent differences in kin distance. This was only partially true in fact. The few middle-class families with *both* parents from Edinburgh did account for most of the middle-class families with relatives as main carers. However, native middle-class parents used street friends for sharing care just as much as incomers did. Another point of interest is that an absence of local roots at the very least did not inhibit the creation of an adequate network for help with child care. Nearly all couples in which both parents were incomers shared care in large carer sets with at least average frequency.

All but a few of the working-class parents were native to the Edinburgh area but on a more local scale they had not been immobile. Although they might have moved less far afield, almost as many of the working-class parents as middle-class parents had moved to their current neighbourhood after marriage and so were newcomers to the district. In the whole sample, only nine mothers and four fathers were still living in the same locality that they had spent their childhood in. Thus even this comparatively 'immobile' sample still included merely a few examples of continuity in residence and community contacts from childhood through to early parenthood. Whitlaw can be seen as a 'traditional' working-class area only in the sense that it has always had a predominantly working-class population and associated institutions. At least as far as these parents of young children were concerned (it may be different for older generations) Whitlaw was a new place for them to live in with a high population turnover. In this respect, though not in its location or urban fabric, Whitlaw resembles more the new housing estates than the inner city 'communities' of sociological studies in the 1950s and 1960s. This meant that most of the working-class parents had to negotiate new neighbour relations just as much as the middle-class families. As they were more likely to have several relatives and old friends elsewhere in Edinburgh there could be less incentive for them to build up social contacts locally.

The influence of the current environment

There were many individual instances where the disposition of space on a common stair, in the street and in the wider neighbourhood affected opportunities for interaction between local adults and play between children. This in turn influenced whether the kinds of social contacts developed which could lead to sharing care. The greater space inside most homes in Milburn meant that entertaining mini-groups was easier than in Whitlaw, where there were usually fewer, smaller rooms. Several Whitlaw parents indicated that confined space at home was a background factor in their desire for group care, because it was hard to amuse children or cope with their energies at home. The large gardens of South Milburn made children highly visible and were a means of facilitating play and hence shared care arrangements. Likewise a large, grassy back green with access from several flats could be a good place for parents and children to meet. The couple who became the main carers for Christopher Hardie had got to know the family after the children met and played together on the green. This was less possible in Whitlaw, where many back greens were very small, hard surfaced and/or poorly kept. A number of Whitlaw parents thought their children especially enjoyed stays with relatives because there was freedom to play in their gardens which was not possible at home.

Although particular families illustrated the influence of the domestic environment on sharing care there was no overall relationship between housing type per se and care patterns. The North Milburn tenement dwellers had patterns which were similar to those of the villa district of South Milburn rather than to the tenement areas of Whitlaw. It might be expected that house dwellers would have less need for group care than families in tenement flats but there was no apparent difference between families living in the two types of housing in terms of their use of group care and reasons for doing so. Even parents with ample accommodation and large private gardens thought that group care offered kinds of equipment and interactive peer play which was difficult for them to provide.

It was not possible to obtain a full picture of the broader local environment in the two areas but parents were asked to name their local area and evaluate its quality for children and for adults. How they described the locality reflected their own values, experiences and knowledge of the area, as well as its more objective nature. In particular, parents were influenced by their own 'reference areas' where they had lived themselves as children or later. In some cases the area of origin remained an important subcentre of family life because of regular contacts with kin there. Some Whitlaw families living in a restricted environment for children did not perceive it as such since they were accustomed to life in a poor inner city area. Conversely, Milburn was seen by most of its inhabitants as attractive, 'with an air of countrification' (Mr Carlisle) but some felt its environment was too restrictive in comparison with rural reference areas they knew well.

Seventy per cent of the couples thought their home area was good or very good for bringing up children. Nearly all those with a negative evaluation of their area for children lived in the main tenement area of Whitlaw. For example:

Mrs Villiers*   There's not really anything

round here for the bairns,
except the nursery. ( ) Mind you,
these houses probably aren't
meant for children.

Mrs Urquhart* I don't think it's an area for
bringing up kids.

Mrs Whigham* They don't cater for children
much. Well, it's not a
residential area, of course. It's an
industrial zoned area.

Some Whitlaw families were content but many were bringing up their children in a district which not only scored poorly on certain objective indices of environmental disadvantage but which in addition they themselves did not see as suitable or intended for young children. In Whitlaw the main disadvantages for children included playspace which was limited in size or dangerous because of broken glass, the general unpleasantness of the neighbourhood and lack of opportunities to mix with other children nearby. In both areas traffic was a major worry. The more extensive open space in Milburn was discounted by some residents on account of dogs' mess. All these factors contributed to a common view of group care as a refuge from a limiting urban environment inimical to children. Besides their low opinion of the physical environment, some Whitlaw families complained about the kinds of people living in their area and the way children were brought up. It is possible that the sense of living in unsatisfactory surroundings where some of the people living round about were seen as lacking responsibility contributed to the strong feelings against stranger care in Whitlaw. It also meant that some parents were relieved to know 'you can send your kids along to nursery in comparative safety' (Mrs Sim*).

As there was such a close correspondence between families' class and area of residence, it was not possible to differentiate between the influences of class and neighbourhood on shared care patterns. Nonetheless, there were some indications that the five working-class families who lived in Milburn resembled Whitlaw families much more than their middle-class near-neighbours. Over the three years, four of these five families had relied mainly on kin as carers unlike most Milburn families. All were against stranger care and none belonged to a circle. On the other hand the influence of local provision is shown by the fact that three of them had used or planned to use a playgroup rather than nursery school, which was the norm among Whitlaw working-class families.

In the next chapter, attention shifts from the physical locale in which the families lived to their social networks.

5 *Families' social networks*

It might be conjectured that care patterns would correspond in a simple manner to the nature of social relationships more generally. This in turn could suffice to explain the class contrasts which have been described. For instance the greater readiness of many middle-class parents to use non-kin for care might be accounted for by the greater likelihood of their having moved a long distance from relatives and the resultant reduced frequency of contact (Hendrix, 1979). Similarly the presence of kin nearby could reduce working-class couples' needs to turn to neighbours for assistance in looking after their children (Lee, 1968). We shall see that there was indeed an intimate interaction between care patterns and network relationships which did exhibit large class contrasts but the differential availability of relatives appeared to offer only a partial explanation for this.

For present purposes the term network will be taken to refer to those people known to the family with whom the children had their main social contacts. Information was gathered about both the structural and interactional aspects which Mitchell (1969) identified as the two main elements of a network. On the whole it was only possible to deal systematically with 'first-order' contacts, i.e. the direct relationships between the family and others. Only very general information was obtained about the connections amongst network members, since detailed investigation of these is very time-consuming and was not warranted in this kind of study (Boissevain, 1974). Social networks change both independently of and in response to shared care processes, so in addition qualitative information was sought about network changes since the child was born. In general, it will be seen that most families had developed and altered their network membership

and contacts in important ways after they had children, sometimes as a result of sharing care. There were three main ways
in which membership of a carer set related to the family
network:

1 Carers were recruited from the prior social network
  (mainly kin and old friends).
2 Shared care and befriending developed together, chiefly
  through interaction with other families who had young
  children.
3 The care function was the prime focus of the relationship
  with the carer, so that social contact was minimal (group
  carers, childminders, some circle members).

First of all we shall examine the kin segment of family
networks and then friends and neighbours. This division lends
clarity to exposition, but is also empirically justifiable. Nearly
all the respondents said that they saw their relatives separately from their friends. It was also rare for a relative to have
independent contacts with a friend. This segregation of contact
was confirmed by the diaries and is consistent with earlier
studies (Bell and Boat, 1957; Irving, 1977). Finally, the nature
of social and care networks will be shown to have implications
for children's attachments and their relations with other
children.

Children's contacts with relatives

All relatives aged over sixteen outside the nuclear family with
whom the child had had contact in the previous year were
counted as 'significant kin'. Using respondents' estimates of
the frequency of the child's meetings with significant kin,
each day of contact with each adult relative was deemed to
constitute a 'kin-contact day'. This is a somewhat crude
measure, as it is derived from retrospective approximations,
tends to undervalue twenty-four hour stays by or with relatives and overvalues contacts at the same time with more than
one relative. Nonetheless, the current frequencies of interaction recorded in the diaries correlated well with the kin-
contact day measure and produced similar groupings of
families.

Most children had between ten and twenty significant relatives. This was nearly always a considerably larger number than had ever shared care. Understandably those children with many significant kin (fifteen plus) and above average frequency of contact with relatives also had a high proportion of kin amongst their principal carers (p = 0.001). On the other hand having a large kin set (fifteen plus) did not necessarily lead to exclusive use of relatives for sharing care. Well over one third of such children had a non-relative as main carer. In all, half of the sample's significant kin lived in Edinburgh but very few children had considerable numbers of kin in the immediate vicinity.

There was a vast range in the number of kin-contact days per child from 0 to 1200. Nine children saw no relatives at all during the diary fortnight and at the other extreme there were nine who spent at least one quarter of the time in the company of relatives. The general picture was one of frequent contacts by most children with at least a few kinfolk. Three quarters of the children saw at least one relative every week. If distance precluded frequent part-day contacts this was often made up for by occasional stays of a week or more. Such factors as personal and genealogical closeness, health, transport and alternative commitments modified any simple direct association between distance and contact.

There was no class difference in the overall size of a child's effective kin set but there were contrasts in location and hence in frequency of contact. Given the marked class differences in geographical mobility, it was not surprising that working-class families usually had more relatives living in Edinburgh, although this contrast disappeared if only families with 'native' parents were compared. One third of middle-class families but only a single working-class family had no significant relatives in Edinburgh (p < 0.01). Twice as many working-class children (one half) had at least one relative living in their local area. Six of these had a relative living in the same street.

As a result of these differences, most of the working-class children saw a wider range of relatives more often than did most middle-class children (p < 0.001). Nevertheless, the stereotyped image of middle-class children as remote from their extended families was not borne out. Half the middle-class children saw at least one relative in the two weeks of the diary record. Some middle-class parents were emotionally very close to their parents or siblings. Mrs Miller described herself as 'very family oriented, actually. My sister is still my best friend.' Furthermore the diaries revealed that most of those middle-class families with close relatives living in or near Edinburgh did share care with them quite often. However, when only those children who saw at least one relative weekly were considered, most of those who were middle-class had a non-kin main carer but just a few of those who were working-class ($p < 0.05$).

Information about the frequency of children's contact with different kinds of kin showed the same hierarchy as care patterns. Mothers' parents were seen most often by more children, followed by fathers' parents, mothers' sisters, and so on. The importance of mothers' relationships with their own mothers and sisters which was found in earlier research (e.g. Young and Willmott, 1957) is clearly seen. But in some instances the fathers' parents and occasionally fathers' siblings were equally or more significant. The bias towards grandparents and to mothers' family which occurred in the selection of carers was apparent but less strong with regard to social contacts. This suggests that the particular intimacy involved in sharing care emphasises predispositions in contacts, especially towards maternal grandmothers.

Grandparents – the primary carers

It has sometimes been thought that grandparenthood is a role of diminishing significance but this study confirmed its continued vitality. For well over half the children the relative they had most frequent contact with was a grandparent. The special importance of grandparents in patterns of shared care is summarised in Figure 5.1. Grandparents were the main carer for half the children in the first two years and for one third of children in the third year, both during the day and in the evening. They were also second carers for nearly as many children. Thus, many of the generalisations made about kin care derive particularly from grandparent care. Many of those grandparents who lived too far away for routine care looked

1 Carer Sequences

Number of Families
(N = 63)

First Carer — Year 1

First Carer — Year 2

First Carer — Year 3

2 Main and Second Carers at time of interview

Main Daytime Carer

Main Evening Babysitter

Second Daytime Carer

Second Evening Babysitter

3 Overnight and Crisis Care

First Choice Overnight Carer

Carer for Short Crisis Care

Carer for Long Crisis Care

4 Persons child is most fond of (outside the nuclear family — adults only)

First Fondness Person

Second Fondness Person

Third Fondness Person

KEY

Maternal grandparent(s)

Paternal grandparent(s)

Either set or both sets of grandparents

Others

Nobody

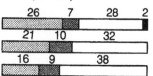

Figure 5.1 *Grandparents in the lives and care of children*

after the children during visits. In about a dozen families grandparents had come from some distance to stay with the family and give support during the period of childbirth. A few couples who made little or no use of grandparents for care were careful to explain that they had used other carers because the child's grandparents were precluded on account of distance, health or age. A comparison of grandparents' names revealed that, contrary to Goody's hypothesis (1962), grandmothers called nanna or nannie – which he took to be etymologically related to child care – were no more likely to be main carers than were grannies and grandmas.

In the social science literature 'extremely little attention has been paid to grandparent-grandchild relations' (Troll *et al.*, 1979: 274). Perhaps this is just because their centrality is so taken for granted in everyday family life. Likewise academics have for the most part subsumed consideration of them within that of kin relations in general. Most research has looked at the grandparents' viewpoint or more rarely the child's (Kahana and Kahana, 1971). In this study, grandparents were considered from the point of view of the middle generation, which has a crucial role in mediating the experiences for grandparents and grandchildren (Hill *et al.*, 1970; Robertson, 1975). In the main, positive attributions and special salience were accorded to grandparents by the people interviewed. These favourable qualities will be assessed first of all, but then it will be shown that there were limitations to parents' expectations about grandparent care, as well as problems which could arise from it. Perceptions by parents of their mutual interests and potential sources of conflict with grandparents often paralleled those which independent studies have observed from grandparents' perspectives.

The primacy of grandparents in choice of carers was sometimes masked, because parents spoke of preferences for 'family' or 'close relatives' in general. However, there were also specific comments about the special desirability of grandparents. This was found in both classes. Of course, most parents liked their own parents as people. Indeed a few wives described their mothers as their main social companions outside the nuclear family. Mrs Weir* looked on her mother as 'a friend as well as my mother, y'ken'. Since many other well-liked people did not share care often or at all, there were evidently other factors which explain why grandparents were so popular for shared care. The four principal ones mentioned were:

1 Their high motivation to be carers;
2 The absence of any required payment in cash, kind or time;
3 Proven competence;
4 The perceived uniqueness of the grandparent-grandchild relationship.

In many cases, grandparents' enthusiasm to be with grandchildren was seen as sufficient explanation for their choice as carers. Asked why his mother was their main carer, Mr Chalmers* explained 'just grandchildren . . . she wants them round there all the time'. Grandparents showed pride in their new status and liked 'showing the bairns off to all their neighbours' (Mr Baxter*). Thus, parents knew that a request for care would not be seen as a burden but would be welcomed. Mr Quinn* said 'if you want them watched, the grandparents are the first to volunteer'. Other researchers' interviews with grandparents have confirmed the alacrity with which many take up opportunities to babysit for grandchildren. It affords occasions for sole access to the child and allows grandparents to be less inhibited than when the parents are there (Robertson, 1977). Normally grandparents feel they have to restrain their natural desire to spend as much time as possible with a young grandchild because they do not wish to interfere (Cunningham-Burley, 1983). Sharing care serves as a way of reconciling these two opposing factors since it provides benefits for the parents as well as the grandparents. Some respondents in this study pointed out that grandparents had the time and interest to play with the child individually, unlike friends with young children. Quite a few grandparents rarely went out in the evening and so were readily available for care. For at least three widows the grandchild had become a major solace and life interest, even substituting partly for the deceased husband. Mrs Spence* said of Virginia: 'Since my Dad died, she usually sleeps beside my Mum (during an overnight stay). She cuddles in beside her and she says "I'll look after you".'

Mr Clark summed up a second advantage of grandparent care: 'you don't have to compensate them'. Several parents remarked that the child's company brought its own rewards so that no additional repayment for care was necessary. Many parents felt inhibited from offering anything directly for fear of giving offence. Even so, the norm of reciprocity was upheld because parents made small gifts or offered help at other times so that they did not feel indebted.

Thirdly, it was understandable that in looking for someone to substitute for themselves, parents often turned first to the people whose parenting they were most familiar with and sure of. Typical comments were 'I think of my mother first, because she's done it, I suppose' and 'They've brought up a family and know what to do'. Mrs Sinclair* thought that 'Most people do not on the whole question the qualities of their own parents. You always think your own mother is capable, because you survived all these years.'

The special qualities of grandparenthood were exemplified by the fact that they were often seen as the people with the clearest sense of duty to act as carers and the only ones to be granted some kind of right to do so. Some grandparents had insisted on giving the parents an opportunity to go out in the evenings or in providing relief care at times of stress. This insistence would be acceded to whereas offers from others might be refused. Grandparents' right to share care was illustrated more explicitly by Mrs Urquhart*, who stated that both sets of grandparents 'are *entitled* to an equal shot of them'. Mr Clark described babysitting as 'a *privilege* of grandparents and we benefit'. Some grandparents communicated their sense of entitlement to care by expressing feelings of hurt at the possibility or actuality of others being asked to babysit when they were available themselves.

The most common image of grandparents as very eager, trustworthy and entitled to care for the children was by no means universally held, nor applied equally to all grandparents. In some cases it was confined to grandmothers. Some grandfathers were less available because of work but also some appeared to be more hesitant or even indifferent about being involved with care of the children. A few brought their wives by car to babysit but did not stay themselves. When grandparents did act as joint carers, sometimes the grandmother monopolised the direct dealings with the child (according to parents' descriptions). Not uncommonly, respondents said that their child had stayed with 'my mum', even though the grandfather was there too. It is possible that this gender difference is exaggerated by social expectations which lead men to express their pleasure and interest in grandchildren in different ways and in different contexts (Cunningham-Burley, 1984). Some grandfathers of the children in this study were very involved in care. Ralph Quinn's grandfather took him to nursery school each day. Mrs Miller's father 'doted on Malcolm, and has always taken him off to the park with him every Sunday morning'. Three families had widowed grandfathers who stayed with them for considerable parts of the year, during which periods they babysat and took the children out.

Even with regard to very willing grandmother carers there was often a feeling that this should not be exploited. In particular it was thought unfair for them to look after the children whilst the mother worked long hours for this would be seen as a second period of parenting. Mrs Ritchie* said 'I don't think they should have to bring up another family.' Mrs Urquhart* opined: 'They have had their share of bringing up kids and it's about time they were enjoying themselves.' It was indicated that ordinary babysitting could be seen as voluntary whereas 'work care' would be an obligation. Interestingly, this corresponds to the findings of several studies that grandparents themselves usually do not want to be overburdened. They are glad that care of grandchildren is more limited in time and in scope of responsibility than parenting itself (Albrecht, 1954; Crawford, 1981).

Now and then reservations were expressed about grandparents' behaviour as carers, mostly by middle-class parents. This partly accounts for the shift away from grandparent care for some purposes which was evident for a number of middle-class children as they grew older. Of course, the majority remained very favourable about grandparent care. For those parents who did perceive difficulties the main problems concerned authority, spoiling, rivalry and intrusiveness. These were all issues which could threaten parents' autonomy to determine how they conduct their own lives and influence their children's behaviour.

In our society grandparents do not have the formal authority over parents that may be found in other societies (Apple, 1956). In rare instances, considerable accountability to the senior generation was apparent. Mrs Robertson* said 'I'm sure my Dad would still leather me, even though I'm married.' Mrs Ormiston's* father was 'terrible protective with us and he's exactly the same with his grandchildren. Before I do anything, I stop and think "Would my Dad approve?".' More usually parents felt independent but retained respect for their parents which persisted from the authority relationship of their own childhood. This meant that there could be much ambiguity when grandparents acted as carers. Their seniority within the family could conflict with parents' implicit expectations that people who acted as carers would defer to their wishes. Most respondents did not find this a major problem. Several acknowledged that their parents were sensitive not to appear as intruding. Non-interference is a widely accepted ideal for the grandparent-parent relationship (Blaxter and Paterson, 1982; Kahana and Kahana, 1970). Nevertheless, there were sometimes different attitudes about discipline and then parents could find it hard to be openly critical, yet felt their own authority undermined. This created difficulties for Mr and Mrs Griffin; Emily's grandmother pampered her during the periods when Mrs Griffin was at work and they felt she disregarded their appeals for her to be firmer. Mrs Spence's* mother 'used to bring up a sweet every day. She started when Virginia was young and I didn't like it.' Delicate negotiations ensued to control this spoiling: 'She said "just a wee sweetie won't do her any harm". I said "I don't want her to have sweets" – a bit joking, but she gets hurt then.' More commonly, spoiling was simply accepted as a characteristic or even a right of grandparents (especially grandmothers) even though the Newsons (1963) showed that most parents are concerned not to spoil their children themselves. For example:

Mr Forbes*	She does get spoilt, but what are grannies for?
Mrs Chalmers*	I think it's a grandmother's privilege to spoil their grandchildren.
Mrs Brown*	Every child should have a grannie who spoils them.

Acknowledgment of grandparents' rights to indulge a grand-child fits with the view of Radcliffe-Brown (1952, 1960) that there exists an affinity between alternate generations which is combined with relaxed rules of interaction when grand-parenthood is dissociated from ongoing responsibility and authority. Grandparents can take pleasure in giving things to grandchildren without having to heed the consequences (Neugarten and Weinstein, 1964). On the other hand the residual authority of grandparents was shown by respondents' hesitation in challenging their own parents when spoiling did create difficulties.

Some parents were aware of the potential rivalry for the child's affection if grandparents were too involved as carers. For instance Mrs Nichols* preferred to use a childminder, because 'they can get too attached to their grannies and then they dinna want you'. Although most respondents whose parents did not live close regretted that they were not nearer, a minority were glad. For instance, Mrs Hardie said that once her mother had a foot in the door she would take over. Mr Balfour and Mr Carlisle both said they were glad to have grandparents fairly near at hand but would be unhappy if they lived any closer. Several middle-class parents complained that grandparent carers did not abide by unwritten rules of shared care. Some altered the timing of care sessions to suit themselves. The Arnots said ruefully that an evening babysit could easily turn into a whole week-end stay. Consequently, several parents preferred street friends as carers because it was thought the implicit contract for care would be more straightforward and reliable. It may be that a larger proportion of middle-class couples are concerned to assert their independence from close kin than working-class parents (Hubert, 1965; Reiss, 1962).

In a few cases, it was apparent that grandparents them-selves dissented from the typical willingness to care. Mr Hardie's mother had made it clear that 'just because she was a grandmother, she wasn't going to be on tap'. Mrs Shaw's* mother was reluctant to babysit because 'she thinks she should be going out, not having to watch him'. Mr Davies and Mrs Traynor* expressed strong disappointment that their chil-dren's paternal grandparents had shown little interest in them, which they regarded as abnormal and puzzling for grandparents.

These interpersonal differences should not be exaggerated, for they seldom appeared to develop beyond minor irritation. Non-use or restricted use of grandparent care was more frequently explained by means of practical difficulties, though this may occasionally have been a rationalisation. It is therefore important to examine variations in grandparents' distance, health and work commitments which were crucial influences on their availability for sharing care.

For only one of the children were all four grandparents dead. Over 90 per cent of the sample had at least two grandparents living. More grandmothers were alive than grandfathers, which is quite natural in view of the later age of marriage of men and their shorter life expectancy. Three quarters of the children had both grandmothers alive and nearly all had at least one. Although there has been a tendency to assume that grandparents are elderly (Cunningham-Burley, 1986) that is not necessarily the case, particularly with respect to three-year-olds. Two fifths of all the grandparents in the current study were aged under 60. In any case 'elderly' grandparents over that age usually give much help to the next generation especially by assistance with child care (Streib, 1958; Townsend, 1957). Nearly as high a proportion of grandmothers who were main carers for children in this sample were over 60 as were under 60. It was poor health as much as age itself which reduced or eliminated involvement by grandparents in sharing care. About one quarter of children had at least one grandparent (usually only one) with a serious health problem. Several of them were therefore considered unable to cope with the demands of a young child, especially if there were more than one, or even to be dangerous in their lax supervision. Sometimes the involvement of an active grandparent in sharing care had to be reduced because of the partner's ill health. On the other hand, sometimes a grandparent who was not fully fit was able to act as a carer with the support of a more healthy partner.

Just under half of the families had both sets of grandparents living in Edinburgh. One in three had no grandparent in Edinburgh, but nearly all of these kept in regular contact with grandparents either in person or by phone. Subsidised public transport made it easier for some grandparents to come and look after the children. Understandably, grandparents in Edinburgh were usually seen most often. Nearly all working-class children had at least one grandparent living in Edinburgh, compared with just under half of middle-class children. Therefore, far more working-class children had weekly or even daily contacts with grandparents. Contacts could be highly regularised:

> **Mr Preston***   My Mum comes up on Monday evenings to look after the kids as I'm working late. She also comes up on Wednesday for tea. And Saturdays, the two sets of grandparents take it in turns.

> **Mrs Preston***   My parents come here every Tuesday night, then I go up there every Thursday during the day.

How far away grandparents lived had an important but not determinant effect on care patterns. Two thirds of the families who had grandparents in Edinburgh did use them as either their main or second carer. There was also a much stronger likelihood of overnight stays occurring with grandparents if they lived in Edinburgh ($p < 0.01$). On the other hand, for only six out of the thirteen families with a grandparent living in the same local area was the main carer a grandparent. Half of the working-class families with both sets of grandparents in Edinburgh had grandparents as both main daytime and evening carers, but only one of the nine middle-class families did so. Moreover, the working-class families with Edinburgh grandparents who did not use them as main carers mostly used another relative who was preferable on grounds of age, health or strong personal tie. By contrast, over half the middle-class families with Edinburgh grandparents had non-relatives (usually local mothers) as both main daytime and evening carers.

It has often been noted that the rapid post-war rise in the numbers of married women working has reduced the ability of older women to look after their grandchildren, especially in order that their daughters might work (Hunt, 1968; Land,

1981). All but nine of the sixty-three children had at least one grandparent who was not working, though of course some of these were infirm or far away. Thus in only a few cases did grandparents' work by itself preclude daytime care. Moreover many of the grandmothers who worked did so part-time and were free to look after grandchildren for considerable parts of the day. Grandparents' work rarely interfered with their availability for evening or week-end care.

Sometimes grandparents' preparedness to act as carers was affected by what might be called 'grandchild status'. By analogy with sibling status (Sutton-Smith and Rosenberg, 1970), this may be defined as the child's combined sex and birth order in relation to the number of grandchildren of a particular grandparent. Grandchild status was often used as an explanation of grandparents' relative willingness to babysit, especially in comparison with the other set of grand-parents. Being the only grandchild, the oldest, the youngest, the first girl or boy, or one of twins were all cited as reasons for special interest in looking after that child. For example Shona Nairn's maternal grandmother had fourteen older grandchildren and was already very committed as a babysitter for several of them. Shona was more special as the first grand-child for her father's mother, who had consequently become her main carer. Several parents noted what Mr Barker called the 'first grandchild syndrome'. Mr Finlayson said that when their first child was born there were 'plenty of offers, but now there are two (children) the offers dry up'. Excitement wore off and two children were more of a handful than one. Both the Baxters* and the Ogilvies* had turned to teenage relatives as babysitters when grandparents shifted their attention to share care for new grandchildren. Indeed it seemed to be generally the case that when parents had several siblings with children they were likely to use younger single relatives for care rather than grandparents who did not have the time to be carers for more than one or two of the youngest generation.

Aspects of the wider kin network

Aunts and uncles usually have many advantages similar to those of grandparents for shared care, such as trustworthiness, willingness and continuity of relationships. For example some maternal aunts attracted such epithets as 'she's like a second mother' and 'she treats mine just like hers'. However, selection or self-selection of aunts and uncles as carers seemed to have a greater element of voluntariness. There was a less automatic expectation that they *should* be carers than was generally true for grandparents. Often only one or two acted as carers out of several who were available, either because they had an especially close relationship with the parent who was their brother or sister, or because they had a particular interest in children.

The different patterns of contact with categories of aunts and uncles broadly concurred with their involvement in sharing care. There was much more contact with aunts or uncles who were related through blood rather than marriage. Some married siblings of the parents were seen frequently without their spouse. William Sim*, for instance, saw his mother's sister 'three or four times a week', but 'he very seldom sees her husband'. As in previous studies (Bowerman and Dobash, 1974; Irish, 1964) there was greater contact *on average* with parents' siblings when they were females and of the same sex. There were many deviations from this generalisation, however. For the sample as a whole, maternal aunts were seen markedly more often than other kinds of aunt and uncle. There was also a strong tendency for single brothers of parents to be seen much more frequently than married brothers. After marriage, it seemed that brothers in particular became more oriented to their new family and to their spouse's family of origin. Nearly all of the uncles who were important carers were single but many married aunts were major carers. Overnight stays of more than one or two nights were primarily with parents' married siblings, whilst evening babysitting was done more by single siblings. Presumably, married aunts are freer in the day and more likely to have children of their own which would fit more readily with taking in a child for a substantial period. They were considered less free to visit the child's home for evening babysitting. Middle-class children, with some notable exceptions, generally saw aunts and uncles much less often than working-class children, which corresponds with the difference in care patterns.

The vast majority of the relatives who saw or looked after the children more than occasionally were members of their parents' own nuclear families of origin (and their spouses). Only one third of the children had more than fifty contact days in the year altogether with any other kind of relatives. The most important of these were grandmothers' sisters. This is consistent with the special importance of the sister-sister relationship already noted, but in relation to grandparents this time. Occasionally, even relatives seen rarely might be important as latent carers. A few parents thought they would call on their aunts or cousins in a crisis, in preference to more local friends known much better. Being 'family' made it easier to ask and more probable that a desire or obligation to help would be elicited.

We saw earlier that kin carers came more often from the mother's side of the family and were most commonly women, although men were better represented than amongst non-related carers. How far does this correspond to sex and laterality differences in network composition and contacts? 'Significant relatives' included only slightly more women than men. Fifty-eight per cent of all kin-contact days were with women and 42 per cent with men. Thus, the bias towards female relatives in contact was much less than for shared care (Table 5.1). Clearly these three-year-olds had considerable contact with male relatives and they provided the main contacts with men outside the nuclear family for most children.

The greater use of maternal than paternal kin for sharing care was striking. This was not explained by differences in accessibility because similar proportions of relatives from each side of the family were living in Edinburgh. Likewise as many children lived closer to paternal grandparents than maternal grandparents as vice versa. There were also no important differences between the numbers of maternal and paternal grandparents who were dead. Contacts with kin did show a definite bias towards maternal kin, although this again was less strong than for sharing care. The mean number of contact days per child with maternal kin was 197, compared with 123 for paternal kin. These averages mask wide variations and there was a significant minority of children whose main

Table 5.1a *Contact and care by male and female kin*

	Females	Males
Mean number of significant relative	7.7	6.3
Mean number of contact days	200	162
Main daytime carers – number of families*	54	1 (7)
Main evening carers – number of families*	38	13 (7)
Second daytime carers – number of families*	45	7 (7)
Second evening carers – number of families*	31	12 (14)

* (Couples are placed in brackets)

Table 5.1b *Contact and care by maternal and paternal kin*

	Maternal	Paternal
Mean number of significant relatives	74	66
Mean number of sessions spent with relatives in diary fortnight	38	22
Main daytime carer* (number of families)	20	8
Second daytime carer* (number of families)	18	11

* (Grandparents, aunts and uncles)

contacts were with paternal relatives or roughly equal between the two sides of the family. More intense interaction with mother's kin was most pronounced when both parents were native to the Edinburgh area. A child's greater contact with maternal kin sometimes resulted from a higher degree of involvement by the family as a whole with mother's relatives. However, in some cases this reflected segregated contact with the father mainly seeing his family by himself whilst maternal kin were seen in the daytime by the mother and child.

It seems, then, that practical considerations did not explain the progressive preference shown by many though by no means all families towards mother's side of the family firstly with regard to contact, and then more strongly in selection of carers. A few mothers did say they chose their mothers as a carer, because of confidence in them derived from their own experience. More usually the bias was tacit, for the side of the family which a relative came from was hardly ever expressed overtly as a factor in the choice of carer. Presumably, the greater prominence of women in maintaining kin contacts and in arranging care meant that a mother would normally feel freer to ask her own mother or sister to share care than an in-law (Rosser and Harris, 1965; Willmott and Young, 1960). Nevertheless, fathers' kin were generally just as acceptable as carers even if less often approached. In most families someone from both sides of the family had been a carer. Furthermore, some parents asserted a value of bilateral fairness, held by themselves or by grandparents. This is broadly consistent with previous research on intergenerational kin relations, which showed a theoretical norm of bilaterality co-existing with a matrilateral bias in practice (Rosser and Harris, 1961; Sweetser, 1968). Mrs Urqhuart* considered both sets were entitled to an 'equal shot' of the children. Mrs Chalmers* averred 'There is no sort of favouritism to my Mum.' Mr and Mrs Allan alternated between the two grandmothers as carers, because of 'family politics, you know, whose turn it is and that sort of thing'. Some parents were at pains to explain that care by one set of grandparents was less than the other only because of practical considerations or grandchild status. Selectivity on grounds of laterality or personality was thereby implicitly denied.

Despite the high levels of involvement which most children had with both sides of their families, the two segments of the kin network appeared to operate independently, as the quotations from Mr and Mrs Preston* illustrated earlier in the chapter. Only rarely did paternal relatives meet with maternal relatives. Few had known each other before the couple had originally become acquainted. This segregation probably served to reduce pressures towards equal treatment in access to the child.

Friends and neighbours

A few families shared care with old friends or colleagues from outside the local area. Some carers were immediate neighbours who were elderly or had grown up children. But in most cases when parents referred to either neighbours or friends in relation to sharing care this meant other parents of young children living close by, especially other mothers. Consequently, it seems sensible to consider friends and neighbours together and employ the composite term 'friend-neighbour', because the distinction is often blurred. Parents themselves showed variability or uncertainty about whether to describe someone as a friend or neighbour when that person lived in the vicinity and had also become fairly intimate. In different parts of the same interview, phrases like 'friends round the corner', 'friends in the street', 'neighbours along the road' or 'the girl across the street' were used to depict the same kind of relationship. Mrs Forbes described Dorothy's carers as 'just neighbours I think – friends'. One of Kerry Edwards's carers was described as 'a neighbour – a friend across the road'. The word neighbour was not confined to people next door but commonly designated people in nearby streets. Furthermore, the most prominent neighbours and the majority who became carers were those who had come to be regarded as 'friends'.

Whereas most families' kin networks were fairly stable in composition and contact frequency, relations with other local parents were much more dynamic. Sharing care may reinforce kin contact and perhaps alter the relative frequency of contact with different members of the kin set, but on the whole sharing care with kin fits into a pre-established pattern of relationships. Contact with friends and neighbours was just as likely to be a consequence or accompaniment of sharing care as the other way round. Therefore, even more than usual, statistical associations between aspects of non-kin networks and care denote reciprocal influences.

Time did not permit a complete mapping of a family's 'friend-neighbour' network. A convenient abbreviation for this was to ask parents to list and describe those friends and neighbours they thought were important to the child. For the sake of simplicity, such people will be called 'significant friends', but this may include neighbours and acquaintances who do not necessarily have all the qualities of friendship. The location, marital status, age of children and relationship to the parents of such friends and neighbours were recorded. It was thought that the record of significant friends would vary a good deal according to parents' subjective interpretations and so be of doubtful validity. However, for the purpose of differentiating families this measure tallied well with the diary record of all contacts with people described as friends or neighbours (p < 0.001).

Most parents listed between four and nine significant friends. In all about half of these lived in the local area. Both the interview measure of contact days and the record of diary sessions showed that some children met parents' friends and neighbours frequently – even daily – whilst others hardly engaged with them at all, like Ross Whigham*. For instance, twenty-two children visited two or more different homes of neighbours or friends during the diary fortnight, but thirteen children went to none at all. Those families in which the child had frequent contact with many significant friends usually had larger carer sets and multiple swop care arrangements (p < 0.01).

Overall, families from the two classes had similar *numbers* of significant friends in Edinburgh, so that it was not a shortage of non-kin contacts among working-class families which explained their much rarer involvement in shared care. On the other hand, *frequency* of contact with 'friend-neigh-bours' was considerably higher on average for middle-class children (p = 0.001). Two thirds of them spent time with four or more different 'friend-neighbours' during the diary fortnight, compared with only one third of working-class children (p < 0.02). In particular, middle-class children visited the homes of friends and neighbours much more often on average (p < 0.001). Even so, the difference in contacts was much smaller than the divergence with regard to shared care by 'friend-neighbours'. Only four working-class families shared care with a 'friend-neighbour' in the two weeks, but three quarters of middle-class families did so, half of them more than once (p < 0.001). Although many of the working-class children did meet neighbours on the street or stair quite a lot or saw parents' close friends at home in the evenings they were looked after by them hardly at all. With a few exceptions, friends and neighbours were normally thought of for sharing care only on the rare occasions when relations were not available. This happened when there was a wedding in the family, for instance.

Much more than was the case with relatives, significant

friends were predominantly women. In all, five out of every seven of the friends and neighbours listed as important to the sample children were women. An even smaller proportion of those seen very frequently were men. This illustrates how the lives of these three-year-olds were commonly dominated by contacts with women. Nevertheless, it was clear that children had more contact than care from male friend-neighbours, because shared care by a male non-relative was rare.

Two in three of the families in the main sample included no unmarried persons in their list of significant friends. This contrasts with the position for kin of the same generation (i.e. parents' brothers and sisters) with whom contact was generally greater if they were single. About 40 per cent of all significant friends were also parents of under-fives. Over four fifths of the people interviewed listed at least one significant friend who had a child under five. This high degree of befriending according to the same life-cycle stage may be termed 'stage-grading', by analogy with the anthropological concept of age-grading.

Most parents' social networks appeared to consist of a small number of sectors comprising people who usually had contact with others in the same sector but seldom knew those in another sector (cf. Cubitt, 1973). The most significant types were local parents (particularly mothers) of young children, parents' 'old friends' and other neighbours. For smaller numbers of families, the father's current work colleagues or their wives, the mother's former colleagues or ex-neighbours were also important. Although a person from each category was an important carer for at least one child, it was clear that 'friend-neighbour' carers were mostly selected more narrowly according to combination of similar life-cycle stage, proximity and personal compatibility. Not many families stated explicitly that non-relative carers should mainly be mothers of young children, but this was an important taken-for-granted factor in choice. Apart from relatives, they had the greatest combination of eligibility factors for care – experience with children; nearness; opportunity to reciprocate; ability to offer peer play for the child; and daytime availability.

Middle-class families were much more likely to name considerable numbers of other local parents amongst the list of non-relatives significant to their children (p < 0.001). Of course working-class families usually did have at least a few good friends living not too far away but more of these were old-established friends living in other parts of Edinburgh. These friendships seldom extended to include sharing care. This arose in part from ideas about the inviolability of other people's family commitments which was noted in the last chapter. Mrs Spence* explained that she did not share care with friends, as 'they are nearly all married with kids of their own'. Mr Nairn* said that people in their street hardly ever went out as couples *because* they all had young children. In Milburn this situation would normally have been seen as a basis for reciprocal care and given rise to a street care network. In Whitlaw there seemed to be less integration of social life with the family and home since most friends were seen in the evenings at a club, pub, cinema or other outside venue. Another important factor was that most working-class parents' friends had regular kin carers too, so they were seen as having no need for reciprocal care. Thus, those few families with no suitable kin carers in Edinburgh were usually not in touch with others in a similar position. In Milburn, the much higher proportion of 'incomers' meant that there was a common need to look outside the kin network for care. The resulting exchanges of care were intimately linked with social contacts. This placed pressures on the families who did have nearby kin carers to become involved with the street care networks and circles or else they would be seen as opting out of the local pattern of friendship and reciprocation.

Styles of neighbouring

The class differences in befriending and sharing care were associated with contrasting ways of perceiving neighbour relationships. This did not apply to those living next door, with whom the kind of relationship depended on the particular individuals concerned. In both classes and in both tenement and villa districts similar proportions of couples described their immediate neighbours as either 'friendly' or 'not close'. The fact that the class differences in neighbour relationships did not apply so close to the threshold fits with the fact that in the few working-class families in which friends or neighbours were important as carers they were mostly immediate neighbours. There were several instances in Whitlaw where a family had minimal local contacts except that there was a very close interchange between adjacent households.

Beyond immediate neighbours, however, contacts were chiefly with other households who were similar in composition and life-stage, as Nahemow and Lawton (1975) have shown. Then there were strong class dissimilarities. With a few important exceptions, the working-class families in the sample seemed less interested or less skilful in making new relationships locally. Three quarters of those living in Milburn described other people in the street as friendly compared with only one quarter in Whitlaw (p < 0.02; Figure 5.2). Not surprisingly then, some working-class parents explained that they did not use neighbours for care 'because we're not very close to them' (Mr Wallace*). Apart from the few families who had achieved close pair relationships with a nearby family or widow, neighbours were generally approached for care in emergencies only, when there was not time to get in touch with kin. With a few exceptions, there was little resemblance to the patterns of friendly integrated stair and street communities found in many early community studies including one in Edinburgh (Hutton, 1975; Klein, 1965). Even when neighbours were depicted as friendly, several parents stressed that there was little or no going in and out of each other's houses. Good neighbouring was defined in terms of the absence of trouble or interference. A general preparedness to help was valued rather than intimacy or mutual aid. This was epitomised in remarks like these:

Mr Quinn*   They don't bother you, don't mind your business or you mind theirs, but they are there when you need them. They are very good.

Mr Vallance* (It's) a good place to stay, because nobody bothers you.

Mr Brown*   I've no problem on this stair – no arguments with anybody.

It is noteworthy that most of such comments were made by

1 Perceived attitudes of immediate neighbours

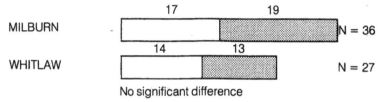

2 Perceived attitudes of people in the street

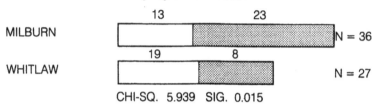

3 Number of friends parents have in the street

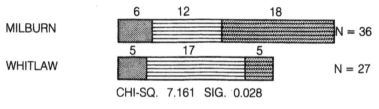

KEY

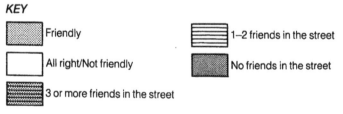

Figure 5.2 *Area differences in neighbour attitudes and contacts*

fathers, as in the case of defensive views expressed about strangers.

On the other hand, the Milburn pattern did fit with that which has been observed before in some middle-class areas with high proportions of newcomers (Seeley *et al.*, 1956; Whyte, 1960). In the majority of the streets where people were interviewed, there were friendly networks, often with routine exchange of services. These feelings of friendliness were generally restricted to other families with children and there were frequent comments about the aloofness of elderly people in Milburn.

Within this study it is not possible to say how far these differing perceptions of neighbouring were particular to the areas concerned or reflected broader social processes. The nature of an area may affect networks not only through the attitudes of the people, but by means of structuring opportunities to meet. There were some sharp contrasts over short distances. Mrs Page described her neighbours as old and unfriendly, whereas her sister round the corner had made friends with several mothers of a similar age in her street. Nevertheless, neighbours were generally seen as very friendly in both the tenement area of North Milburn and the villa area of South Milburn, whereas there was a lack of closeness and fewer 'local friends' in most parts of Whitlaw. One or two streets or stairs were exceptional. Shona Nairn* and Susan Vallance* both lived in low rise housing with friendly families whose children often played together. Even so there were no regular shared care arrangements with neighbours. This provides some further if limited evidence that the patterns of social interaction were attributable in part to class or the general character of the area and not only the immediate physical environment. In addition, there was some suggestion from the working-class families in Milburn and the six interviews with families who had moved to other parts of Edinburgh that the differences in neighbouring style had much to do with how class *in general* affects people who move from their home area and not simply differences between two particular areas. The three families who had moved from Milburn to other middle-class suburbs had soon encountered similar street networks to those they had known before whilst the families who had moved from Whitlaw were isolated and largely reliant on kin from elsewhere for contacts and shared care.

All this should not be taken to imply that the working-class families were less friendly. Rather it seemed that once working-class people had moved away from the area they had grown up in they had inhibitions and notions of privacy which meant that a more favourable set of opportunities was needed in order to foster a network of street relationships. Distrust of stranger care and high involvement with kin also reduced the stimulus to interaction. This may have historical origins in that past immersion in extended kin networks living close together perhaps made it less necessary for working-class people 'to learn the arts of social intercourse' (Hoggart, 1973: 305).

Besides the differences in neighbouring which happened when people close by had similar socio-economic positions there were also processes which served to keep apart those who by and large belonged to different social classes. In particular, perceptions that surrounding people were snobbish or offhand helped to keep those working-class parents who lived in Milburn or on the better-off fringes of Whitlaw from becoming part of the prevailing social networks. As a result they did not have access to membership or even knowledge of social institutions like swop networks and babysitting circles. Four mothers had withdrawn from mother and toddler groups as they were uncomfortable at what they felt to be the social exclusiveness of others there. Mrs Taylor* had heard of a circle through the playgroup, but stated 'I wouldn't like to leave the kids with them. I think they are kind of snobby.'

Likewise, contacts in the street foundered on apparent rejections of attempts to be friendly:

Mrs Brown* They get quite taken aback that you made an attempt to speak to them.

Mrs Traynor* They think they are better than us. ( ) You couldna get too friendly with them, because I've tried . . . I've tried, but they just pass by you without even looking at you.

Both the Lauries (who were of working-class origin) and the Baxters* considered their Milburn neighbours unpredictable – sometimes they would talk, sometimes not. Families in Whitlaw were very aware of Milburn's reputation as a 'more

snobby area' (Mrs Ogilvie*), where 'they seem to have the idea
they are better than us' (Mrs Reynolds*). These quotations
illustrate how factors other than housing and income serve to
keep even quite prosperous working-class families from social
acceptance. It corresponds to the relational aspect of class
identity and differentiation described by Goldthorpe and Lockwood (1963). This may in turn contribute to middle-class
families' confidence in the fact that members of circles or other
street carer networks would be similar to themselves.

Network development and change

So far we have considered networks in a somewhat static
fashion, but they are dynamic in ways which affect and are
affected by care sequences. Well over half of all the parents
thought that since having children they saw at least some of
their former friends less often. One quarter said there had
been a big decrease in contacts. The main kinds of friendship
affected were those with friends living at a distance, single
friends, and mothers' former work colleagues. One reason for
seeing people less often was the difficulty of travelling with
young children. Just as important were the differing time
structures, interests and orientations compared with those of
old friends who had not started a family. Both single friends
and former colleagues who still worked would not be free
during the daytime, so that mothers at home with young children became more interested in contacts with those people
who were at home then, i.e. grandparents, other local mothers
and elderly neighbours. Mothers found it easier to maintain
contact with those women who had had children at roughly
the same period because those friends who were in a different
life-cycle phase could be still at work or perhaps have returned
to work when their children started school. Drifting apart from
old friends was not just a matter of practical difficulties or
confined to mothers. Mr Powell said 'People who don't have
children have strange ideas about what to expect and what
not to expect.' Mr Arnot thought 'We just don't talk the same
language anymore.' However, a few parents made special
efforts to keep in touch with single friends, who might even

be major evening carers as was the case for Eleanor Buchan and Lisa Jamieson*.

This reduction or loss of the 'old friend' segment of parent's networks was usually compensated for by the growth of a new segment which was locally based and stage graded. Only seven families reported both a decrease in contact with old friends and no development of new friendships since having children. The children themselves were often the sources and focus of these new relationships. Sixty-five per cent of the parents said they had made new friends through their children and a further 15 per cent felt that their children had reinforced certain of their previous friendships more than others. This apparently strong influence of children on their parents' friendships contradicts the earlier finding of Babchuk (1965) and has received little attention in the relevant literature (Duck and Gilmour, 1981). Sometimes stage-grading was very precise in that parents of children whose age differed by only a year or two were likely to link up. There were several examples of families becoming friendly as each had two children of similar ages and spacing, such as a three-year-old and a toddler or a five-year-old and a brother or sister two years younger. Matching in this way occurred partly because mothers with children of similar ages were likely to meet at such places as clinics or toddler groups which cater for quite narrow age bands of children. In addition, having children of similar ages meant there was a greater likelihood of a common interest and shared needs, as well as a high probability of being home during the day. Mothers who only had children aged under five might belong to different networks from those with school age children. Mrs Boyd illustrated this distinction when she described how hard it was to break into an established clique at nursery school of mothers who had got to know each other through their older children. They were 'chit-chatting, obviously known each other for ages' and apparently uninterested in someone coming with a three-year-old for the first time. Others whose oldest child was also aged three were more open to the possibility of forming new acquaintances.

Usually, initial befriending through children was by mothers rather than fathers, but quite often families then became joint friends. Occasionally, the children met first, by playing on the back green or in the park for example. Many mothers had begun talking to each other because they saw that they both had similar aged children when out walking or because they met at the same place for the same purpose with children. Being a mother (or expectant mother) is a highly visible category, with positive associations and assumed common interests, so it provides a more legitimate justification for starting to talk to a stranger than is normally the case. One third of families had made friends through children by meeting in the street, at the park or out shopping. Group care and school had also been important ways of making new friends. For some people, group care provided the first opportunity of making new friends through children whereas others had built up a sizeable network before the child was three. A smaller but significant number (thirteen) had made friends by meeting at maternity hospital or at a children's clinic. Befriending was assisted if mothers met in more than one context, for then recognition of a common link elsewhere helped the initiation of conversations. For instance, Mrs Gunn met another mother from along the street at the clinic and because they recognised each other they stuck up conversation and soon got to know each other well. Local acquaintanceships made through children usually started with limited functions in one context but could then diversify and intensify. Mrs Spence* described how one such relationship developed with 'We were like sisters. ( ) Everywhere we went we used to go together.' The Buchans became intimate friends with the family across the street, so there was daily contact and Eleanor was happy to stay there frequently without her parents. Dorothy Forbes called the woman across the road 'Mummy'. She became her main carer. On the other hand several mothers reported relationships which involved frequent contacts and maybe shared care but which remained superficial or functional.

Such factors as the length of residence in the street, the ages of the older children and the mother's personality affected how a family interacted with others round about. Broadly, four main kinds of disposition to neighbouring were identified:

1 **Autonomous** The family is inward looking or oriented to kin outside the area.

2 Insufficient	More local social contact was desired. This was most likely when the three-year-old was the eldest and there had been little opportunity to get to know people through a group.
3 Interactive	There are some local friendships and the family is open to new ones.
4 Satiated	The family has enough social contacts and would be reluctant to spare time for new befriending. This applied especially to those who had made many contacts through older children.

There was a marked class contrast in befriending patterns which helps explain the differences in contacts and sharing care with non-relatives. Similar proportions of working-class and middle-class parents reported diminished interaction with old friends after having children but far fewer working-class parents said they had made new friends through their children (p < 0.02). It was mainly middle-class parents who had made friends through group care and by initiating contacts with local parents in the street or park. These are the situations which perhaps require more social confidence and openness towards strangers. As a result, most of the families who had autonomous or insufficient local network relationships were working class. Of course, often this was compensated for by kin contacts. With befriending as with sharing care it was more characteristic for a working-class mother to pair up with one other, whereas typically middle-class mothers joined or developed a network of local friends.

The interviews with middle-class couples revealed individual and group mechanisms for getting to know people which were hardly evident amongst working-class families. Many middle-class parents actively sought out peer contacts for their children from an early age. For instance Mrs Edwards said she made friends, because 'you tend to cultivate them at the time the children are wee to give them company'. Most working-class parents identified a need for peer contact only after their children were aged two or three and then they expected this to be achieved with the help of a nursery school or playgroup rather than by means of street networks. New neighbours were invited in for tea or coffee in both areas, but in Milburn there was a much more extended expectation that people encountered casually in the street could be invited back home and that routine, reciprocal contacts might well ensue. Working-class mothers appeared to have greater difficulty in diversifying a relationship from one context to another. Mrs Spence*, who seemed by no means a shy person, explained why it was hard to get to know other mothers in the area:

> I don't know ... even walking up the road with one or two of them from the nursery, you walk as far as their street and then they go off. They stop a minute at the corner of the street, and then they say 'I'd better get on with the housework'. There's no way of saying ... there isn't even ... There's a cafe down the road, but the first thing in the morning you don't want to say 'Come and sit in a cafe'. If (the nursery school) just had a room they could sit in, it would make a big difference. You wouldn't need to do anything, but just stay there for an hour with a coffee before you went home, and then you could get to know them.

Several of the working-class mothers welcomed the opportunity to meet others at the group care coffee mornings but typically 'that's as far as it has got' (Mrs Whigham*). It could be that relationships would develop later but few working-class mothers had made friends through their older children's nursery school or playgroup unlike many middle-class mothers. Others found it hard to make friends in the street because there was no 'going into each other's houses' (Mrs Robertson*) and 'there is not really a meeting place' (Mr Wallace*). Allan (1979) has drawn attention to the fact that working-class people seem less prepared or able to make use of their homes for social purposes. There certainly seemed to be less preparedness to invite people home so that relationships might be developed. This may partly be due to the more limited space for mothers and children to congregate. On the other hand, old friends did visit the home quite often. It was not the case that all non-relatives were denied access to the home but normally a greater intimacy was necessary before people were entertained at home. A number of parents commented that neighbouring was more difficult in comparison with their childhood reference areas simply because people had not been brought up together in Whitlaw so that trust had not been established. In contrast, middle-class families invited others home as a means of furthering a relationship, rather than as its culmination.

As well as the more routinised expectations about individual contacts, Milburn and the other middle-class suburbs to which three families had moved also contained institutionalised groups which facilitated befriending. In particular there were circles and coffee gatherings which helped to integrate newcomers and served to make good the deficits in friend and carer sets resulting from departed families. On moving to a new area, several parents had been asked to join circles or had actively asked around to find one. It was seen as a natural part of settling into a new neighbourhood. Indeed, there could be pressure put on mothers to join a circle or take part in reciprocal care. Mrs Christie had to keep refusing such overtures. Furthermore it was common to invite other circle members round so that the child could get to know them before they babysat and this promoted parental befriending too.

'Coffee mornings' or 'coffee gatherings' as named institutions involving several sets of families appeared to be confined to middle-class families, well over half of whom mentioned them. Although some were restricted to a few people who were already well acquainted others had open membership and it was generally accepted that mothers moving into the street would be invited to them. Mr Finlayson said 'When a new neighbour has got established, they tend to hold a coffee morning to introduce her to the community.' Thus newcomers had less need of social skills to make friends for they were automatically invited to join in. Some of them introduced innovations learnt in their previous home area – such as the idea of a mini-group or a street party. Coffee mornings also extended the relationships of those already in the area and increased network connectedness by introducing people to friends of friends. Although the gatherings mostly involved women during the daytime, some streets also arranged evening parties of social events in order to involve the fathers.

Some had an overlapping membership with other kinds of groups which had been set up to co-operate in such activities as swimming, music and book-lending. The larger gatherings usually acted as or arose from the 'business meetings' of circles. Smaller ones developed as mini-groups for sharing care or from subgroups of the larger coffee gatherings. Mrs Johnstone set up a 'run' to nursery school with three other mothers and they then began to hold a weekly coffee morning. The smaller groups were often organised ostensibly just for the children to play. As Mrs Henderson said 'they are *supposed* to be for the benefit of the children'. However, there were social benefits for the mothers and commonly sharing care was arranged too. The Arnots described how, once children were happily playing together, mothers had begun to take it in turns to pop out to the shops, although Mrs Arnot insisted that this was very much not the reason for coming together. Such incidental arrangements became regularised means of sharing care in several cases.

Children's overall relationships with adults outside the nuclear family

In spite of the general separation between the two main segments of social networks (relatives and non-relatives) it is important to compare them and see how they add up within the total pattern of a child and family's social contacts. There was little difference between a child's mean frequency of contact with friend-neighbours and with relatives, despite the fact that most of the relatives seen lived elsewhere in Edinburgh whilst many friend-neighbours lived close by. It must be remembered that group care and paid childcarer contacts are excluded from consideration here and this would boost the amount of contacts the children had with non-kin considerably. Only a slightly higher proportion of relatives seen in the diary period (17.5 per cent) acted as carers than was the case for friend-neighbours (12 per cent).

High levels of kin contact were not necessarily inimical to the development of non-kin relationships. Interview and diary data showed that the amount of contact with friend-neighbours varied independently of the frequency of interaction with kin except inasfar as it was unusual to have very frequent contacts with large numbers of both. When the total number of adults seen by individual children was added up there were no class differences revealed because the more frequent interaction with relatives by working-class children was balanced by their more restricted interaction with non-kin. Indeed there was a tendency for working-class children to spend somewhat more time with other adults present because individual relatives were seen on somewhat more occasions than non-relatives on average (p < 0.02). Clearly, it was not paucity of contacts which inhibited working-class parents from sharing care as frequently as middle-class parents.

The way in which members of a family's social network did or did not know each other independently of the family (i.e. the 'connectedness' of the network) could influence shared care. A close-knit Edinburgh kin network or a street non-kin network provided easy interchangeability and substitution of carers if that was needed. There were also greater opportunities for replacement if a key carer moved away or otherwise became unavailable. Moreover, reliance on particular individuals would be reduced. Connectedness could make arranging shared care easier as there were communication channels for establishing who was available. Sometimes 'linked' people combined to provide care, as when two or more relatives kept each other company or divided up periods of shared care to suit their own convenience. When Mrs Forbes went into hospital for a week several neighbours arranged care of Dorothy between them. In similar circumstances two aunts did the same for Tammy Robertson*. People linked in a set of friends or carers also transmitted information and evaluations about particular group care facilities as well as more general values about group care or other forms of shared care. When people moved house then friends of relatives or of friends sometimes provided useful contacts for incipient social relationships and potential carers. Sometimes a carer's network extended the range of a child's contacts. Some children had a close relationship with the neighbours of relatives with whom they often stayed or with the friends and relatives of a childminder.

Following Bott (1957), connectedness has mostly been

viewed in terms of connections which are independent of the focal person. But connections which are made deliberately may be important too. Coffee mornings, circle meetings, parties and other kinds of social occasion could be used to link friends. Some connections arose concurrently, often through a common group membership or function, as at work, in a circle or at church. Moreover, the origins of independent connections between families (say B and C) known to the key family (A) can arise in various ways with differing implications:

1 B and C knew each other before either met A
2 B and C met independently after one or both had met A
3 B and C were introduced to each other by A
4 B introduced A to C
5 A, B and C all got to know each other through common membership of a group

These variations in the tempo of connectedness affected which families were focal in arranging care and which ones were newcomers fitting into an established care arrangement. The latter might simply fall in with established practices of the 'old hands' or might contribute innovative ideas about organising reciprocal care. Some network members actively set out to link up other people known to them.

So far we have largely considered the child's contacts with members of the parents' networks, without taking account of the subjective importance to the child of those concerned. In order to obtain a picture of children's attachments and friendships some studies have asked parents to name people in relation to whom infants or toddlers exhibit specific overt behaviours, especially separation distress (Schaffer and Emerson, 1964; Tizard and Tizard, 1971). This seemed to have less value in relation to children aged three, who may express attachment more variously, positively and verbally. Therefore, it was decided simply to ask parents which people they considered the child was most fond of. Two separate lists in order of closeness to the child were made for adults and children. This has the merit that parents are in a position to make overall judgments about their child's feelings about others, but there may be distortions produced by the subjectivity of the parent's viewpoint and differing interpretations of what 'fond of' means. In practice, most parents indicated that they inferred fondness from just a few criteria: children were thought to be fond of people if they were notably relaxed, pleased or excited to be in their company, talked about them positively and frequently, or showed signs of missing them when apart.

Most of the children had lists of seven to twelve adults including parents of whom they were said to be fond. As with choice of carers, it was grandparents, street friends and to a smaller extent aunts and uncles who dominated the majority of fondness lists. As many middle-class children were said to be most attached to grandparents as working-class children, despite the differences in distance, kinds of contact and availability as carers. The main class differences consisted in the much higher numbers of friend-neighbours for most middle-class children and the high representation of aunts and uncles for working-class children. Nineteen middle-class children but only five working-class children had a friend or neighbour amongst the three adults apart from their parents they were said to be most fond of. A consequence of the greater predominance of kin amongst the attachments of the average working-class child was that 70 per cent of working-class children had four or more men in their fondness list, but only 25 per cent of middle-class children ($p < 0.01$).

Normally there was a high degree of overlap between a child's carer set and fondness list. It was generally the case that the child's main carers were selected from people of whom they were already fond or else the child became fond of them partly as a result of being looked after by them. The main lack of correspondence between the ranking of carers and attachments was that many children were thought to be more fond of some relatives who lived too far away to act as carers (except on visits) than they were of major local carers. By contrast, there was no instance in which a child was said to be most fond of a friend or neighbour when the main carer was a relative. In consequence far more working-class children were said to be most fond of their main carer than middle-class children, who were often thought to be more attached to a close relative than a non-relative main carer. This was especially true with respect to evening care, because of the greater middle-class openness to care by paid non-relative babysitters and circle members, some of whom were not very familiar to the child.

Relationships with other children

There is an important interaction between sharing care and what may be termed children's 'child networks', as opposed to their 'adult networks'. Children of carers were often present when shared care took place as sometimes were other children. This could lead on to close relationships amongst the youngsters concerned. Conversely, amicable associations with other children could give rise to shared care, as when children asked to play in a friend's home.

An important influence on child networks is evidently the density of children in a local district and particularly in nearby streets. Information from the previous Census (1971) suggested that there was little overall difference between Milburn and Whitlaw in this respect. However, the parents interviewed tended to see things differently, perhaps because the situation had changed in the previous few years. Nearly all the parents in Whitlaw thought there were few young children in their street but over half of Milburn families thought there were many in theirs. Those parents who perceived their locality as having a high density of young children usually also had children with more than the average number of friends living nearby ($p < 0.001$). There may have been real differences in the number of children in the two areas because some Milburn parents thought there had been an influx of younger families in the previous few years. On the other hand several working-class parents seemed less aware of other families with children under five even when they did live nearby. Mrs Tervit* said 'there is nobody in the same position as us in this street' (i.e. with a young child, but the Traynors* lived just up the road. The Sadlers* and the Scotts* lived opposite each other, but both contended there were no other young children nearby. Mrs Brown* thought their children lacked friends because there were few children in the area, but 'We were surprised when Emma started school. There were 90 children started at the same time and we didn't think there were that many children in South Milburn.' The majority of children in both areas did play with other children from the same street but about 40 per cent of the working-class children (twelve) apparently never did so, compared with only about 10 per cent of middle-class children (three) (p < 0.05). This made group care especially important for such families. Mrs Sim* said 'It's helped him going to nursery, because there's no kids round here. I think if there had been other kids, I might not have bothered putting him to nursery.'

More detailed information about the amount of contact with other children outside group care came from the diary (Figure 5.3). Of course not all playmates can be regarded as friends. There is much uncertainty about the meaning of friendship and the significance of mutuality for pre-school children (Mannerino, 1980; Vandell and Mueller, 1980) but the term friend was commonly used by parents to describe those whom their child especially liked. Therefore, it seems legitimate to use children's fondness lists as some measure of friendship patterns.

Ignoring brothers, sisters and other children seen at group care, the number of children with whom the study child spent time in the diary two weeks varied greatly, from none to over twenty. The number of reported attachments to other children ranged less widely. The mean figure was 4.7 excluding siblings, considerably less than the equivalent for adults excluding parents (7.7). This may simply reflect an adult (parental) viewpoint but is consistent with the greater amount of contact with grown ups than other children which occurred before starting group care. Whereas children who had frequent contact with many relatives had the longest lists of adults they were fond of it was mainly those who spent a lot of time with friends and neighbours who had a long list of children they were fond of.

As a result of their limited mobility pre-school children tend to become acquainted with other children who live in the immediate vicinity (Bigelow and La Gaipa, 1980). Hence it was not surprising to find that the majority of children's 'friends' in this study lived in the few streets surrounding the child's home. There were eleven children who apparently had no friends living nearby and these were mostly working class. For instance, Ross Whigham* 'doesn't really know any chil-

1 Contacts with non-kin children in the diary fortnight

	Middle Class (N = 30)	Working Class (N = 28)	TOTAL (N = 58)	%
NONE	0	4	4	7%
1 — 8	16	20	36	62%
9 — 22	14	4	18	31%
	CHI-SQ = 9.943		Sig. = 0.007	

2 Contacts with kin children in the diary fortnight

	Middle Class	Working Class	TOTAL	%
NONE	27	14	41	71%
1 - 8	3	14	17	29%
9 - 22	0	0	0	0%
	CHI-SQ = 9.337		Sig. = 0.002	

3 Number of sessions spent with non-kin children in the diary fortnight

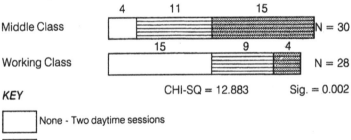

CHI-SQ = 12.883   Sig. = 0.002

KEY

☐ None - Two daytime sessions

▤ Three - Seven daytime sessions

▨ Eight or more daytime sessions

NOTE: These figures *exclude* contact at group care

Figure 5.3 *Contacts with other children*

dren, apart from the ones he's met at playgroup'. Mrs Tervit*
said that Yvonne 'hasn't got any children that she really
knows. None really of her own age group. That's why she's at
nursery.' Indeed, social class proved to be closely linked to
differences in children's contacts with and attachments to
other children (p < 0.001). Nearly half of the working-class
children saw fewer than four other children in the diary two
weeks outside group care, whereas all but four middle-class

children saw more than that. Just as working-class parents typically had less contact with other local parents than was the case for most middle-class couples so their children generally knew fewer children and saw them less often. Indeed there were indications that middle-class three-year-olds were already demonstrating some of their parents' skills at developing and formalising relationships at home and in different contexts by asking their parents to arrange meetings for lunch and tea. This finding contrasts with repeated conclusions that middle-class parents are more sheltering about children's external relations whilst working-class children engage in more outdoor play and interaction with others of similar age (Newson and Newson, 1970a; B. Tizard *et al.*, 1976). The patterns in Whitlaw and Milburn are more consonant with the view of Turner (1969) that there has been a shift in middle-class values in favour of encouraging children to mix from an early age, as exemplified by the playgroup movement.

Relatives were less prominent in child networks than was the case for adult contacts. Whilst kin contact compensated for the less frequent meetings with friends and neighbours of working-class children, this was not the case with respect to child-child relations. Only three middle-class children met a cousin or other relative aged under sixteen during the diary fortnight compared with half of the working-class children (p < 0.01). However, the frequency and numbers of individuals concerned did not usually make up for the excess of middle-class contacts with non-kin children. A relative aged under sixteen (usually a cousin, but occasionally a young aunt or some other kind of relation) was the 'best friend' of one in three working-class children (nine) but no middle-class child. The importance of cousin contacts may not persist into adulthood for hardly any of the parents saw their cousins very often.

Most studies of pre-school friendships have involved observations in some kind of nursery with an age range of a few years at most. Unsurprisingly they revealed that there is a close matching of age between friends (Allen, 1981; Green, 1933). Diaries from the current research demonstrated that even outside group care there was a strong bias towards contact with peers (defined for present purposes as other children aged between two and four). Most children had spent time with between one and five peers in the fortnight. The average number was three. Nevertheless, thirteen children apparently had no peer contact in that period except at group care. The fondness lists revealed an even greater peer dominance than the diary record of actual contacts, presumably because the latter was more influenced by quite frequent interaction with the friends of older brothers and sisters. Only five children had no peer they were fond of and for many children the majority of their friends were aged between two and four.

The peer concentration in child networks did not appear to result from group care attendance for there was no difference between attenders and non-attenders with regard to the proportions of peers they were fond of and the number of children seen during the diary fortnight. In any case most of the peer friendships had been established some time before the children went to a playgroup or nursery school. Children who had many friends and frequent contacts with peers tended to have higher care frequency and larger carer sets. Those cared for by childminders or au pairs had large child fondness lists, so they were not apparently handicapped in making friendships by lengthy substitute care. However, the highest levels of peer interaction and fondness were associated with weekly rather than daily shared care, within a large carer set of friends and neighbours.

It is probably true that mixed age playgroups are much less prevalent in our society than elsewhere (Konner, 1975) but the diaries showed that in this sample a fair amount of cross-age interaction occurred. The vast majority of the child relatives that were seen in the diary two weeks were of school age and all of those on the child fondness lists were aged over five. The literature on children's friendships has tended to assume that friends are non-kin and mainly peers but over one third of the children were said to be most fond of another child aged six or over (excluding siblings). Some children were also said to be very attached to older friends of a brother or sister.

By and large middle-class children, whether living in the tenement or villa district of Milburn, saw more other children of both pre-school and school age than working-class children with the exception of teenagers. The average middle-class child had more peer friends (mean = 3.5) than the average working-class child (mean = 1.9; p < 0.01). Especially striking is the more accurate age matching amongst middle-class children: 80 per cent of them had contact in the diary fortnight with another child aged three but only 40 per cent of the working-class children (p < 0.01). The best friend of half of the middle-class children was aged exactly three, and for three quarters was aged below six. This is understandable in view of the common stage-grade befriending by middle-class parents, usually in association with some form of reciprocal shared care arrangement. It is also consistent with the fact that more middle-class children knew another child when starting group care. In contrast, for half the working-class children the child they were most fond of was aged six or over. Cousins and occasionally other kinds of relative constituted a major source of contacts with teenagers for working-class children.

This chapter has illustrated the ways in which children's relationships outside the immediate family were closely linked to the kinds of contacts developed by their parents both in the past and as a response to the transition to parenthood itself. Our focus now narrows to concentrate on relationships, roles and perceptions within the nuclear family itself.

6 The effects on shared care of parents' life experiences, activities and ideas

Parents' life experiences and adjustments to parenthood

Previous experiences in parents' lives are likely to be important in shaping their attitudes and practices in relation to shared care. They may wish to repeat, modify or react against what happened to them in their own childhoods. Once confronted with their own real children in day to day situations they may well change or develop their ideas about what are the desirable or acceptable ways of being a parent. That does not necessarily happen in a clearly thought out fashion. This study largely concentrated on parents' current descriptions of how and why they did what they did, so that the evidence about the influences of the past on present care practices was more superficial. In a single interview it was possible to ask specifically about only a few aspects of parents' experiences and opinions. To supplement this respondents were encouraged to give their own accounts of what they thought had influenced their attitudes about sharing care.

On first consideration it might be thought that parents of three-year-olds would not vary much in age. In fact there is quite a wide spread as a result of differences in the timing of people's marriages and variations in the number and spacing of other children in the family. Parents in this sample ranged in age from 22 to 52 years. Nevertheless, about half were in their early thirties and it was not possible to detect any systematic ways in which care patterns varied with parents' age.

It seems plausible that adult attitudes and behaviour in relation to sharing care are affected by their own childhood experiences of attachment and separation. As yet little is known about such influences over the life-span (Antonucci, 1976; Spanier et al., 1978). It was not possible to examine this in depth but parents were briefly asked about major separations and losses they had experienced as children. Twenty mothers and twenty-seven fathers recalled a major childhood separation from one or both of their own parents for at least some weeks. There was a definite tendency for those parents who had had a childhood separation to be married to others who had also had separations ($p < 0.01$). There were weak trends for couples who had both experienced major childhood separations to be high sharers and to make greater use of non-relatives for care. Half of the mothers who had a major separation as a child had started their own children in group care before the age of three, compared with only one in six of other mothers ($p < 0.02$). In individual cases the same kind of separation could lead to different inferences being made. Both Mr and Mrs Balfour remembered how traumatic they had found episodes in hospital when they were young children. As a result Mrs Balfour did not want her children to stay with grandparents overnight as she feared they would be upset in a similar way. Mr Balfour had reached the opposite conclusion that an overnight separation now would help his son be more prepared in case he suddenly had to go into hospital unexpectedly.

Parents' recollections of their own experiences of shared care may not have been very accurate but they indicated some differences compared with the current generation of children. A higher proportion of middle-class parents recalled their main carer as being a relative than was the case for their own children. Interestingly, a considerable number of parents from both classes said they did not recall their parents ever going out together without the children. A typical comment was that of Mrs Balfour: 'I honestly don't think they used babysitters.' Like many working-class respondents Mrs Shaw* had a strong recollection of home-centred life twenty to thirty years ago: 'I can't ever remember my parents going out together. I mean one of them might go out – like my mother would go to the pictures, but I don't think they both went out. It was really for the family. They were all for the family.' Some parents believed that values have altered somewhat in favour of greater entitlement for women to be apart from their children. Growth in real incomes and wider leisure opportunities may also have played a part in these changes. Mrs Urquhart* said 'I think it's all right to go out maybe for an afternoon, whereas my Mum wouldn't. I think my Mum should have gone out more.' Mrs Raeburn made a similar comment and added that 'Now there is a different attitude towards the family. A lot of people feel they have a right to children but also the right to have freedom and a social life.' However, several working-class parents had opposite recollections of more shared care in the past when economic pressures had made it more necessary for both parents to work. Those from rural backgrounds or old established working-class districts remembered more brief sharing of child care amongst neighbours in the past or spontaneous groups of children at play without the dangers from modern traffic. The big increase in the number of cars on the roads and reduced neighbourliness were seen as contributing to the present-day need for special supervised settings in which children can play.

Fewer than one in four parents had been to any form of pre-school group as far as they could remember. This provides a marked contrast with their own children, all of whom would be having pre-school group experience. This demonstrates in individual terms the effects over a single generation of nursery school expansion and the playgroup movement on children's experiences before school. Wadsworth (1981) reported a similar change.

Parents were asked about the extent of their general contacts with children and of looking after children before they had their own. Considerably more of the women had had more 'practice' in both respects, but quite a few men did have some expertise and there were some women who had very little. For instance, about half of the mothers (thirty) and fewer than one quarter of the fathers (fourteen) described having done a fair amount of looking after other people's children before they had any of their own. More working-class women had done a lot of babysitting (mostly for relatives) than middle-class women. In about half the families in both classes neither parent had done any significant babysitting before having children, so their ideas about sharing care may well have been unformed when they came to make arrangements for their own children.

In spite of women's generally greater readiness for dealing with children, more mothers (twenty-two) than fathers (fourteen) felt that they had had some difficulty in adjusting to parenthood. This is not unexpected for women have more emotional, physical and practical adjustments to make (Dominian, 1982; Richman, 1978; Rollins and Galligan, 1978). The following extracts illustrate the differences:

1	**Interviewer**	How did you find it adjusting (to parenthood)?'
	Mrs Griffin	Pretty horrible, I think. Pretty awful.
	Mr Griffin	For you.
	Mrs Griffin	Well, I hadn't any great positive feelings about having kids, and I didn't really like stopping work. Not because I was so involved with my work, but because I didn't really know of any other way of life, because of the way I had been conditioned actually. So that it was difficult for me to adjust to being at home doing domestic things for a start and to have this baby who was very demanding.
	Mr Griffin	I don't think I had so much adjusting to do. I must say I enjoyed it, but then I don't have to do the bulk of the heavy, messy stuff. I'm not a complete male chauvinist pig – I did help a bit.
2	**Mrs Purdie***	Three children in five years. That's a lot!
	Mr Purdie*	A great experience.
	Mrs Purdie*	Tiring!

Two thirds of the mothers who had found it hard to adjust to parenthood had children with problems in adapting to shared care, compared with only one third of other mothers ($p < 0.02$). Mothers who had had their first child comparatively late included a higher proportion who had adjusted poorly to parenthood. Also more of them shared care infrequently and had children who reacted badly to separations.

Parental anxiety and pressures

The arrival of young children has been shown to reduce marital satisfaction and increase stress for many parents. This is particularly true for mothers (Burgess, 1981; Hoffman and Manis, 1978). The term 'stress' is used here as a shorthand to represent the felt anxieties or pressures which arise in response to internal and external stressor events or circumstances (Cox, 1983; Levine and Scotch, 1970; McGrath, 1970). The assessment of parental stress was approached in a number of ways. The Malaise Inventory or MI was borrowed from earlier studies of children (Osborn, 1981a, 1984; Rutter et al., 1970). This uses the sum of various physical and psychological symptoms to give a numerical indicator of stress for particular individuals (see Appendix). In order to gain some idea about stressors, too, parents were asked separately about what they regarded as pressures and sources of unhappiness for them in their current situation. None of these measures revealed class differences in this study.

The MI scores for the sample are given in Table 6.1. Normally, a total of seven or more positive replies to the questions is considered to indicate high anxiety or stress. In this sample only five mothers and three fathers recorded an MI score of 7+. This proportion is much lower than has been found for mothers in the other studies, which is doubtless partly due to the lack of single parent and mobile families in the sample. In view of this, a further subdivision was made between 0–2 and 3–6. Parents who scored 3+ will be referred to as 'more anxious' but this need not imply a high level of stress.

No other study I am aware of has administered the MI to men but most research has found that mental stress in the form of depression and anxiety occurs more commonly among married women than married men (Gove, 1972; Taylor and Chave, 1964). Although married people generally show a lower incidence of stress than single people it seems that the greater

Table 6.1 *Parental stress – malaise inventory scores*

Absolute numbers	Mothers	Fathers	
Score of 0–2	44	43	
Score of 3–6	13	14	
Score of 7+	5	3	

Percentages	Mother	Father	CHES* Study (mothers only)
Score of 0–2	71%	72%	37%
Score of 3–6	21%	23%	39%
Score of 7+	8%	5%	24%
	N = 62	N = 60	N = 12,942

Combined scores		
Families with both parents scoring	0–2	30 (50%)
At least one parent scoring	3–6	22 (37%)
At least one parent scoring	7+	8 (13%)
		(N = 60)

* Child Health and Education Study

the family obligations of couples the larger is the difference between the rates of stress for men and women (Aneshensel *et al.*, 1981). In this sample however the range of scores was very similar for fathers and mothers. Cullen (1979) likewise reported a project which discovered similar amounts of distress for mothers and fathers in families with young children. On the other hand, when asked what pressures they felt as parents, nearly half of the mothers in the present sample named two or more but only one quarter of the fathers. For both mothers and fathers the most frequently cited kind of pressure concerned interruptions of sleep by children who were crying or who wanted attention. Children's wakefulness is evidently a major problem in early parenthood whose impact is perhaps underestimated outside the families concerned (Jenkins *et al.*, 1980; Richman *et al.*, 1975). A few parents confessed they were not far from child abuse when exhausted and trying to settle a crying child in the middle of the night. Mrs Hunter recalled 'I really felt I knew what it would be like to shake her to death. She screamed and screamed for three months.' Mr Forbes said 'You come very close to understanding the thin line between a normal baby and a battered baby.' Other important pressures arising from parenthood included:

Limitations of interest for mothers   boredom, isolation, limited conversation.

Worries about the child's health   concern if the child was very ill, fear of a cot death.

Competing demands   (a) between different children and (b) between housework or one's own activities and the child.

Constant demands   repetitive requests, interruptions or need for amusement by the child.

Tensions   tiredness, needing to control or remonstrate with the children.

Only a minority of families admitted to things which led to unhappiness in the family. However, amongst these the most common complaints were about the high demands of the husband's work or about the wife's restricted life at home. In other words the man's breadwinner role interferred with his involvement at home whereas the wife's domestic role prevented greater opportunity for fulfilment outside the home.

MI scores were not related to any of the indices of social contacts but did vary with shared care frequency. Families in which at least one parent was 'more anxious' usually had small carer sets made up primarily of kin; they shared care infrequently ($p < 0.05$). Such families made up only half of the sample but they accounted for nearly all of those children who were mainly upset by shared care ($p < 0.02$). Higher MI scores for both mothers and fathers were associated with generally poor reactions to shared care by their children. Considered together with the link between mothers' difficult adjustment to parenthood and children's negative reactions to shared care, these findings could be explained by inheritance of anxiety (Scarr, 1969). Alternatively it is possible that anxious parents give their children less preparation for shared care and/or communicate their own worry to the children who respond accordingly (Gewirtz, 1976).

Pressures can be eased in many ways but a number of parents had found sharing care helpful – directly, indirectly or as a by-product. Several grandparents had taken out or cared for children in order to relieve the strain on a mother or both parents at times of difficulty. Mrs Buchan found Eleanor's crying and clinginess as a baby very stressful. She therefore welcomed a break yet was reluctant to ask anyone to look after Eleanor as she would be difficult to deal with. Fortunately Mrs Buchan's mother-in-law offered to look after her grand-daughter and did so in a very sensitive manner. Mrs Christie described problems she had had in coping with tantrums, getting up at night and meeting the constant demands of their children. She concluded 'I'm lucky having my mother and John's mother coming over every week and giving me a break.' Mrs Powell on the other hand regretted that she had no close relatives to help when she had been very depressed after Peter's birth: 'I needed to share him more – I wasn't prepared to go to the extent of sharing him with somebody outside the family.' Similarly, a number of mothers in street networks commented that regular swops helped prevent pressures becoming unmanageable. When things got on top of them they could leave their children with someone else at short notice. More indirectly, going back to work and thereby getting out of the home afforded a welcome relief for several mothers. Mrs Baxter* typified this: 'If I've had a hard day with the children, I've got three hours to unwind at my work and sort of charge my batteries again, when I come home. It does make me feel a lot better.' Similarly many mothers felt they benefited once their children were at group care which permitted them to increase their range of activities and contacts. Mrs Traynor* said this helped her become much less depressed than she had been when alone at home with her young daughter.

In contrast, some parents resented the implication that sharing care was a solution to pressures they felt. Mrs Robertson* denied vehemently that 'getting rid of the child' was an answer to the restrictions of being a housewife. Mrs Sinclair* was angry about her health visitor's suggestion that occasional separations at a group might help her difficulties with her son. Sometimes stresses were felt to be inherent to parenthood so that 'you have got to come to terms with them'

(Mr Raeburn). Askham (1984) observed how problems seen as deriving from marriage and parenthood tend to be accepted as an integral and expected part of that relationship.

Parents' paid work

Patterns of both internal and external sharing of childcare are crucially affected by the varying ways in which the time of both the mother and the father is distributed between paid work and domestic or social activities. Work in the sense of employment has conventionally been seen as different from the work done to maintain the home and look after children. Feminists have pointed out that from several points of view, not least the efforts entailed in performing these tasks, this is a false distinction. Child care and housework can be shown to have certain formal and functional similarities to paid work as normally understood. They can also make comparable personal demands (Gardiner, 1975; Oakley, 1974b; Secombe, 1974). From this perspective mothers not in paid employment may be described as 'economically active in unpaid jobs' (Nissel, 1980: 12). Child care, like other domestic tasks, often becomes paid work when done by people other than the parents. However, to show that an activity resembles paid work in some ways and that it sometimes becomes paid work does not mean that it is the same thing, because there are distinctive financial and cultural connotations. Stacey (1981) argues that it is misleading to apply ideas from the public market place to the private domain of life at home. New means are needed to conceptualise the division of labour at home. Boulton (1983) observed that the 'domestic labour' model does not do justice to most mothers' own experience and perceptions. The traditional idea of work as something performed for financial gain was the sense used by all the respondents. Hence it seems legitimate to persist with conventional usage, as indeed do several feminist writers (see the titles of books by Mackie and Patullo (1977) and Rapoport and Rapoport (1978) for example).

So far in this book the relevance of parents' paid employment to sharing care has been relatively underplayed in order to emphasise that care patterns are related to much else besides. For the majority of families, reasons other than both parents working at the same time were most important for explaining shared care. It is nonetheless true that when both parents worked at the same time this led to the greatest frequency and duration of shared care. In our society it has become the normal expectation that mothers stop work to care for young children whilst fathers continue working. Hence it was mainly decisions made about when or whether the wife should return to work which had its main impact on care patterns. For many couples making choices about this was difficult, even agonising, in a way that was evidently not the case for the men. Nevertheless there were differences in the length, timing and flexibility of fathers' work hours which had significant effects on how far their wives' routine activities like shopping or special appointments could be fitted in with care by their husbands or were seen to 'need' external sharing. Most fathers in this sample were working a 'normal' 9–5 day, sometimes supplemented by considerable overtime. Only two were unemployed. There were seven fathers currently doing shift work and a few others had worked shifts in the past. All these were in working-class families. Several were home to look after the children quite a lot during the daytime so that their wives needed to share care less than average or not at all for everyday activities like going to the shops. Three of the eight fathers who regularly took their children to or from group care did shift work.

Of the twenty-four couples who admitted to a source of unhappiness in their family eleven complained about the way in which the man's absences at work or other demands from the job reduced his involvement in family life. To avoid such strains a few working-class fathers had changed their jobs partly so that they could spend more time with the children. For some men with manual occupations the lack of career structures and lower training investment meant they felt more able to alter the overall timing of their work by changing jobs. Middle-class fathers would stand to lose pay, seniority and accumulated benefits so that their work hours and timing had usually remained stable or else increased in length since they became parents. On the other hand, middle-class fathers generally had more flexibility to adjust the day to day work timetable of their present job. Some had taken time off when their wives had to attend an appointment whereas factory workers did not have such freedom.

Given the comparative uniformity of fathers' work hours, it was the variations in mothers' work which led to larger differences between families in their need to share care. For a number of reasons it was not possible to identify two sharply defined groups of working and non-working mothers. Firstly, there is some uncertainty whether activities like child-minding, studying or typing at home constitute 'work'. For this research it was decided to include all paid activities as work. Secondly, there was a wide continuum of hours worked. Several women did so for only a few hours a week. A third consideration was that mothers often moved in and out of the labour market so that adjudication to a category of 'working' or 'not working' at any one time would misrepresent their situation over a period. Not infrequently mothers seemed to have been neither totally committed to working or not working. Some said that requests from employers or offers from friends or relatives to look after the child(ren) had tipped the balance when they were uncertain. For others, strains, dissatisfactions or complications in child care arrangements had brought a spell at work to an end. The most common reason for stopping work again was the birth of another child. For all these reasons it is necessary to consider changes in mothers' work patterns over time rather than present a static picture.

Eight of the mothers had stopped work only briefly for the birth of their first child and then returned to work. The rest were asked how they had reacted to giving up work. Nearly all recognised both gains and losses but it is noteworthy that two thirds said they missed companionship. Well over half the mothers (thirty-eight, i.e. 60 per cent) had done some form of paid employment between the birth of the key child and his or her third birthday. Of these, twenty-four were still working at the time of interview (38 per cent). Fewer than half of those who had worked before the child was three said they had intended doing so at the time of birth. There was wide variation in the timing of the return to work, although the peak age was in the second half of the first year. Very few mothers had gone back to their previous job within the seven months post-natal period for which the Employment Protection Act was relevant (Daniel, 1981; Elias, 1980). Overall five main types of work sequence were identified. They are described in Table 6.2. This shows the importance of evening and night work particularly for working-class mothers. At the time of interview fewer than half of the mothers who worked did so outside the home in the daytime and so required an external carer. In addition, nearly half of the non-working mothers said they were interested in doing evening work but could not find a suitable job or were prevented from doing so by their husband's evening commitments.

Table 6.2 *Mothers' work sequences*

	Middle class	Working class	Total (N = 63)
1 Never done paid work since first child was born	15	5	20
2 Brief or locum work only	6	5	11
3 Worked between children but not subsequently	2	3	5
4 Regular work at home OR outside the home in the evenings, at nights, or at the weekend	5	10	15
5 Regular daytime work outside the home	5	7	12

Note: These groupings refer to work patterns *after* the birth of the first child in the family.

Rather more working-class than middle-class mothers had returned to work but more had stopped again too, so that the proportion of mothers working at the time of interview was similar in both classes (two fifths). Several working-class respondents who had previously been clerical workers had taken on lower status jobs (chiefly cleaning) so that their hours fitted with their child care commitments. By contrast, middle-class mothers normally considered only work of equivalent status when assessing whether to return to work or not. A few middle-class mothers had 'converted' leisure or voluntary activities into work by pursuing it in a more structured way for reward (e.g. keep fit teaching, sale of handicrafts).

Only four mothers were working full-time according to the usual definition of over thirty hours per week. It was therefore more helpful to distinguish fifteen mothers who were working 'short hours' (under twelve hours per week) from nine mothers who worked 'long hours' (more than twelve hours per week). The high proportion of mothers who worked short and/or un-social hours reveals how difficult it is for mothers to obtain a 'normal' work pattern which is compatible with their domestic responsibilities. For similar reasons half of the mothers worked in their local neighbourhood compared with only one in six fathers. Several mothers worked at home or alone and few of the others had significant contacts with colleagues outside work unlike most husbands.

There have been many studies which look at the reasons why mothers work. It is assumed that fathers do so because they are expected to. This study fitted with the general findings that mothers give a combination of explanations for working (Ginsberg, 1976; Moss, 1980; Siegel and Haas, 1965). Most working-class mothers stated that they returned to work mainly for financial reasons and/or to have more social contacts. Such factors were important for middle-class mothers too, but some also mentioned the inherent satisfactions of the job or career commitment.

In about half the families in which the mother had worked care of the child had been retained within the nuclear family while she did so. This is consistent with other research but runs counter to the common stereotype of the 'working mother'. A few middle-class mothers did things like typing or giving lessons at home so that there was no need to ask someone else to look after the children. A couple of working-class mothers were able to take their children with them on their cleaning jobs. The most frequent arrangement of all was for the father to look after the child. Over a quarter of all the families (eighteen) had used regular internal sharing at some time so that the mother was able to work. Nine were doing so at the time of interview, i.e. one in three of those with an employed mother. It was more common in working-class than middle-class families for fathers to care for the child while their wives worked. This was because fewer men in manual occupations had work commitments in the evenings and their wives were generally more willing or able to take on the kind of work available in the evening or at night. Nursing was an important source of such work for women in both classes however. Couples who preferred the wife to work whilst the husband was home explained that this had the advantages of maintaining responsibility for the children within the marriage and minimising changes in the child's routine. Therefore the mother was able to work without deviating much from the child care patterns or values of non-working mothers.

At the time of the interviews only twelve of the twenty-four working mothers shared care externally for this purpose. Most of these worked 'long hours'. Over the three years the main work carers had been grandparents, childminders and au pairs. Nearly one fifth of the total sample had used grandparent carers while mother worked at some time. The fact that women often work part-time or episodically meant that quite a few mothers and grandmothers had dovetailed their arrangements. Although friends and neighbours provided frequent, brief care for other reasons, there were very few instances of sharing care with them for mothers' work. This resulted from doubts about imposing and the difficulty of reciprocity.

One third of the children with a working mother (eight) were at group care while she was working. Six of these spent time before or after the group session with other carers because group care hours covered only part of the time that the mother worked. All but one of the mothers concerned had been working well before the child started at group care and had not been influenced to work by the prospect of using group care. Although a place at nursery school or playgroup had sometimes made mothers' work arrangements easier or cheaper, on the whole entry to group care occurred subsequent to and independently of mothers' return to work. Children went to group care at a similar age and for similar reasons whether they had 'protective' mothers, working mothers or high sharing non-working mothers.

Mothers who were not working in the daytime were asked what they saw as the advantages and disadvantages of doing so, in the same way that working mothers and fathers had been asked this in relation to their work. The majority of mothers at home (thirty-eight, i.e. 69 per cent) cited the child's happiness or security as a benefit. A similar proportion (two thirds) mentioned advantages to the mother from being home. The most important of these were the wish to be with the child and pleasure from observing details of the child's development. Some extolled the satisfactions of the housewife-mother role. Mrs Edwards said 'I enjoy doing the things you have to do at home, looking after children and doing the cooking and sewing.' Mrs Boyd felt 'privileged that one can be a full-time housewife'. There were fewer complaints than perceived benefits of being home but three quarters of the mothers did see disadvantages. Working-class mothers were more likely to complain about lack of company or loneliness whilst more middle-class mothers said they were bored or understimulated.

Just as 'working mothers' are often assumed to be an undifferentiated group so are non-working mothers but they also show significant variations. Comments about the disadvantages of being home were used to distinguish a group of mothers at home who acknowledged some form of boredom, loneliness or tension. Since they often recognised benefits from being at home too, these will be referred to as 'partly-dissatisfied' and the others as 'satisfied'. Both types of mother had similar levels of social contacts and comparable amounts of time spent alone with the child on average, so that their feelings of dissatisfaction could not be explained simply in terms of isolation. A significantly higher proportion of the satisfied mothers had shared care at least weekly, however.

Several writers have depicted employment as one way to reduce the strains of motherhood (Brown and Harris, 1978; Marsh, 1979; Mostow and Newberry, 1975). On the other hand, some surveys have discovered no differences in stress between groups of employed and non-employed mothers (Roberts and O'Keefe, 1981). It may be that relief of stress by employment applies particularly to single parents or those with several social problems but makes no differences for ordinary two parent families (Osborn, 1984). In the present study most of the mothers who mentioned a pressure or source of unhappiness did *not* work in the daytime ($p < 0.05$). Mothers' MI scores were not clearly related to hours of work, however.

Parents' domestic roles and social activities

We shall now look briefly at the extent of fathers' single-handed care of their children and compare the amounts of time children spent with their mothers and fathers. This will lead onto a discussion of how tasks, responsibilities and rights to be absent for social reasons were apportioned between husbands and wives. Most research has shown that even so-called highly participant fathers do relatively little primary caring of children compared with mothers (Lamb, 1976). It seems that even when both parents are at home most fathers spend less time with their children and take less direct responsibility for practical child care than their wives (Clarke-Stewart, 1980; Pedersen *et al.*, 1979). There is a fair amount of indirect evidence that fathers are now more involved with child care than in the past, as is illustrated by the recent upsurge in attendance at childbirth (Beail and McGuire, 1982; Parke, 1981; Pedersen, 1980). In this study, both the interviews and the diaries gave information about the frequency with which children were looked after by their fathers while the mothers were not there. About half of the fathers (twenty-nine) were said to care for the child alone at least once per week whilst thirteen (21 per cent) did so less often than once a month. According to the diary the mean number of sessions for which children were cared for by their fathers alone was approximately two out of forty-two. This compares with a mean of 6.5 sessions for group care attendance and of 2.5 for other types of external sharing. Most commonly fathers looked after their children on their own so that their wives could pursue an evening social activity or attend an evening class. Other important reasons were to allow mothers to shop, work, recover from night work or study. Fathers sometimes took their children out or played with them, partly because both would enjoy this but also in order to give the mother a break.

It has become a commonplace generalisation that marital roles tend to be more separate amongst working-class couples and overlap more in middle-class families (Aldous *et al.*, 1979;

Newson and Newson, 1970b). It was pointed out by Lee (1979) that this applies particularly to social activities and the contrast is by no means so clear cut for domestic tasks. This study bears out the importance of that distinction. It was not the case that middle-class fathers looked after their children more. To be sure, the working-class families did include a higher than average proportion of fathers who hardly ever looked after the child on their own but also a greater percentage who looked after the child for the longest and most frequent periods. This was either because their wives were working in the evenings or because they themselves did shift work and so were home when their wives wanted to go out in the daytime. The increase in part-time work by working-class mothers while their husbands are at home would appear to have been an important factor in modifying traditional marital segregation in relation to child care.

It is now three decades since Bott (1957) put forward her famous hypothesis that families with segregated conjugal roles are more likely to have close knit networks. She suggested that this pattern was typically working class, whilst most middle-class couples were thought to have less connected networks and greater jointness in marital roles. This supposition was subsequently tested and modified. It became apparent that role allocation varies from task to task and that network connectedness may differ with respect to kin and non-kin or males and females (Bott, 1971; Irving, 1977; Platt, 1969; Toomey, 1971; Turner, 1967). Although the details of Bott's original hypothesis have been shown to be oversimplified, it remains important to consider the interaction between a couple's inward and outward relationships. With regard to child care, the current sample revealed no statistical association between the frequency of internal and external sharing of care. This was because each of the four possible combinations of high or low rates of internal and external sharing were well represented. The diaries also showed a variety of patterns (Figure 6.1). Some couples said that they deliberately used care by the father to avoid external sharing but in other cases these two alternatives to mother's care were supplementary or complementary.

Care of children by mothers is the background against which

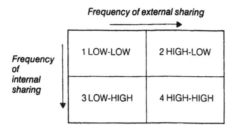

Types of family

A number of families showed each of the combinations shown in the figure and, of course, there were also some intermediate frequencies. The four standard types were well represented in the sample in the following ways:

1 *Low-Low* Both parents were home-centred. The children were rarely apart from the mother at all. The father was seldom away from the family except at work. Hence there was little need for either internal or external sharing.

2 *High-Low* The father did not look after the children on his own at all or only occasionally, either because of his heavy work commitments or traditional role expectations. However, the mother went out on her own a fair amount or worked. Then she shared care with people outside the nuclear family.

3 *Low-High* The family was reluctant or unable to use carers. There was a deliberate preference for the mother to go out or work at times when her husband was home.

4 *High-High* Very active families where the mother often shared care with relatives or local friends in the daytime. Both parents went out often separately and together in the evenings.

Figure 6.1 *The relationship between internal and external sharing*

the less common and more differentiated features of external sharing and sole care by fathers stand out. During the diary fortnight children on average spent three quarters of all the sessions with their mothers present. Over half the sessions away from mother were spent in group care so that the predominance of mother care would have been even greater before children started going there. There were seven mothers who had no break at all from their children's company apart from group care in the two weeks. All of these were working class. On average, fathers spent just over half as many sessions with the child as did the mothers (seventeen as opposed to thirty-one sessions), although more of that time was in the evenings when the child was asleep. Most of the fathers in 'protective' families were home with the child more than average. Curiously perhaps, there was no correspondence between the amount of time a father spent with his child and the extent of his sole care of the child.

A thorough analysis of marital role allocation was not possible since that was not the focus of the study. As an admittedly imperfect shorthand, parents' agreed statements about the husbands' contribution to several housework and child care tasks were rated and summed to form indices for comparison (Table 6.3). Scores on individual tasks conformed to the hierarchy of relative father involvement which has been found in other research (Herbst, 1960). Men tended to engage most in those activities which are more pleasurable (playing with the child) or more obvious (like washing up). They contributed least to the more long term or distasteful tasks such as washing clothes and cleaning. Contrary to some assumptions (Rapoport and Rapoport, 1982; Young and Willmott, 1973) quite a few fathers contributed very little to all the tasks assessed and they were as likely to be middle class as working class. Edgell (1980) and Pahl and Pahl (1971) likewise discovered marked segregation amongst certain kinds of middle-class couples. Even when fathers did housework it was sometimes as mothers' assistants or back up, rather than on their own initiative or in their own right. Thus, some mothers described their husbands as being good 'because he helps me'. Others talked of their husbands doing something 'for me' or 'when asked'. A few mothers had a clear sense that they did not want the man to be involved in their domain. Mrs Purdie* asserted 'I don't like to see men doing housework.' Several other women spoke proprietorily of it as 'my work'.

There were a number of evasive techniques employed by fathers to justify not doing certain things. These mechanisms were voluntarism, incompetence and distaste. Voluntarism meant that fathers felt entitled to exercise an option about whether to do something which for a mother would be obligatory. For example, Mr Munro* said he always bathed his daughter as 'it's a labour of love for me' but his wife did the ironing because he did not like doing it. Opting out was sometimes justified by the father's actual or assumed poor performance. Mr Villiers* confessed 'I never got (nappy changing) right – it would fall down, so I'd just leave him.'

Table 6.3 *Domestic role scores and maternal exclusiveness*

Family category	Description	Number in sample (N = 62)
A Exclusive Mothering Family	Low sharing care sequence and Low father's role score	12
B Intermediate Parenting Family	Medium sharing family OR Family where either the father or outside carers make important contributions but not both	34
C Inclusive Mothering Family	High sharing care sequence and High father's role score	16

Explanation of Categories

1 Low sharing = child apart from both parents only a few times a year in 2 out of first 3 years.
  High sharing = child apart from both parents weekly or more often in 2 out of first 3 years.
  Medium sharing = other frequencies of sharing care.
2 Father's contribution to several tasks (shopping; washing-up; washing clothes; cleaning the house; cooking; changing nappies; getting children ready for bed) was ranked according to both partners' agreed statements on a 5-point scale:

    1 Never
    2 Occasionally
    3 Sometimes
    4 As often as mother
    5 More often than mother.

The scores on all the tasks were added together to form the overall role score.

There might be collusion by partners which preserved the woman's sense of expertise. Mr Purdie* said 'She's moaning all the time I do (the cleaning) and then she does it again.' In relation to nappy changing some fathers felt able to excuse themselves out of distaste for the task, a choice not available to mothers some of whom found it similarly unpleasant. Here are quotations from two fathers who had messy jobs in garages but would not change a dirty nappy:

Mr Johnstone I've not got a very strong stomach. Wet ones, yes, but the other ones, no.
Mr Baxter* My stomach doesna take it.

By combining measures of sharing care and father's role scores it was possible to distinguish three types of family (Table 6.3). Terminology used by Holman (1980) in relation to foster parents has been borrowed to apply to the couple's apparent receptivity towards the performance of child care and domestic tasks by persons other than the mother. In particular, twelve 'exclusive' families were identified in which the mother seldom received relief from the husband or people outside. Six were middle class and six were working class. 'Exclusive' families tended not to have the typical care patterns of their class. For instance, children in exclusive middle-class families had rarely been looked after by non-relatives whilst those in working-class exclusive families had not had any overnight stays. Children from exclusive families had fewer friends and less frequent contacts with peers than average.

In most families, parents went out in the evenings more often separately than together. Twenty-five mothers and thirty-four fathers said they went out on their own once a week or more. This usually meant that one went out while the other was home with the children but some couples went out to different places at the same time. In contrast only eight couples said they went out jointly at least once a week, thereby requiring external sharing. Mothers who went out quite often alone also usually went out frequently with their husbands, but men's outside leisure time seemed to be more independent of joint activities. When only one partner went out weekly this was normally the husband. Twice as many working-class fathers (two thirds) as middle-class fathers went out alone each week for social reasons ($p < 0.01$). Over three quarters of middle-class couples went out together at least every six weeks, compared with fewer than half of the working-class families ($p < 0.02$). This is consonant with the higher rates of evening shared care for middle-class parents in this study. As a result it was mainly the women in working-class families who went out least often whether alone or as a couple. It appears that not only were mothers the main caregivers, but even at times when both parents were not working many men felt more free to pursue leisure activities while their wives looked after the children than vice versa. This is also reflected in the fact that most mothers' interests were solitary or else could be done with the family around. The main ones were reading, knitting, sewing and swimming. Far more of the fathers' leisure interests were based outside the home and so required someone else to look after the children, usually their mother. For instance Mrs Miller complained that 'Michael goes to karate on week-ends. The family priority is still mine. He can still do what he wants to, so it doesn't affect him so much.'

Furthermore making arrangements to share care was also mainly looked upon as the woman's responsibility. This occurred even at times when fathers were home too. Contacting a babysitter so that both could go out was typically done by the wife, except sometimes when the carer was the father's own mother, sister or brother. It is well known that communication amongst relatives tends in any case to be maintained by the females. Moreover, local friends who acted as carers were usually women who knew the mother much better than the father from daytime contacts. Some men assumed that it was up to their wives to arrange about the children, as they were the main beneficiaries. Mr Crawford said 'She has to get a babysitter, if she wants out', though he was referring to them both going out in the evening. Many fathers did take considerable interest in decisions about the best kind of group for their children and about what age they should start but normally the wife did the preparatory investigations and booked the place. The typical pattern was summed up like this:

Mrs Miller	Arranging nursery, that's me. We discuss it, but I do it.
Mr Balfour	Maureen did the research, and then it was talked over.

A small minority of the fathers had taken more initiative in arranging about group care, because they had relevant work contacts or because English was their wives' second language.

Parents' beliefs and values

In the introductory chapter it was stated that parents' choices and decisions about sharing care are not simply a product of the opportunities and limitations of their personal and social circumstances. These also depend on how they as individuals perceive and respond to relevant features of family life and of their particular environment. We have already seen that parents react differently to such 'objective' facts as having grandparents living close by or receiving offers to look after a child from elderly or teenage neighbours. It is time to examine parents' thinking more closely with special reference to their different understandings of the rights and responsibilities involved in parenthood and of children's needs and behaviour. The following analysis is largely based on themes which emerged during the general discussions which occurred within the interviews and from reading transcripts of the conversations later. This was supplemented by examination of spoken and written answers to standard questions (see Appendix).

Before describing what was said, it is useful to look briefly at how things were said. This can be just as revealing about the ways in which certain lines of thought either lead to different practices or are used to explain and justify actions after the event. In the social sciences much attention has been given to the measurement of attitudes and opinions by obtaining responses to specific questions on standardised scales. There has been comparatively little guidance about how to make sense of people's ideas as they present them more naturally in open conversation (Mostyn, 1985). Interpretive sociology has produced a number of terms like 'typifications', 'assumptive worlds', 'ideologies' (Giddens, 1976; Schwartz and Jacobs, 1979; Young and Mills, 1978). These rightly emphasise that our ideas are often implicit, generalised and taken for granted, but they were too global and imprecise for present purposes. Therefore, a framework was developed by classifying the ways in which parents expressed their ideas about sharing care with the help of some important distinctions made by several previous writers on the family. Backett (1977) suggested that people have images of children and of parenthood which guide and explain their behaviour. She recognised several different types of image according to their source and content. She called 'grounded images' those which are based on personal experience and 'abstract images' those which are developed from general knowledge diffused in society. From a somewhat different perspective, Stolz (1967) divided parents' statements about children and parental behaviour into three main types based on their form and function. Firstly, she distinguished beliefs from values. Then she divided beliefs into descriptive and instrumental types. An instrumental belief may be seen as a special kind of causal belief which expresses a relationship between *two* objects, persons or events, whilst descriptive beliefs are simply propositions about one thing or person. This corresponds with the contrasts noted by Fishbein and Raven (1967) between beliefs *in* the probability that something is the case and beliefs *about* the likelihood that two phenomena are associated in some way. The transcripts suggested two further categories depending on whether a causal belief explains something which has already happened or is happening; or whether it makes a prediction about a future event. The following fivefold classification combines these distinctions with examples concerning children from the present study:

Descriptive beliefs – these assign attributes to individuals, behaviour or events. They include images of children.

e.g. 'I think for his age, he is still on the clingy side.'
'Three year olds don't play with each other.'

Explanatory beliefs – causal associations in relation to past or present events or characteristics.

e.g. 'I think she takes after her father.'

Predictive beliefs – casual beliefs about what will or may happen in the future.

e.g. 'I think that once Yvonne settles down she
      will assert herself.'

Instrumental beliefs – these assert a relationship
between an action and a goal or value.

e.g. 'I wouldn't say she mixes too well, but I'm
      hoping nursery will bring that out of her.'
      'We thought nursery would calm him down a
      bit.'

Values – these ascribe (dis)approval or
(un)importance to individuals, behaviour, events
etc.

e.g. 'You shouldn't palm them off to someone else
      so that you can work. You should still be
      there for illnesses.'
      'I'd like them to get as much education as
      possible.'

Some beliefs were 'individualised' according to the kind of
person, time and/or context referred to. It must be emphasised
that many parents' ideas were expressed in relation to specific
situations and kinds of shared care. The same individual could
hold very different opinions about brief daytime care, work
care, group care or overnight care, for example. Other beliefs
were 'generalised' to cover all or most persons or situations.
A third distinct form consisted of 'comparative beliefs', which
noted similarities and dissimilarities between two individuals
or contexts. Comparative beliefs were most commonly made
about siblings, as would be expected. During the interviews
in families with more than one child the focus of conversation
frequently shifted from one child to another, comparing and
contrasting them. Occasionally parents were confused about
which child had done what. Quite often ideas were also shaped
by comparisons with cousins, friends' children or others at
group care. By this means parents framed explanations of
their own children's behaviour and sometimes developed more
generalised beliefs about 'all children' or 'every parent'.
Comparisons outside the family also served as standards to
judge one's own child by or as confirmations of one's own
actions. Some parents opposed to frequent sharing cited
instances of children they had seen made unhappy by it. In
contrast, those people who were more favourably disposed to

sharing care provided examples of children they knew who they thought had been made anxious and dependent by low sharing parents.

Although Rokeach (1973) regards values as just one type of belief, it seemed useful to maintain Stolz's distinction between matters of fact and of evaluation. The latter have frequently been divided into attitudes and values. Attitudes refer to specific dispositions towards some kind of thing or person whereas values denote broader moral orientations (Kluckhohn and Strodtbeck, 1961; Reich and Adcock, 1976; Warren and Jahoda, 1973). Important though this distinction may be, it did not emerge as very pertinent in the present study, so that the word value will be used to depict all 'concepts of the desirable' (Kohn, 1969:7) whether they are broad or narrow in scope. Like beliefs, values may be individualised, comparative or generalised. It is also possible to distinguish values which are ultimate in that they simply state an objective and those which are instrumental since they include the means of achieving the objective (Rokeach, 1973). All the parents supported ultimate values along the lines that children need loving care and should not be harmed. However, some thought that this inevitably entailed instrumental values, like loving care is only possible from the family, or that mothers should refrain from working in order that their children should not be harmed. Others disagreed and believed that there were alternative ways involving people outside the family which could achieve the same end.

On most issues there were a variety of opinions, sometimes even within the same family or individual. It is therefore important to understand how these relate to each other. Some were compatible, some conflicted. Here are a few of the ways in which they did so:

A Conforming ideas

1 **Combination** This is a set of beliefs and values which reinforce each other. Most couples gave a combination of reasons for using group care or for a mother to work.

2 **Ideology** This word has become much diluted in recent sociological writings but it seems best to retain the notion

that it comprises a *coherent* set of beliefs or values. Thus, ideas about children's needs and development could be seen to form an attachment ideology or a social exposure ideology.

3 **Specification** This gives the conditions under which a wider value operates. For instance, a value that carers should be competent becomes relevant to teenage carers only when there is a specifying belief that teenagers cannot look after children properly.

4 **Merged ideas** These describe expressions in which a value contains an implicit belief or vice versa. For example, the idea that neighbours should not be imposed on by asking them to look after your child implies the belief that the neighbours would see sharing care as an imposition. Many beliefs were implicitly evaluative, because it was taken for granted that the state of affairs referred to would be approved of or not. Especially common was the tendency to express values in the form of descriptive beliefs about what children need such as peer contact or constant parental care.

B Non-conforming ideas

1 **Differentiation** Many ideas were expressed by parents not as absolute rules but as conditional upon such factors as the child's age, the nature of a carer, the context of care, and the timing of care.

2 **Hierarchy** Where values are in conflict they may be ranked such that a higher order value takes precedence (cf. Rokeach's value system). Normally, the happiness of the child was seen to outrank the mother's wishes if they were incompatible. Father's work commitments were generally seen as paramount, but could be overriden by a child's urgent care needs.

3 **Neutralisation** Matza and Sykes (1961) introduced this term to further the understanding of delinquency but it would seem to have wider usefulness. It covers situations where one idea cancels out another or makes it inoperative. Matza (1964) pointed out that many norms have widely accepted exemptions. For instance, violence is

normally disapproved of but may be justified in self-defence. People who appear to deviate from the expected pattern of behaviour may appeal to such exemptions when accounting for their apparent non-conformity. Thus some people believed that neighbours should not normally be asked to look after a child but that could be neutralised by saying it was justified in an emergency. Neutralisation may be seen as part of a wider category of 'aligning actions'. Stokes and Hewitt (1976) defined these as mechanisms which smooth over inconsistencies between actual and ideal behaviour or between the views of two individuals.

4 **Contradictions**   An individual's ideas usually include some incompatibilities. These may be maintained by compartmentalising thought. The view that a mother working full-time cannot form a close bond with her child is widespread yet people commonly accept that most children are closely attached to their fathers who also work full-time. Mrs Christie argued strongly against using strangers as babysitters and against leaving an upset child at nursery school, yet in another part of the interview she indicated that her son Adam had been looked after by strangers and been distressed in a church creche which they continued to use.

5 **Disagreements**   These are differences of opinion between people. Within some of the couples in the study partners disagreed about such matters as the ideal frequency of shared care, about care by strangers or about when a child was ready to start going to nursery school.

Values about care of children

There seemed to be a number of important values used by nearly all the families, either to follow or to use as reference points when deviating from them. In our society there are two major responsibilities placed on parents of young children which have important implications for children's care and social relationships. Firstly, parents are expected to ensure adequate care and supervision of their children. There is an associated ideal of close attachment by young children to their parents. Secondly, there is a legal obligation for children to begin formal education at the age of five. Normally this means that a child has to be able to adapt successfully to a large, strange environment with an unknown supervisor and a large group of children. For most of the respondents these goals were reflected in two dominating values that children should have security in their family relationships yet should also develop the capacity for independent action. However, there were marked divergences of opinion about when and how the balance between these two aims should be achieved.

The parents were asked to complete the following sentence on one of the attitude forms they were given – 'What I feel most strongly about in relation to the care of young children is. . . .' The most frequently occurring words or phrases in the responses concerned two main dimensions:

1 love-affection-happiness
2 security-stability

Individual attention, understanding and stimulation were also mentioned quite frequently. The statements were sometimes ultimate values which simply declared what was desirable such as warmth or constancy but often they took the form of instrumental values specifying the centrality of close, warm relationships in the nuclear family (e.g. 'a stable home', 'loving parents'). In the interviews, there was also a common presumption that love and security could only be provided by parents looking after children virtually unaided. A few respondents did give the contrary opinion that it was possible for stable, loving care to be given by a combination of parents and other caregivers. Although a loving secure relationship in the family was the supreme value at this stage, most parents also agreed with a global statement that children should become independent of their parents. There is a potential tension between these two major values (love-security and independence) which was recognised by Erikson (1965) who depicted the contrasting tasks for children at this age as basic trust and autonomy. There are also parallels with sociological observations that there are expectations for family members to act together and be sensitive to each other's emotional needs, yet also to take responsibility for preparing children to cope with the more practical, individualistic values of the outside world (Busfield, 1974; Parsons and Bales, 1956).

On the whole there was a remarkable uniformity in the general values about care of children despite a wide range of sharing care practices. Partly this resulted from vagueness in the expressions which parents used. Furthermore, a fair degree of consensus was possible because parents' specifications of how they applied these values in practice involved contrasting instrumental and explanatory beliefs. For example, low sharers believed security came from almost exclusive care by the mother or parents, whilst high sharers sought security by careful selection of who looked after the children. Mrs Green said it was important that her daughters should have love, stability, fun and stimulation, but she thought this could be provided by a combination of herself, her husband, the au pair and several local friends. It did not require the constant maternal presence which she correctly believed many other mothers regard as desirable. There were also differences of emphasis and timing. Some thought that a long period of security with minimal shared care should precede attempts to encourage independence. Others considered that early sharing with trusted carers could help a child gain more independence at the same time as ensuring a sense of security. They could both be aimed for concurrently. Sometimes, shared care was deliberately arranged with this purpose in mind. Both Mrs Urquhart* and Mrs Inglis concluded when their children were in their second year that they had been unwittingly encouraging their sons to be too dependent, so they began to leave them more with others in order that they would get used to operating without a parent around. Mrs Reid and Mr Crawford had also tried to develop their children's self-confidence, but with less success. Mr Sadler* said 'We try to bring her out of herself, we talk to her and that, but (it doesn't work).' These last remarks indicate a lack of effective instrumental beliefs to achieve the aim of greater independence. Of course children can be helped towards independence in ways other than sharing care. There were some parents who did not share care much but involved the children in many activities and gave them plenty of opportunities to mix with others.

Ideas about parenthood and family life

Evidently, issues of child care are intimately linked to expectations about the nature and implications of being a parent. In many societies, responsibilities for children are distributed within a wider kin structure but in the West they are largely vested in parents alone. Therefore, shared care patterns tend to be judged according to values about what kind of delegation are thought to be compatible with the proper exercise of parental responsibility. Many of the families in Milburn and Whitlaw adhered to a view that parenthood and especially motherhood should involve almost total care of the child. 'Protective' parents and even some medium and high sharers thought that more than minimal sharing (based on their particular idea of a minimum) contradicted the nature of parenthood itself. Mrs Ormiston* expressed that as follows: 'I have this thing, that they are my children and basically I ought to look after them. It has to be something special for me to hand over that responsibility.' The identification of parental responsibility with near-total care was particularly incorporated in disapproval of families who shared care for the mother to work. Sometimes mothers' wishes simply to have a 'break' from children were viewed negatively, too. Many comments were not confined to the speaker's own situation but were generalised to others by means of references to 'they', 'you' or 'people', as in the following quotations:

Mrs Elliott If people want to follow a career, then they shouldn't have children.

Mrs Booth (explaining why she did not take part in weekly swops) I reckon you've got them, so you look after them.

Parenthood was seen as voluntary, with predictable care obligations which ought to be accepted – at least by women, as we shall see in a moment. Mrs Robertson* explained why she hardly ever went out since having children: 'Well, if you plan children, it's your responsibility. They are not forced on you – not nowadays, anyway. So, if you want them, it's up to you to look after them.'

It was noteworthy that many of the statements about

responsibility referred to parents rather than mothers, even though in practical terms it was the mothers who looked after the children for most of the time so that *maternal* responsibility would have been a more accurate term. Thereby the differing implications for men and women were disguised. The use of joint terms like 'we', 'both of us' or 'a parent' served a similar purpose. Examples included 'at least one parent should be available when illnesses and problems occur' (Mrs Raeburn) and 'It is necessary for one or other parent to be there when children are not at school' (Mr Morrison). Explaining why Shona was rarely looked after by others in the daytime, Mr Nairn* said 'It's our responsibility, so we should look after them.' Mr Preston* was very hostile to the possibility of his wife working in the daytime. He said '*I'd* not want to be a week-end parent' although his contact with the children would have been unaffected.

Some respondents did talk about the particular duty of mothers to provide most of a child's care but this chiefly occurred in individualised expressions unlike the generalised values about parents just discussed. Mrs Morrison linked such personal feelings to childbearing: 'I feel it's my duty. I brought them into the world. ( ) You make up your mind that you're going to have children and you look after them.' For some mothers constant availability became less important once a child was attending a pre-school group or school itself but others believed it was still essential to be home in case of illness or to prepare for the child's homecoming. Mrs Preston* stated: 'A mother's place is in the home. Even now he's at nursery, I still need to be here, in case I'm needed.' Associated with such values was the implicit idea that overall care responsibility for the child has to stay with one person, except when neutralised by clear gains for the child, as in group care. Several parents felt that children needed a 'single constant focus' (in Mrs Jackson's words). There could be disagreements about this. Unlike his wife, Mr Jackson had doubts about the benefits to children of having what he called 'a totally dominant mother-figure'.

Most high sharing couples did not feel they were abrogating parental responsibilities, although some thought that their own parents, friends or colleagues held this view. Mothers who did share care comparatively often had two main ways of neutralising the norm of maternal responsibility which none of them could ignore even if they disagreed with it. The first method was to cite justifications. According to Scott and Lyman (1968: 47) these are 'accounts in which one accepts responsibility for the action in question, but denies the pejorative quality associated with it'. The common assumption that children are harmed by more than minimal separations from their mothers was refuted. Instead parents pointed to advantages for the child such as greater confidence, learning from others and more variety of experience. A second and stronger neutralisation took the form of 'counter-claims' that parents and mothers have rights as well as responsibilities and these include independent interests away from the child. Mrs Carlisle argued vigorously that she was entitled to breaks from the children. For her a major benefit of group care 'was to get a bit of *personal space*, which if you are making a record put in triple underline'. Indeed sharing care was sometimes described as improving and not contradicting parenthood. As Mrs Sim* declared 'It makes us better parents when you have a bit of free time to yourself.' She and others believed that children benefit indirectly from improvements in their mother's morale.

Even though parental responsibility was mostly applied in practice to mothers, there were also implications for fathers. As some fathers specifically stated, the idea of joint responsibility meant that they exercised this in relation to the child's general upbringing rather than actual care. The father's right or duty to work and the mother's major duty to provide care was hardly questioned. This issue of the division of labour with regard to tasks inside and outside the family has become of major importance in public discussions in recent years. Certainly a good many mothers did feel that fathers should do more at home and that women's rights should be given more public recognition. On the other hand, only three mothers expressed interest in their husbands' modifying their work patterns in a major way in order to share care more equally. Some mothers evinced strong animosity towards what Mrs Davies disparagingly called 'these libbers' (i.e. supporters of women's liberation).

Nonetheless, most families did clearly feel a limited form of interchangeability in that fathers were just as acceptable to look after the children as the mother although in practice they did so for much less of the time. Sometimes parents' spontaneous comments emphasised family togetherness and joint activities. Fathers' absences at work could be compensated for by a strong concern to do things together in the evenings and week-ends, either very deliberately or as a matter of course. Mr Ferguson* said 'We tend to do things as a family, like going to the baths, playing badminton – things that the children can do along with us.' Mr Irvine said that he had hardly ever gone out in the evenings or week-ends except with the children, because 'we believed that the parents' place was in the home and not to palm her off to someone else'.

Backett (1982) showed how middle-class mothers tempered their ideas about responsibility towards their children with the knowledge that this would be a relatively brief part of the life-cycle. In this study, parents of both classes expressed this idea. There might be stresses and sacrifices but these would soon be over. With regard to staying home until her children started school, Mrs Whigham* said 'Five years of your life is not a lot to sacrifice.' Mrs Robertson* described how restricted her social life was, then added: 'And then your kids will be grown up soon. You'll be getting out when they are grown up. So it's only for a short time of your life really.' In contrast, others definitely regretted the brevity of the child-rearing period. These beliefs were mainly expressed by low sharers and those who preferred their child to stay for short hours at a playgroup. When the child started at group care, some of these mothers felt a sense of mourning the end of the child's dependence. The children had provided company, a sense of purpose and time-structuring. For instance:

Mrs Kerr	I felt slight withdrawal symptoms the first week he was there and sort of thought – Goodness me, what's going to be my role in life now?
Mrs Hardie	It was a wrench when he went. It was pointed out to me that he wasn't a baby

any more. ( ) I was a bit annoyed that he
didn't mind me not being there.

In consequence children's moves towards independence might
be experienced as a personal loss:

Mrs Vallance* Once they are at nursery, you tend to lose
them a good bit, anyway.

Mrs Laurie Once they are at school, you've lost them
to the teachers.

Attitudes and beliefs about working mothers

Ideas about parental responsibility were intimately linked
with attitudes towards working mothers. It was often assumed
that mothers' work required non-parental care on a scale
which was bad for children. Many people made generalised
assertions about working mothers as if they all worked full-
time, probably using a childminder or day nursery. In fact,
this image applies to only a small minority of mothers who
have worked, both in this sample and more generally (Fonda
and Moss, 1976). Only slightly fewer mothers than fathers
approved of daytime working and many women expressed
great hostility to the idea. The majority of mothers and fathers
agreed with a statement that it harms children if both parents
work full-time, although twice as many mothers as fathers
disagreed or had mixed feelings. Parents usually invoked the
needs of the child in arguing against working mothers. Mrs
Laurie asked rhetorically 'What affection is (the child) going
to get? (The mothers) are not really going to know the child.
To me, that's cruel.' Mr Davies thought that 'being a parent
is a career in itself. And the children need you most when
they are young. And going out to work involves dereliction of
your duty.' Despite the ambiguous references to 'parent' and
'you', this was meant to apply to mothers only.

In practice a much less negative picture emerged from the
replies of mothers who were actually working about the effects
of this on their children. Only one reported that her child was
adversely affected. Eleven said there had been no significant
effect and twelve thought the child benefited. Mothers who

worked in the evening or at week-ends while their husbands were home were pleased to see their children become closer to their fathers. For instance Mrs Brown* considered that 'they've got to know their Dad much more, because he's the only one here on Sunday'. People who used carers outside the family whilst both parents worked had observed benefits similar to those noted by Mrs Green above or Mrs Hunter in chapter 2. They thought the child had gained in independence and had received extra love or stimulation from an additional person.

There were several neutralisations which even respondents who expressed disapproval admitted could sometimes justify mothers' work. These included:

1 Financial necessity
2 Single parenthood
3 Taking advantage of child care arrangements established for other reasons (normally this meant group care or times when the father was home)
4 Short working hours or brief work episodes

Several husbands whose wives were working emphasised that they did so only because of the extra money. The men often held traditional attitudes in other ways so it might have been thought that they would not offer a financial explanation because this could be seen as diminishing their position as breadwinners. Probably this kind of explanation appealed because it implies that deviating from the norm of maternal care is involuntary. Were it not for the 'necessity' for extra cash the family would conform to the ideal. Besides, to admit that a wife's motivation to work is mainly personal or social undermines the cherished notion that full-time motherhood provides its own adequate rewards. Some wives disagreed with this financial version of the reasons for their working. They asserted that company, interest in the job or getting away from home were more important factors for them.

Values about sharing care

In chapter 3 some of the immediate reasons for sharing care were listed. In this section I shall indicate some of the more general beliefs and values which underlay parents' varying dispositions to share care. Of utmost importance were ways in which parents categorised situations and people as desirable/undesirable or as safe/risky for the care of children. Understandably parents were concerned to adhere to a generalised value that children should not be harmed by care arrangements but they varied in their specifying beliefs about what kinds of care would harm a child. Some parents saw frequent sharing even among relatives and friends as detrimental to children whereas others might think it helped children's confidence. Mrs Christie held a generalised belief that it was always harmful for mothers to work but her husband qualified that it depended on the family circumstances and the particular care arrangement.

Concern about possible harm to children from shared care meant that there was a strong 'child primacy' value, which meant that sharing care should only occur when it was 'necessary' or for the benefit of the child. Otherwise, it would be seen as selfish. There was disapproval of those who shared care 'just to get time to themselves' (Mrs Arnot). Even high sharing parents might say they 'had to' or 'needed to' leave the child in order to pursue an activity which others would have seen as voluntary and avoidable. 'Protective' families tended to justify instances of shared care by emphasising that they were exceptional. The child primacy value acted as a restraint on mothers' sense of entitlement to time for themselves. Mrs Gunn remarked that Jackie's playgroup hours were short: 'It isn't very long, if you want to do something. But I think it's probably long enough for the child, and it is the child you really must consider, not the parent. . . .' Those mothers who did not acknowledge their own rights to share care would only feel entitled to do things without the child when the child was already being looked after by someone else partially or wholly for a 'good reason'. Similarly, some mothers felt they could work or have a break only when their husbands would be looking after the child anyway or after the child had started at group care for his or her own benefit. Mrs Ormiston* had a job waiting for her but felt she could not start until her son was at nursery school, so that her parents and sister would not think she had sent him there in order to work. A related norm expressed by a fair number of respondents was that nursery schools should not be used 'as a babysitting service' for mothers to work. This would offend the 'rule' that care arrangements should be for the child's sake.

Whether a particular form of shared care was seen as in breach of the child primacy principle or not affected how the arrangement was described. There were a small number of neutral terms employed by parents to describe sharing care. They spoke of 'leaving children' or of children 'staying with' other people. In both classes, carers were said to 'look after' children, but working-class parents often used the word 'watch' instead. Forms of the verb babysit were common, mostly but not always to describe evening care. In some circles the word 'sit' had acquired new grammatical forms and meanings. Thus, someone could 'do a sit', 'sit for' somebody, or 'be sat for'. There were long sits, short sits, late sits and last minute sits. These terms appeared to reflect a perception of sharing care in a circle as a separate formal function in contrast to care by friends and relatives which is rooted in everyday interaction.

Besides this neutral terminology which described sharing care done by oneself or in an approved manner by someone else, many respondents used more pejorative words and phrases. These usually expressed disfavour towards some other people's pattern of sharing care. These expressions will be called 'rejection labels' because they impute inconsiderateness towards the child and evasion of parental responsibility. Such labels were mostly directed against mothers not fathers. They designated the boundaries of legitimate kinds of shared care and thereby expressed a pressure to conformity. A search through the interview transcripts revealed that well over half of the families had used rejection labels. By far the most common was some form of the word 'dump'. There were at least twenty examples of this, as in 'she's not dumped on different people' (Mrs Green) and 'I'd rather struggle for the benefit of every one than dump them as soon as I've had them' (Mrs Henderson). Other rejection labels were 'palm off', 'get rid of', 'farm out' and variations to do with children being 'pushed', 'shunted' or 'shoved' out, around or away. These all contained a suggestion of children being treated like an animal or inanimate object. It was implied that the parents who 'dumped' or 'palmed off' children were abruptly dispensing

with them in some kind of care vacuum, rather than respon-
sibly making a care arrangement with another person who
had a positive contribution to make. It is likely that children
are aware of the widespread use of rejection labels. They may
internalise the underlying attitudes and so perceive some
forms of shared care as rejecting which they might not do if
sharing care was more generally approved of.

Rejection labels were used equally in both classes, and by
mothers and fathers. Commonly but not invariably they
referred to working mothers or the use of childminders or day
nurseries. Mrs Christie described her weekly swop as 'having
a break', but referred to working mothers as 'dumping' their
children. In fact, the implication of remarks like this that
working mothers did not care about their children was far
from accurate. Working mothers shared the common value
that children should not be harmed by care, although they
held more individualised beliefs that the effects of shared care
depended on the particular arrangements. For them frequent
shared care took place not in spite of harm to the child but on
condition that there was no harm to the child. Talking about
her work, Mrs Quinn* said 'He's never bothered, because if
there had been any trouble I obviously wouldn't have left him.'
Sometimes a label was applied with respect to parents who
used group care in ways or for reasons which differed from
the speaker's. Other people (though never the speaker) were
described as using nursery schools 'as a dumping ground' or
'just to get them off their hands'. On the other hand labels
occasionally expressed acknowledgment that parenting may
legitimately contain feelings of wishing to be apart from a
child. Mrs Miller said 'It doesn't matter how doting a parent
you are, it's nice to get rid of them (now and then).'

Of course, there were many parents who did not see frequent
or extended shared care as negative. Mrs Edwards said in
relation to regular swop care 'I don't think it does them any
harm being left.' Quite a few parents thought that fairly
frequent shared care helped the child by giving them extra
attention and stimulation, assisting their development or independence, or simply giving them additional company and fun.
It could also be seen as preparing children for later or unexpected separations, as at group care or in hospital. Some

mothers also emphasised that it made the mother-child relationship less intense and enhanced mutual pleasure after reunion.

Whilst rejection labelling reflected a normative concern to restrict the extent of shared care, there were also negative connotations ascribed to the opposite extreme of 'overprotectiveness'. Here are some examples:

Mrs Laurie   I think I'm, well, overprotective.
Mrs Taylor*   Doesn't it sound awful – sheltering him.
Mr Finlayson I don't wish to sound overprotective, I
                            know they are very resilient.

Whereas rejection labels were normally directed at other people, these phrases occurred mainly in the form of apologies or denials about oneself. They seemed to represent an indulgent disapproval which contrasted with the vehemence towards others which sometimes accompanied rejection labels. A few mothers felt somewhat defensive that their concern to be with the child as much as possible was 'old-fashioned'. Others regarded it as a widespread attitude. For instance, Mrs Booth said 'I suppose I always had a fear I mollycoddled him, but I'm sure every mother thinks the same.'

As there is a widespread belief that to share care of children more than a minimum is not good for children, the enterprise is imbued with uncertainty. Therefore it was usually important that only trusted persons should be allowed to look after the children. However, the criteria for trust varied considerably. Earlier we saw that the main elements of trust were competence, reassurance, reliability and conformity. Trust was partly related to individual's personal qualities, but also to more generalised descriptive beliefs about different categories of people. Parents set boundaries of trust at differing social distances. Most people took for granted the trustworthiness of close relatives unless there had been a particular interpersonal problem or there were difficulties due to ill health. Some set a firm boundary of trust around the (extended) family and would hardly ever share care with others. These were mostly working class. A much higher proportion of middle-class families, although by no means all, extended their boundaries of trust more widely to include non-relatives and even people whom they did not know well before-hand. However, willingness to use previously unfamiliar people as carers did not mean a lack of discrimination about the carer's qualities. Usually there was felt to be some kind of guarantee of trust from official approval (group care, child-minders), contractual employment (au pairs) or access procedures (babysitting circles).

Trust was usually a necessary but not a sufficient condition for sharing care with someone. Trusted people might be used not at all or less often than desired out of concern that care of the child might be burdensome. For instance, Mrs Booth said 'I'd take the children with me, and sort of lumber them, you know. It's me, I don't like using people.' Conversely, a person of uncertain trust might be used because of their clear willing-ness to be 'imposed on' (e.g. childminders, au pairs). The possi-bility of imposing introduced another form of uncertainty, which concerned the reaction of the carer rather than that of the child. Fear of imposing was also connected with a concern about family autonomy. Parents' sense of indebtedness to those who shared care for them could make them feel that carers had a reciprocal claim on them. Hence the avoidance of imposition protected parents as well as carers from unwelcome feelings.

Like their grounds for trust, parents' fears about imposing upon people comprised several elements. These included taking up their time, distracting them from other commit-ments and giving them the physical demands of child care. Mrs Balfour would not leave her son with friends if she thought it interfered with what they would otherwise be doing but she did share care with them when she felt it fitted in with their existing arrangements. Even if someone took the initiative in offering to act as a carer, parents sometimes suspected that really they did not want to be imposed on much or even at all. Mrs Ormiston* remarked that her best friend 'only asks, because she knows I won't take her up on it'.

As in the case of trust, the location of boundaries of impo-sition varied considerably from individual to individual. So did factors which might soothe worries about imposing. One of the advantages of group care for nearly everyone was that it was not seen as involving interpersonal impositions and had clear cut obligations. Otherwise there were two main ways in which uncertainty about imposing was neutralised. These were kinship and reciprocity. Some couples did not like sharing care much even with close relatives because imposing was thought to begin outside the nuclear family. Most extended their boundary of imposition to include grandparents and perhaps aunts and uncles because they were seen as enjoying the experience for its own sake. For many working-class families in particular, the boundaries of imposition like those of trust were drawn tightly around close relatives. The crucial importance of grandparents was very much strengthened by the fact that they combined high levels of both trust and imposability.

Many people were reluctant to impose on friends or neighbours. Those who did so mainly felt free to do this when there were opportunities to reciprocate by looking after the carer's child in return. Several parents were reluctant to accept offers to share care from non-relatives with no young children because they felt this was a 'favour' which they could not return. The imbalance of exchange evoked feelings of indebtedness which parents preferred to avoid. In addition neighbours were likely to be less well known to the parents than kin, so there was more doubt about how genuine was their willingness to be imposed on. As regards 'local people' with young children, ideas about imposition were linked to class. Most middle-class parents readily accepted that sharing care was a 'natural' response to a mutual need by parents for carers and a mutual advantage to children of playmates. Working-class parents were more likely to define this situation more problematically as one of potential intrusion or obligation.

Besides kinship and reciprocity, imposition could be neutralised by exceptional circumstances. Mrs Villiers* and Mrs Laurie had seldom shared care, and always with close relatives, but they both felt able to call on a neighbour they did not know very well when they had to go to hospital unexpectedly. Conversely, feelings of imposition might be intensified if the carer was more vulnerable (e.g. elderly, unwell) or if the care demands were greater than normal (e.g. more than one child, a difficult child, a long period). Carers were perceived as having different satiation levels of preparedness to look after someone else's children. This sometimes affected choice within a child's carer set on a particular occasion. Sometimes secondary carers were approached when a main carer was seen to have reached their current limit. Several middle-class parents thought that a major benefit of a street network was that imposition could be spread amongst several people. On the other hand, kin carers usually had higher individual satiation levels than non-kin so there was less need to call on other carers.

Two other important matters emphasised by many parents were consistency for children and the opportunity for gradual adaptation to change. For this reason, new carers were usually recruited from those already familiar to the child. Often the absence of the mother might be the only alteration in a setting which the child had experienced previously many times. If the carer or place of care were unfamiliar, mothers usually went to considerable trouble to help the child become familiar with them before the child was left. For the majority of parents continuity had to be provided essentially by parents, with occasional interruptions. But for working mothers it could be just as important that the child had a reliable and familiar substitute care arrangement. This was seen by Mrs Green as a major advantage of using an au pair rather than friends or childminders. Although some parents preferred two or three changes of group care and then school others valued the continuity of environment provided by a nursery class attached to the school the child would go to. Mr and Mrs Tervit* found Yvonne's nursery class unsatisfactory but placed her there because she would be going to the attached school when she was five. The desire for continuity could mean that too many changes at once were seen as undesirable for a child. Several parents pointed to the problems for children of having to adapt to group care at the same time as either the new arrival of a younger sibling or the departure of an older sibling to start school.

Sometimes continuity of peer relationships was thought to be important. Thus parents chose a playgroup or nursery school partly because their child knew others who were going there. Some chose a group where it was expected that friendships could develop with other children who would later go to the same nearby school. By contrast, both Mrs Johnstone and

Mrs Kerr said that this did not matter. They believed children's friendships are superficial and readily changed. Two other mothers commented that continuity in the child's relationships reassured parents more than it affected the child. There is some empirical support for the transience of early friendships although the involuntary ending of a friendship can be sad even for a pre-school child (Dickens and Perlman, 1981; Rubin, 1980).

A linked concept to that of continuity (minimising change) was that of gradualness (extended opportunity to get used to change). Mr Buchan thought it was essential for children to be gradually familiarised with the practice of staying with people they knew well. This idea seemed to be especially prominent among middle-class families, whose statements and care practices indicated a preference for several graduated steps of frequency, group size and formality. Thus, occasional sharing would build up to regular swops and then mini-groups or multiple swops, which were themselves partly intended as preparations for group care and school. Parents believed that such successions of care arrangements helped children adjust to progressively more structured settings. Some parents were undecided about their plans for the child at four, because they were unsure whether continuity of placement should prevail or whether a move to a more formal setting would help in gradual preparation for school. Combined centres might help resolve this dilemma.

Previous research has shown that issues of control and discipline are very important to parents (Kohn, 1963; Stolz, 1967). Surprisingly perhaps, this was not prominent in most parents' discussion of shared care. Some did express concern about carers spoiling or being unable to handle the children. This applied especially to grandparents and teenagers. It is probably a sign of how careful most parents are about sharing care that it was very rare indeed for anyone to refer to ill-treatment of their child by a carer.

Influences on parents' sharing care attitudes and practices

Parents were specifically asked how their own childhood had influenced their views about sharing care. It was much more common for parents of both classes to feel influenced in the direction of following their own upbringing than to react against it. This conforms with empirical findings of a considerable degree of continuity in major values from one generation to the next (Hill *et al.*, 1970). Most parents felt influenced towards family closeness and restrictiveness in relation to care frequency and choice of carers. Fewer than one quarter of the parents thought that their childhood had swayed them in favour of involving other people in the care of their children or fostering greater independence for children. By far the most common references were to the closeness of their family of origin which parents wanted to reproduce. Nearly half of the working-class parents made almost identically worded remarks to the effect that 'My mum was always there' or 'We were never left.' Mrs Ritchie* expressed a typical explanatory belief: 'Your Mum and Dad was always there – you feel that you should always be there.' On the other hand, several mothers who worked in the daytime said they had been affected by the example or encouragement of their parents away from a conventional housewife role.

Some parents did differ from or even react against their own early experience. Mrs Nichols*, who had used childminders and paid stranger babysitters, described how 'My mum always says she never had a babysitter – she didna believe in babysitters.' A small number of parents felt that their own upbringing in a close-knit nuclear family with minimal shared care or social contacts had inhibited their self-confidence and personal development. They wanted their own children to have wider and more independent experiences. Conversely, quite a few parents cited negative experiences in their own past which they said had led them to circumspection about sharing the care of their own children. Several respondents said they had suffered from a breakdown in their parents' marriage or from their mothers working which meant they were all the more determined that their own family should be close.

Parents were not specifically asked about how they had adjusted on entry to school, but during the questioning about the growth of pre-school provision fourteen different parents spontaneously recalled that they had been very unhappy when they first started school. It would seem that a generation ago when there were far fewer pre-school groups the transition from home to school was often painful and became seared on the memories of many. Nearly all who had suffered in this way thought their children would avoid this by attending group care.

Respondents were asked to say what apart from their upbringing had influenced their attitudes about sharing care (Table 6.4). The most frequent replies concerned the direct experience of their own children. This replicates Backett's findings (1980) that parenting is seen to be learnt largely through trial and error. On the other hand external influences were important too: many respondents said they had gained from watching and talking to their friends, brothers and sisters who had children. Finally quite a few people had been affected by their training and work. These were nearly all middle class.

Table 6.4 *Influences on attitudes to sharing care*

	Parents' report of main influence on their attitude apart *from their own upbringing*	
	Mothers	*Fathers*
Work/training	15	6
Experience with own children	14	15
Other parents	14	10
Books	5	0
Media	3	1
Money/environment	3	4
General education	2	2
General life experience	2	0
Spouse	1	6
No comment/unable to say/other	(1)	(10)

This chapter has concentrated on the parents' role in sharing care. It is time for the children themselves to come to the fore.

7 *Parents' perceptions of children, children's characteristics and shared care*

Care patterns and processes are affected by the way adults perceive and react towards both the general characteristics of children and a particular child's individual nature. We shall consider first the main kinds of ideas used by parents to organise their thinking about children in relation to shared care. Then we shall discuss some specific attributes which children have. A child's sex and birth order provide a natural bridge between these two types of information for they constitute objective 'facts' about the child but were also major elements in parents' interpretations of children's behaviour.

Images of children

Bringing up children in general and sharing care in particular depend on judgments which parents made about what their children are thinking or feeling in a given situation or about how they might react to a possible situation. Many parents acknowledged that children's internal processes can be difficult to discern. Typical comments were:

> I don't know how kids of that age perceive.
> You never know with a fourteen-month-old – they can't tell you.
> It's difficult to know how aware he was.

Mrs Clark delayed sending her older son to nursery school because she was unsure how he would react to leaving his mother at home with the new baby: 'He was very jealous of Alexander and I wouldn't have liked him to have gone – not really knowing how their minds work. And maybe brooding on the fact that Alexander was at home.' It may be hard to choose between several competing explanations of children's nature or behaviour. Mrs Buchan said of Eleanor's crying when she stayed with a friend: 'It's quite difficult to know whether it was just a way of getting attention or whether she was feeling a genuine sense of loss or whether it's a moment of boredom.'

Especially before children reach the age of two, parents receive much less verbal information to assist them in working out what is going on in a child's mind than is true for adults and older children. They rely heavily on their intimate non-verbal knowledge of the children. This can lead to false predictions about how they will respond to separations from their parents. Referring to two periods when his wife was in hospital, Mr Balfour said 'On neither occasion was he as bothered about it as we thought he might have been.' There may also be a temptation to project one's own feelings. Elizabeth Johnstone had spent two days with an aunt she hardly knew when she was about fifteen months. Her mother said of their reunion: 'To me she was happy to see us, but whether it was just my imagination or me wanting her to feel that way?' Parents may go a step further and substitute their own interpretation for the child's. For instance, Mrs Buchan described Eleanor's separation crying as 'quite an act on her part'.

Since it is hard to know accurately what a young child thinks or means, it is tempting to draw on a supply of common-sense explanations of children's behaviour to supplement one's own intuitions. These help reduce uncertainty about what is the best way to deal with a child. In addition parents in this sample had developed explanatory beliefs from reflecting on the ways a single child changes from time to time and context to context and from comparing the actions of brothers, sisters and other children. These two methods are less systematic versions of the ways in which psychologists also develop and test hypotheses about children's behaviour. Parents realised that children can be very different depending on the context. Several commented that their child was reserved with other people, but talkative or boisterous at home – 'Jekyll and Hyde' as Mr Sadler* depicted his daughter. Pauline Purdie's* parents had regarded her as a gregarious child because of her engaging manner with relatives and close friends. Once she started nursery school, however, they had to revise their image of her because she was very withdrawn in that unfamiliar context. Parents were well aware of the many differences between individual children but they also held generalised beliefs which applied to all children. The main ones relevant to shared care involved children's degree of rewardingness to the parent(s), their emotional make-up and their cognitive or social qualities.

Some parents expressed the view that children were so valuable or rewarding that the need to share care should hardly ever arise. Mrs Davies described children as a 'precious gift' to parents, whose care was therefore not to be lightly transferred to anyone else. Mr and Mrs Munro* had their only child unexpectedly late in life and felt she was too special to them to consider letting her stay with neighbours who had offered to babysit. Sometimes children became almost inseparable companions for their mothers. Mrs Laurie described how 'I feel so lost when I'm on my own, I feel as if I should be looking round for my wee one'.

Different parents held quite contrasting views about children's emotional resilience. Ideas also changed. For instance a generalised image based on a first child's characteristics was modified into a comparative one when a second or later child turned out to be markedly different in adaptability. Some parents, especially those who stressed the importance of security for children within the nuclear family, had images of young children which emphasised their immaturity and vulnerability. To some a three-year-old was 'just a wee baby' (Mrs Robertson*). Mrs Traynor* said 'I don't think they are ready for nursery before they are three, because let's face it they are still babies even at three.' Others gave greater recognition to children's adaptive capacities. Then the child care value of independence was more likely to be stressed. Several parents thought that children were fairly unconcerned by changes in carers and environment or even that they positively enjoyed them. Normally, it was couples who shared care frequently and had large carer sets who regarded their children as being resilient. But it could be that a perception of the child as adaptable meant that the child would be taken along to places like the dentist's or busy shops, whereas parents with a view of the child as more delicate might prefer to share care so as not to expose the child to such places. The degree of fit between what parents expect and the nature of the child can be crucial (Thomas and Chess, 1977). Those children who adapted contentedly to the care arrangements made for them seemed unproblematic to their parents. Difficulties arose chiefly when children resisted early attempts to share care or when babies with little experience of shared care became unacceptably clinging later.

As important as parents' general notions about children's adaptability were the ways in which they interpreted and dealt with particular separation reactions. Nearly all the parents showed great sensitivity to possible ill-effects of shared care on their children. Usually arrangements were prepared for well in advance and adjusted subsequently in order to minimise the chance that the children would be upset. Of course, children were often happy or even enthusiastic to stay with a familiar person. When the carer was less well known some parents perceived their children as having a strong curiosity and attraction to novelty. Even so, many children had at some time cried or been otherwise upset at the prospect or actuality of parental separation. Psychologists have observed that individual children possess contrasting propensities to cry from an early age (Dunn, 1977; Korner, 1974) and this was evident to parents, too. Mrs Henderson had looked after babies 'who didn't know me and they didn't mind in the least'. Yet when she left her own son with his grandmother or a close friend for brief periods so that she could go to study at the library 'he would literally scream all the time',

It has also been demonstrated that crying in protest at the short term departure of familiar adults is different from and largely unrelated to the less consolable distress which follows prolonged separation (Weinraub and Lewis, 1977). Whether crying expresses a transient complaint or more prolonged unhappiness may vary according to the child and the circumstances, but it also seemed to be the case that some parents were predisposed to define a child's negative separation response mainly in one way or the other. High sharers were inclined to see it as ephemeral, whereas low sharing parents tended to define any negativity in the child about sharing care as severe. Similarly Hock (1978) concluded that full-time working mothers observed less separation distress and were less anxious about it than non-working mothers. Mrs Green said that Alison

> used to cry when I went out (to work) in the morning, from about one to two (years). But I think that is the sort of howls for a few minutes that are forgotten very quickly. (Now) she just waves good-bye.

Mr Miller described how his son 'had the usual two minutes after we left, because he didn't want us to go, but after that he had forgotten'. Such crying was ignored because it was thought that it did not represent true unhappiness and would soon subside. Some mothers felt very guilty or anxious about such ideas until they were told later that the child stopped crying shortly after they left and then played happily. When Mrs Villiers* first left Simon at nursery school 'I thought "Oh what a terrible mother going and leaving him crying", but he was soon all right.' By contrast several parents expressed a predictive belief that separation distress could lead to long term damage, especially if it was repeated. This merged with a value that it was incumbent on parents not to leave a crying child. Whilst discussing Alexander's start at nursery school Mrs Clark argued that it would be wrong to 'send him as some mothers have done crying in someone's car or to leave him crying'. She believed that could do long term harm:

> A lot of mothers say 'Oh, he'll get over it', but I think it can take quite a long time for them to get over it. They can overcome it but I think in the long run it can do something – maybe retard them. I think it can have some long term effect.

Similarly she had stopped leaving Alexander with his grand-parents as a baby when he started to cry if she attempted to do so.

The two differing perceptions of distress were associated not only with differing value emphases (security or independence) but also dissimilar instrumental beliefs. Thus, crying defined as protest was usually seen as best dealt with by unambiguous preparation and firm departure. The child's uncertainty was seen to be reduced by the clear communication and expectations. Some emotional reassurance might be given initially, as well. By contrast, crying which a parent believed to represent intense suffering was best overcome by avoiding shared care or by staying with the child as long as possible until the child accepted the situation (hopefully). Several parents with this viewpoint had decided not to take their child any longer to an individual carer or group where the child showed initial distress. However, the same people were more inclined to persist if it seemed important enough. Far more mothers had withdrawn their children from miscellaneous groups than from nursery school or playgroup, because the former were seen as more marginal to both parents and child.

Parents also differed in their opinions about who should determine the outcome of separations – the parents or the child. This was a matter of degree, but parents who shared care less would normally stress that the child's expressed wishes should be paramount, so that it would be wrong to leave an upset child. With regard to his son going to nursery school, Mr Tulloch* averred 'if he didna want to go, he wouldna be there'. Mrs Jamieson* had taken her daughter out of playgroup because she was unhappy. Conversely some respondents thought that it was a parent's responsibility to make a decision about what was right and then adhere to it. They thought children should and generally would accept this and get over temporary difficulties. Mrs Buchan considered it wrong to withdraw an upset child from group care as that would only reinforce the child's fear that he or she could not cope. This illustrates a common belief that parental anxiety or confidence communicated itself to the child. Mrs Balfour said she would like her son to be less dependent but felt that she had transmitted to him non-verbally her own anxiety about separation. In a more general way, some parents thought that their expectations and preparations could shape how and when a child was ready for group care. Mrs Davies suggested: 'There is a particular time they take them in, so you get them ready for

that, don't you? I mean Donald was just three when he went
and he was ready because he had to be.'

The sample was almost evenly divided between two opposing
viewpoints about the best way to help children settle in at
group care. The first view was linked to the belief that the
child's crying was a sign of acute distress which should be
avoided. The continuing presence of the mother was seen as
necessary to help the child become familiar with the group
and feel secure. The second view corresponded with the perception of a child's crying (if it occurred at all) as a short-lived
protest. From this perspective a parent who stayed a long time
might inhibit the child from mixing with others and collude
with the child's reluctance to separate. Quick departure was
thought to convey a clear understanding that the child was
going to be left and so help the child accept the situation. It
was evident from parents' descriptions that playgroup leaders
and nursery school staff also had varied opinions about the
best way to help children settle. Some group leaders expected
all children to be treated more or less the same. They advocated a standardised gradual increase of the time spent there
by the child, first with the parent and then alone. Other groups
had a more individualised approach in which the teacher or
supervisor judged when the time for departure of mother was
ripe. Sometimes parents' own ideas about the appropriate
procedure were taken into account but some groups appeared
to be more inflexible. Many parents welcomed or simply
adhered to the group carers' advice. In a few instances group
care staff had intervened to persuade a mother to leave a
resisting child and weather the outburst. One or two mothers
had found relief in such assistance which had overcome an
impasse with their children, who afterwards settled well. A
handful of parents disagreed with their group's particular
policy about settling, although from opposite angles. Mrs
Tervit* insisted on staying with Yvonne at nursery school
until she was happy to be left, whereas the staff had urged a
swifter departure. In contrast, the staff policy at the nursery
schools used by Mrs Reynolds* and Mrs Purdie* was to
encourage the mothers to stay a long time, which they both
thought only prolonged the agony of separation for their
children.

In a number of families, attitudes about their child's nature had been much affected by 'crucial incidents' which several respondents described at considerable length. Several cited an episode when the child had been unexpectedly and acutely upset, so that they grew much more circumspect about sharing care. Some simply suspended the particular arrangement but others became loath to share care at all. Mr and Mrs Forbes exemplified the first type of reaction to a crucial incident. Dorothy had disliked intensely going to a church creche so they simply stopped taking her, but they continued to leave her regularly with local friends as before. Other parents generalised their response. It may be recalled from chapter 2 that after Ross Whigham* cried continuously in a holiday camp nursery his mother and father became reluctant to leave him with anybody. Likewise, Mr and Mrs Booth hardly shared care at all after Fraser was extremely distressed at a church creche when he was a baby. Crucial incidents were most noticeable when they produced negative reactions from the child, but positive examples occurred too. Mrs Forbes had asked her own mother to look after Dorothy now and then when she was a baby but had not shared care with anyone outside the family. At short notice she had to go into hospital for a week. Dorothy, by then aged twelve months, stayed happily with three different street friends. Mrs Forbes was encouraged by this so that from then on Dorothy went to play once or twice a week with the same friends.

The absence of crucial incidents might also reinforce beliefs. Protective parents were confirmed in their view that shared care was upsetting because they did not risk situations when the contrary might prove to be the case. From an opposite standpoint several working mothers said that their uncertain beliefs about sharing care so frequently had been strengthened when they found that their children were happy to stay with carers. Mr and Mrs Balfour said they had no qualms about using unfamiliar people as evening babysitters because Anthony 'never' woke up. They were content to ask unknown circle members to babysit but said they might feel differently if he did not sleep so soundly. In fact, they revealed in another part of the interview that he had awakened once but had simply chatted with the babysitter and gone back to bed. This was therefore a potentially crucial incident which had little effect because of its positive outcome.

Parents' accounts of sharing care also revealed implicit or explicit beliefs about how children's understandings of situations affected their reactions to them. It was often stated that a child would be upset by shared care if he or she could not understand that the parents would return. Mrs Reid said: 'when they see you going out, they think you won't come back'. However, ideas about what children knew or could learn were highly variable. Mr Whigham* had thought that Ross would soon realise that his parents came back each time he was left in the holiday camp nursery at seven months. His wife disagreed, saying that babies get alarmed because they think that any departure by the parents is permanent. Most parents were of the view that a child's increased understanding between two and four made it easier for them to comprehend and accept separation from their mothers. A few thought an older child would be less willing to be left because of greater awareness of the implications of what was happening. Another reason why some parents did not like leaving their children for long was that they perceived them as having a short attention span. Children's short attention and memory spans were seen by some as reasons against a long stay at group care or at least as necessitating plenty of time for the child to become accustomed to the routine. An alternative view was that young children 'don't have any conception of time' (Mrs Ormiston*). Therefore they would not be bothered by a long stay in nursery school since they were absorbed in the here and now.

Parents had different methods of preparing to leave children, depending on their beliefs about how a child's factual knowledge of what was going to happen influenced the reactions to shared care. Dilemmas about this arose in relation to evening care when the babysitter was going to arrive after the child was asleep. Should the child be told beforehand lest he or she wake up or could they be safely left in ignorance of their parents' impending absence? In relation to daytime care mothers also had to decide whether to make their departure obvious or to leave unobserved. Some considered that prior knowledge dispelled uncertainty for the child. They believed in telling the child details of where they were going, when they would return or who an evening carer would be. This could be a long term strategy. It was realised that the child might be upset at first but honesty would eventually pay off by increasing the child's trust that he/she would not be deceived. Mrs Powell said 'I never tried to sneak out. I always told him I was leaving, even if he cried.' Other parents did indeed 'sneak out', however. They argued that doing so caused less alarm since the children did not have to anticipate all the implications of the care arrangement. Slipping out of group care or a carer's home unnoticed while the child was absorbed in play was seen as making the parting process less prominent and so more acceptable to the child. Sometimes experience had tutored this approach. Mr Crawford recalled that 'if we just said good-bye to him he'd be very upset, so what we had to do was sneak out without him knowing'.

Parents' actions were much affected by merged ideas about the nature of 'children's needs'. Making a statement about what children need was often a way of expressing personal values in the form of a factual proposition. For instance, parents with protective care patterns thought that children require constant or near constant care by their mothers. Mothers who worked in the daytime did not reject the idea that children need a close bond with one or both parents but this was accompanied by an image of children as also needing variety, independence and/or stimulation. A child's need for stability could still be achieved by the same familiar person looking after the child when both parents were not there. Many parents thought that children's needs expand after they are two or even earlier to include wider play experience and contacts with peers. Hence social contact at a playgroup or nursery school was not just something parents wanted but was 'necessary' for the children:

Mrs Sadler* (explaining why Nicola liked nursery school) She needed something, she needed other children.

Mrs Brown* I don't know if it is too young to be at nursery, but he desperately needs company, desperately needs his own peer group.

The child was seen to need something additional to what home life could provide:

Mrs Traynor*   She was fed up with just me for company in the house. ( ) She needed other children's company – more than I could provide for her in the home.

Mrs Crawford   He does demand a lot of attention, which I do give him, but I also think he needs something else.

This view of children at this age as intensely social in their interest is at odds with some expert opinion. There were also a few parents in this sample who asserted that three-year-olds lack social interest. Mrs Cairns remarked 'Andrew does not associate with other children, only with adults. I think this is true of a three-year-old. They are all like that.'

Parents had differing ideas about learning and play which were of particular relevance to group care. Some saw these two activities as separate whereas others thought they were intimately linked. Several people emphasised that children learn in important ways through play but others thought that learning comes only from formal instruction. Some playgroup users said that under-fives should 'only' play when they are three or four years old since serious learning began soon enough at school. Mostly it was thought that children have a natural inclination to play but some saw social play as involving skills which themselves needed to be learnt. Mr Crawford referred several times to the fact that his son had not learnt how to play because 'he was not exposed to other children – he doesn't know what to do with them'. Likewise Mrs Brown* thought that her son needed to go to nursery school 'to learn to play, because he doesn't know how to play with other children'.

Explanatory beliefs about children

Besides descriptive images of children, parents also had explanatory beliefs about what affected children's general nature or specific behaviours. The most important of these were environment/heredity, and the child's age, sex and birth order. Parents were asked directly what they thought to be the main influences on a child's personality and what age (if any) is most crucial for a child's personality. There was a predominance of environmentalist beliefs, which stressed the importance of parents' behaviour and the general home or family setting. When asked to comment on the relative importance of heredity and environment in affecting children's personalities, only one quarter of the parents (mostly middle class) stated that heredity was of equal or greater significance. Inheritance appeared to be used most often to explain otherwise 'inexplicable' differences between brothers and sisters.

Parents also took into account the importance of maturation, for their actions and explications in relation to sharing care were much influenced by the age of the child. It was most common to believe that the impact of the environment was critical from birth onwards, but some working-class parents asserted that a child's surroundings and treatment only begin to impinge at a later age once the child has become more obviously aware of what is going on. A characteristic contention was that of Mrs Nichols* that the basis of personality was laid when children began to watch and imitate others at the 'impressionable age' of three. Similarly Mrs Reynolds* said 'It's nearly two before they understand anything. Something drastic would probably affect them younger, but just everyday life – they don't seem to pay much attention to that.'

Ideas about universal regularities in children's development were central to many parents' explanations of children. There seemed to be two aspects to this. Firstly, there were 'thresholds', before which children were seen as too young to handle certain situations like an overnight stay or starting group care. For instance members of babysitting circles usually recognised a threshold after which telling the child about the arrangement became desirable, but for some this occurred well before the child was three, for others not:

Mrs Jackson There comes a time when I feel you've got to tell them you are going out and who the babysitter will be ( ) but we haven't got to that stage with the twins yet.

Secondly, there was a common perception (shared with nearly all psychologists) that children pass through limited periods during which particular behaviours or capacities stand out. Parents themselves tended to use the words 'phase' and 'stage' interchangeably to describe such periods. However, it may be helpful to distinguish fairly brief periods not specially linked to a particular age (a 'phase') from those which are more precisely connected with a certain age-span (a 'stage'). The following passages refer to a phase:

Mr Christie Jane went through this bad patch, but has since settled down with people she knows.

Mr Forbes She's been saying 'No' a lot. It's just something they grow through, testing you out.

From different points in the same interview come examples of descriptions which are more age-specific:

Mrs Arnot She went through a very negative stage at about two and a half. If I asked her to do anything she would say 'No'.

Mr Arnot I would have said that two to two and a half is a sudden changing point. They start becoming little people. That seems to be a sort of developmental stage.

Let us examine threshold and phase/stage concepts in a little more detail. Many parents identified thresholds after which certain kinds of care became justifiable as no longer emotionally threatening for children. Mrs Christie had shared care regularly with Diana's grandmothers and great aunt from her second year onwards. She believed it would not have been right to do so earlier: 'Diana would have been too young to leave earlier than that. I think she had to be of an age that she recognised them.' Several middle-class parents explained their unwillingness to consider overnight care in terms of children being too young to understand why they were away from home or whether they would return home. Threshold beliefs were most evident in relation to group care, however.

Some parents held to a firm generalised belief that children were too young for group care before a certain age, usually three. Others held more individualised beliefs that their own child would (or would not) have benefited from earlier group care, although others might be different. Threshold concepts could be useful in compartmentalising values which might otherwise be difficult to reconcile or balance. Many families concentrated on achieving security for the child before three (or five) and regarded independence as something to be tackled later.

A recurring motif in discussions was that children became 'ready' for more activities and interaction outside the home at a particular time, normally between two and three years. This represented a threshold view of children's needs. Signs of 'readiness' for group care took several forms. The child might be a handful for the mother, be bored with activities at home, show interest in other children or seem receptive to different company and activities. Many parents recognised not just a new capacity to manage prolonged separation but also an impulse towards it. Here are some examples:

Mrs Forbes	(talking about Dorothy at playgroup) She was ready to go. She was a very sociable child and enjoyed going out to play.
Mrs Finlayson	By the time he got to two and a half, he was ready for playgroup, he was ready for something. He was bored round the house and was asking to do things outwith the house.

Several parents considered that children's 'readiness' develops earlier now than it used to. As Mrs Spence* put it aphoristically, 'kids are getting older younger, nowadays.' Mr Allan said 'Children are developing at a faster rate now, so I think it's a good thing for children to get stimulus for learning sooner than schools provide.' Mrs Arnot regarded the expansion of pre-school groups as 'a change for the better. Children grow up so much more quickly these days.'

. All parents notice that their children's capacities and behaviour change as they grow older, but it seemed that the use of the concept of a progression of separate stages and the possibility of regression to an earlier stage were more developed in middle-class families. Typifications such as the 'terrible twos' were mentioned mainly in Milburn. They helped explain (away) behaviour as simply a characteristic of that age. Consequently individual parents or children were not to blame for a period of difficulty which all children are thought to pass through. The 'stage' concept also provided parents with an explanation for behaviour which could otherwise be frustratingly difficult to explain. Since a phase or stage is by definition something which children grow out of parents were exempted from the need to take action. Mrs Baxter* thought that nothing could help with the daily strains of child care: 'It's just that they are at a difficult age. There's nothing that you can do. You've just got to go through it.' This helps resolve the dilemma that parents (especially mothers) are held responsible for their children's actions (Kellerman and Katz, 1978) yet may find adequate explanatory and instrumental beliefs hard to come by. Moreover, anxiety is attenuated by the knowledge that something worrying about the child will not last. A friend along the street complained to Mrs Kerr about Ben's aggression. The friend saw this as part of Ben's personality but his mother regarded it with more equanimity as simply a phase he would soon pass out of.

Parents varied considerably in their beliefs and values associated with particular ages or stages. In addition, different values (e.g. imposing, security, independence, child primacy) might have different weighting at different stages. Broadly speaking, parents' ideas showed that children were seen to be progressively easier to leave as they grew older. The literature suggests that young babies are little affected by separation (Gudat and Permien, 1980; Schaffer, 1971) but some parents averred that infants are vulnerable to distress from separation much earlier. Mrs Christie stated that 'babies can be very upset and uptight leaving them with people they don't know and I really don't approve of it'. Mr and Mrs Clark cited a crucial incident when Alexander had cried constantly in response to separation at only two months. On the other hand some thought much older infants were unaware of even long separations. Mrs Balfour was normally opposed to overnight care of young children but had been happy to leave her son overnight at six months as 'he didn't show signs at that age of being upset when he wasn't with me'. Mrs Morrison thought her daughter was 'too young to notice' a two week absence by her parents on a holiday when she was eight months. Mrs Edwards felt her daughter was too young at twelve months to be aware that her mother was in hospital and that someone she did not know before (a friend's au pair) was looking after her.

Most care sequences indicated less frequent shared care of babies than later. Reluctance to risk upsetting the baby was one influence on this but not the only one. It could be easier to take along a sleeping baby to some places or activities than it would be when the child was older. Other factors included general worries about trusting an apparently vulnerable infant to the care of others, concern about imposing on others the nappy changing and feeding, and a desire not to disrupt an infant's sleep or feeding routines. The first time someone else looked after the baby was sometimes recalled by mothers in particular as an occasion of much anxiety and even doubt about whether it was really possible for another person to look after the child properly. All these factors help explain why mothers' own mothers were especially important as carers in the first year, when such a high degree of trust was usually necessary to overcome worries about sharing care. Some working-class parents appeared to make less distinction between babyhood and later as regards the frequency of shared care. This was partly because they had a stable carer set of relatives whom they trusted with a young baby.

Many mothers became more willing to leave children in the second year. Paradoxically this is the time when many experts think children are most vulnerable to separation distress (Kagan, 1979). In his second year, Thomas Urquhart* began to cry a lot when his mother wanted to leave him while she went to the shops. According to attachment theory this would be seen as a universal development of normal bonding (Bowlby, 1973). Mrs Urquhart* however regarded it as a product of his particular experience; she thought he was insufficiently familiar with being left so she deliberately began to share care more often with both relatives and neighbours.

She said he soon accepted this and gained in self-assurance. Mrs Inglis took similar action to increase Barry's independence. Mrs Reynolds* said 'The second year, he was left a wee bit more', and her husband added 'you don't want him to get too tied to us, like'. By the time the child was three most parents felt more able to insist on sharing care, even if the child was not happy. It was regarded as more in the child's interests to do so and mothers' rights were given greater weight than earlier.

Parents' beliefs about stages tended to go together with their values about security and independence such that implicit models of child development could be identified. These may be seen as ideologies comprising a number of beliefs and values which are mutually sustaining. The two main types can be called attachment and social exposure models. Of course some parents combined aspects of both but low sharers tended to have an ideology which included most of the features of the attachment model whilst high sharers' ideas emphasised social exposure much more. The attachment view gives greatest weight to maturation as affecting children's capacities and relationships. It depicts children as needing to pass through a sensitive period in a secure relationship to the parents before they have the emotional security and cognitive abilities to cope with extended separations from the parents. Mr Griffin said 'I don't know how much the Bowlby stuff plays, but I'm not happy about children under three having extended contact with other people'. The social exposure view contains alternative predictive and instrumental beliefs. Children were thought to be able to adjust to care by other people without distress if they are gradually accustomed to this. Learning to manage separation experiences was seen as beneficial in developing the child's independence and coping skills. This could then prevent misery if it suddenly became necessary for the child to be away (e.g. to go into hospital or start school). Some partners in a couple disagreed in their implicit models. For instance, Mr Sadler* thought that an earlier start to group care would have helped their daughter to cope better but his wife considered it best to wait because she believed that Nicola's understanding and confidence would automatically increase with age.

Whilst the two main models were represented in both Milburn and Whitlaw, a third modified attachment model seemed to be expressed mainly by working-class parents. Before about three, separations were seen as potentially threatening to a positive attachment to the mother. After that there was a risk that overattachment would perpetuate children's vulnerability, so it became important to have regular experience away from parents in order to prevent them becoming habituated to dependence. The idea of an optimum period for separation at three was probably affected by the availability of nursery school places at that age, which made a shift in orientation possible.

The majority of parents indicated that their patterns of shared care had been affected by some form of attachment ideology. It was the experience of a few that their efforts to minimise early separation had indeed contributed to the child's willingness to stay with others later. Similarly, some parents believed that crucial incidents had predisposed their child to later upset, in accord with attachment theory. Mrs Morrison thought that her older daughter's early start at nursery school had made her more anxious at school. Nevertheless, it was common for people in the sample to attribute children's general manner of responding to separation as largely a result of their previous social experience rather than as an aspect of maturation. Many respondents made unprompted remarks which attributed poor reactions to separation directly to a lack of experience of shared care. This occurred in statements of an individualised kind given by several protective parents even though this contradicted their more generalised beliefs and values about attachment. Here are a few examples:

Mrs Traynor* They seem to be upset to leave me. Perhaps it's because I don't leave them with people very often. They are with me the whole time.

Mrs Taylor* (to her son, who was highly resistant to being left with anyone else) I never used to leave you. Maybe that's what's wrong.

Mrs Raeburn He was very tied to me, because we never

	had people we could leave him with during the day.
Mr Crawford	He's not got used to being with others much, which is maybe not a good thing. ( ) The few times we did leave him with grandparents, he was a bit difficult, because he just wasn't used to it.

Furthermore, difficulties in adjusting to group care were explained by several parents as resulting from insufficient prior sharing:

Mr Purdie*	We are partly to blame – we keep our children to us.
Mrs Jamieson	Really it took a bit longer (for her to settle in) than a child who's been left quite a lot, you know.

Correspondingly, a number of high sharing parents said that their children were self-confident because they were accustomed to being away from them. In particular, a number of parents gave this as the reason why their child had settled well in group care. For example, Mrs Quinn* described Ralph's start at nursery school: 'He's just settled fine. I think it's because he's always been used to being with other people.' When Craig Allan was suddenly admitted to hospital, his mother declared 'Thank God he's been used to being away from me.'

The child's sex

Whether a young child is a boy or girl may have a direct influence on parental attitudes and behaviour or on the child's befriending patterns. According to Block (1976) parents are least likely to treat their children differently on account of their sex at a very young age, but stereotyped attitudes are already at work then. Gender is also an important element of sibling status – the combined sex and birth order of the child. For instance a girl's experience in the family may be very different if she is the eldest with two younger brothers compared with someone who is the youngest with two older sisters. There are many possible combinations, further complicated by the effects of age spacing. This means that the whole idea of a child's position in the family is much more complicated than appears at first sight (Kammeyer, 1967; Sutton-Smith and Rosenberg, 1970; Warren, 1966). A study with a small sample such as this cannot handle such refinements – indeed few large surveys do so either. However, it is important to bear in mind that the apparently small influence of sex and birth order on sharing care found in this study may reflect not only insufficient precision in analysis but also the cancelling out of the effects of different sibling statuses. More importantly, gender and birth order derive their meaning and influence partly from the reactions to those characteristics by family members and others. Such adult responses may be important yet not in simple ways which give rise to straightforward statistical associations.

The sample contained thirty-six boys and twenty-seven girls. There were fairly similar though not identical proportions in Milburn and Whitlaw. There have been suggestions in the literature that parents may be more loath to share care of girls than boys, perhaps because mothers are more reluctant to separate from girls or find boys more difficult to cope with (GHS, 1979; Stevenson and Ellis, 1975). On the other hand, it has been conjectured that some mothers are more protective towards young sons than daughters (Blomart, 1963). Hardly any of the parents interviewed here expressed an opinion that care frequency should differ according to the child's sex. Comparisons of the care patterns for boys and girls also showed no major contrasts. Both interview and diary data showed a weak tendency for higher proportions of boys to have experienced both high and low sharing, whereas more girls experienced medium frequencies of care ($p < 0.1$). There was a similar slight trend for more boys to have large or small rather than medium-sized carer sets.

Although sex differences appeared to have little direct impact on sharing care, it could be that there were indirect influences operating via network contacts. Boys and girls had similar ranges of adult contacts but significantly more girls had long lists of other children they were said to be fond of (p < 0.02). The diaries showed that a high proportion of these three-year-olds' friends were of the same sex. Only 30 per cent of the children's best friends were of the opposite sex (p < 0.01). Other research has found that sex-matching in children's friendships occurs in nurseries (Challman, 1932; Hutt, 1972; Maccoby and Jacklin, 1980) but in this sample it clearly applied to relationships formed largely outside and prior to attendance at formal groups.

Sometimes ideas about sex differences did affect detailed processes of shared care. The Powells had been concerned that Stephen had been surrounded by girl playmates in his street 'mini-group'. They hoped he would benefit from seeing more boys at playgroup. Sex-typing also entered into Mr Baxter's* explanation of why Derek would benefit from going to nursery school. He said that Derek was bored at home because boys are uninterested in helping mothers whereas girls are content to assist with domestic tasks. Mr Baxter* was glad Derek was going to attend a different nursery school from his older sister, so that 'he'll maybe meet a wee boy he likes, his pal (and) learn to do things that boys do'. Mrs Arnot explained her caution about sharing care of her two daughters by the generalisation that girls are more easily upset than boys. Mrs Ogilvie* thought that it was important for children to learn to stand up for themselves at nursery school, 'especially for wee boys', who might get more involved in fighting and bullying. A few families also suggested that the interest of relatives in sharing care might be affected by the child's sex. There was a direct preference for a boy or girl, or perhaps a special interest in the first girl or boy after several grandchildren, nephews or nieces of the opposite sex.

Birth order and sibling spacing

We shall first consider the statistical associations between birth order and care and network patterns. Second, parents' beliefs about the effects of birth status will be discussed.

There were nine children in the sample who had no brothers or sisters at the time of interview. Most of the remainder had just one or two siblings. There were twenty-three first borns, twenty-six second borns and fourteen later borns. Altogether rather less than one third (eighteen) had a younger sibling. If this sample is typical, then it appears that it is most common for a three-year-old to be currently the youngest member of the family. Girls were significantly underrepresented among second borns, two thirds of whom were boys. This may partly account for the fact that this group differed from first borns in ways which sometimes contradict the birth order effects found in other research. A further important distinction was whether a child was 'closely spaced' or not: forty children were classified as closely spaced because they had at least one brother or sister who was either older or younger by fewer than three years.

In each of the three years a high proportion of second borns had infrequent care (less than six times a year) whilst above average numbers of later born and only children had experienced frequent care (at least once a week). This pattern was confirmed by the diaries. In addition, markedly fewer closely spaced children (13.5 per cent) than others (47.5 per cent) had high shared care frequency in the two weeks of the diary record, despite the fact that more were middle class (p < 0.02). All but one of the protective families had closely spaced children. Probably parents become less willing to share care when there are two under-fives, especially when one is a baby. A number or parents said that they had cut down on sharing care after a new baby was born. Another possibility is that 'child-centred' families who are reluctant to share care may be more likely to plan to have children close together in age.

With regard to overnight care, it is easier to put up and maybe put up with one child than two. Therefore it was not unexpected to find that first borns and only children had been away from their parents overnight more often on average than the rest of the children. About half of the first borns (including seven out of nine only children) had been away for nine or more nights in the three years, but only one quarter of second borns and an even smaller proportion of later borns (14 per cent). Several families had split the children for week-ends or holidays away. They either took the key child away with them and left older siblings with an overnight carer, or vice versa.

Far more second borns than either first or later born children were reported as having found separation from both parents

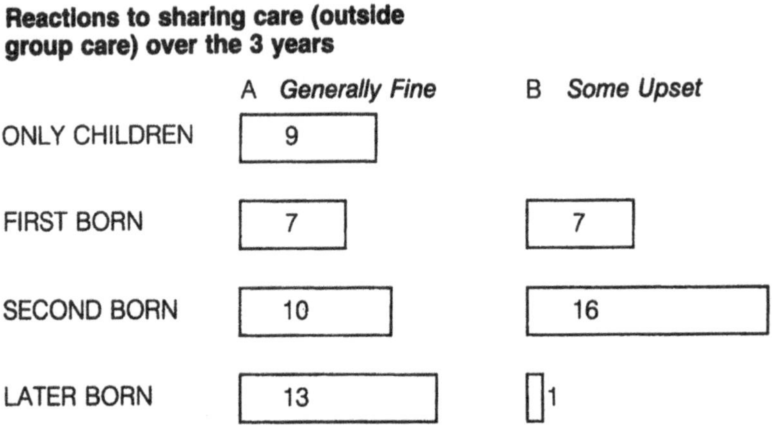

Reactions to sharing care (outside group care) over the 3 years

	A *Generally Fine*	B *Some Upset*
ONLY CHILDREN	9	
FIRST BORN	7	7
SECOND BORN	10	16
LATER BORN	13	1

Note: Several of those who were only children at the time of interview would subsequently have younger siblings and so become first born.

CHI-SQ. 12.319   SIG. = 0.002

Figure 7.1 *Birth order and reactions to care*

with individual carers distressing (p < 0.01; Figure 7.1). At group care too, a higher proportion of second borns (43 per cent of attenders) were withdrawn or playing on their own rather than mixing well compared with only 7 per cent of the others. Closely spaced children included most of those who had been upset by sharing care.

The amount of contact which the children had with different kinds of adults did not appear to be influenced by the child's gender or birth order but relationships with other children were affected. It might be predicted that first born children would have fewer playmates than others. We have already seen that a fair number of three-year-olds' contacts are with friends of older brothers and sisters. This is a possibility not open to the first child in a family. In addition, both first borns and their parents are often building up peer contacts for the first time whereas second and later children inherit contacts with families already befriended through elder brothers and sisters. Understandably then, second and later borns did have more contact with primary school age children outside the family. On the other hand, those children who had few friends were mostly second borns. In working-class families second borns seemed particularly lacking in friends of the same age, but for middle-class families a high proportion of second borns had many peer friends. This is interesting because several middle-class parents thought that their second children tended to be more friendly by nature, which was contradicted by the overall results in this study. It could be that among middle-class families, second borns did acquire peer friends and social confidence helped by street contacts established through their older siblings, but this happened much more rarely for working-class children.

Although birth order did not yield strong and regular associations with care patterns in the way that social class did, it was nonetheless a prominent element in the beliefs which parents volunteered about children. To be sure, some parents explained contrasts amongst their children in reactions to shared care by referring to sex differences, heredity or dissimilar early experiences. However, it was some kind of birth order effect on the child's social environment that was the most common kind of explanation given for such differences. The conclusions reached were not always the same. One person's strongly held beliefs about the typical consequences of being a first born or second born child could be the exact opposite of someone else's.

Psychologists who have analysed the effects of birth order on children have for the most part simply contrasted first borns with others. The differences which have been discovered have usually been ascribed to the ways in which parents react differently to later births and alter the way they treat children in the light of their earlier experience. Sears (1950) and McArthur (1956) concluded that these processes generally lead parents to be less anxious and more encouraging of independence with second and subsequent children, although Lasko (1954) noticed more protectiveness towards later borns in the form of 'babying'. Another important factor involves rivalry and jealousy with regard to parents' attention (Dunn and Kendrick, 1979, 1980). The parents in this sample also made use of explanations based on changes in parent-child interaction but in addition they put greater emphasis on the direct effects of one child on another and indicated that changes in the family's external relationships were important too.

A widespread observation was that the parents had reacted less well to the first child. Many mothers in particular recalled worry, depression, isolation and feelings of great responsibility. The second time round parents usually felt more confident, relaxed and knowledgeable. As Mrs Sinclair* said, 'Everybody learns by their mistakes, don't they?' This applied to fathers too, for Mr Sinclair* added 'With the second one ( ) you are more at ease. You are always panicking with the first child.' People also became less cautious and less involved with every detail of development. As a result many parents said they were much more willing to share care with their second or subsequent child. Their earlier worries had been allayed and in some cases they had concluded that minimal sharing with the first child had led to overdependence. Mrs Kerr admitted:

> I wouldn't have left a nine month old baby with a friend
> had it been a first one. ( ) You think, if it's your first,
> that if it's away from you for two hours some desperate
> damage will happen. You think some psychological
> damage will be done, but by the time the third one arrives,
> you realise it's really quite good for them to get away
> from you for a couple of hours.

Similarly Mrs Balfour remarked 'I think with the first child you're probably overcareful.' She planned to start Anthony's baby sister in a weekly swop or mini-group earlier than had happened in his case, as she believed this would increase her self-assurance. Mrs Sinclair* generalised from her experience as a playgroup committee member that first borns adapted less well to the playgroup because they had been apart from their mothers less often than later children who thereby became more independent. She herself went out more often after her second child was born because she was less worried about leaving him with his grandparents.

Many of the respondents noted the importance of the direct effects of one child on another. In particular, older siblings were described as helping the younger one to do things. Some parents thought that a younger child was held back by not needing to find out how to do things for him or herself, but a more common causal belief was that a second child's capacities developed more quickly through observation and imitation of an older brother or sister. It was a popular belief that younger siblings are highly motivated to do the same things as their older siblings. They wanted to play along the street with friends in the same way, join in an overnight stay or start attending the same group. They wanted both to be treated the same and to avoid losing the company of the older ones. Several parents said that their younger child adapted better to group care because they had become familiar with the place and routine through accompanying and observing older siblings. Likewise Aidan Hunter was quite used to the idea of going to his childminder because his sister had done the same. Several respondents observed that siblings provided a source of comfort for each other during shared care. This view is supported by research (Burlingham and Freud, 1943; Stewart, 1983). Different parents described how an older child reassured a younger child or assisted a carer if the younger one was troubled. This was an important factor in reducing concern about stranger care for a few parents.

A number of parents merged the social exposure explanation of personality with a birth order explanation of differences between children. They commented that a second or later born child acquired a ready-made network of social contacts which had been developed in relation to an older sibling. The later born child was therefore able to mix earlier with other children and so gain practice in social skills. Similarly, a younger child could simply join in or take over from a sibling in a swop care arrangement at an earlier age. Mrs Vallance* summarised several of these points in contrasting Susan and her older brother:

> I know they are differing natures, but when he went along to nursery, he found it a lot harder, because he's been, well you know, just a baby, whereas she had more contact with other children. And her going along to the nursery before it even started, she took to it a lot easier.

Aspects of child development and behaviour

As this was not primarily a developmental or medical study, only a limited amount of information was obtained about the children's personal history and characteristics. Partly as a result of this but also because the sample excluded single parent families and mobile families, few major problems were identified. In all, fifteen couples admitted to their child having some kind of behavioural or social problem. These were for the most part comparatively minor things like eating difficulties, nailbiting or clinginess. Quite a few parents thought that group care had helped sort out a problem. Mrs Gunn believed that the intense, provocative relationship she had with Jackie had improved markedly since she started going to playgroup. Several other children had become less boisterous or aggressive at home when they went to a group. Curiously, in six working-class families it was noted that children who had previously been very resistant to eating a full meal had changed dramatically when they saw this was a normal expectation for their nursery school lunches.

Accidents, illnesses and other 'life-events' had had a vital impact on shared care in a few cases but were too infrequent or diverse in their impact to show consistent associations with care patterns. Therefore they will not be referred to here. From this it cannot be inferred that they are irrelevant to sharing care, but rather that a different kind of sample and study would be required to ascertain their significance in a larger population.

Systematic information about early feeding was obtained from two thirds of the sample. This revealed a higher proportion of mothers who had breast fed (over half) than were reported in studies ten years ago (Leach, 1974: 73). It could be that breast feeding has increased, that there are differing definitions about brief breast feeding or that chance factors explain the difference between small samples. As in previous research (Blaxter and Paterson, 1982; Newson and Newson, 1963), most middle-class mothers had breast fed longer than most working-class mothers. Three quarters of the working-class mothers had bottle fed from the start or after only a week or two. This was the case for only one quarter of the middle-class mothers. This may be an additional factor why working-class mothers could contemplate overnight stays from an earlier age. Mrs Robertson* only began overnight stays when Tammy was weaned at six months. She also stopped them again for six months after Tammy's younger sister was born. Quite a few mothers who had subsequently become high sharers said that they seldom shared care until they had finished breast feeding. The restriction could work the other way, however. Mrs Carlisle said she had to share care because of prejudice about breast feeding in public places where she would otherwise have taken her baby. The comparatively prolonged period of breast feeding did not apparently prevent more daytime sharing care by middle-class families in the first year than by working-class families. Much of the sharing that occurred at that age would have been for only an hour or two and so could be fitted in between feeds. Mrs Green was able to work thirty hours a week whilst breast feeding up to eighteen months, demonstrating that shared care of considerable duration could be managed around feeds and with a bottle as standby.

Systematic observations carried out from birth onwards have shown that many children tend to be consistently either 'good' or 'bad' sleepers. Moreover children's sleep patterns are connected with other aspects of development (Dunn, 1980b; Moss, 1967). Contrary to what people often think, there is good evidence that night waking is normally the product of a child's arousal characteristics which are present from birth or earlier. By and large it does not result from 'wrong' handling of the child by parents (Bernal, 1973; Blurton-Jones et al., 1978). Half of the children (thirty-two) in this sample had apparently been good sleepers since birth. A further six children (all boys) stayed up very late, but then slept well. This meant that they went to bed well beyond the normal time of 7–7.30 in working-class families or 7.30–8 in middle-class families. Twenty-one children (fourteen boys and seven girls) had presented significant night waking difficulties at some time. Of these, seven had persistently woken and cried a lot at night through all of their first three years. These patterns fit with the findings of Moss (1967) that more boy than girl infants slept for shorter periods and cried more. However, Bernal (1973) found no sex differences in night waking in the first year. The majority of the children in this sample who had eating, nailbiting or clinging problems were also poor sleepers. A high proportion of second borns (52 per cent) were poor sleepers, perhaps because more were boys.

Understandably parents with children who often woke up tended to have shared care less frequently in the evenings than those whose child slept soundly. Richards *et al.* (1977) reported that mothers of children who were poor sleepers went out without the child less frequently than others in the daytime too. Several parents explicitly stated that they did not like to leave their children in the evening in case they woke up and were alarmed or the carer could not cope. When a child did have sleep difficulties, specially trusted carers like grandparents assumed particular importance. The Christies had stopped using a babysitter except for Mrs Christie's mother during periods when their children had woken up frequently and cried. Ralph Quinn's* grandparents looked after him more than usual during a spell of particularly high activeness and disturbed sleep in order to give his parents a rest.

Several studies have demonstrated that children vary almost from birth in their degree of calm or restlessness. Some respond to environmental change and stimulation with relative calm, others find it hard to deal with (Carey, 1970; Dunn, 1980a). Mothers tend to find this second type of child more difficult to leave even with people they know well (Barnes, 1975). In the present study it was not possible to distinguish actual differences in the children from parental perceptions. In any case, it was the latter which affected parents' actions. Some parents clearly felt that from a very early age their child was particularly resistant to being left with someone else. This is illustrated in the following:

> **Interviewer**   How did you first notice that she cried a lot when left?
>
> **Mrs Buchan**   When she was born, she screamed, and she screamed fairly considerably. She had colic severely until 3 months. She's a child who still will cling onto you very hard . . .

	will go to some other people with some willingness, but on the whole she wants to be with me.
Mr Buchan	Yes, in her first year, she wanted to be with you.
Mrs Buchan	Yes, to the exclusion of everybody else.
Mr Buchan	It was quite difficult for me to have her for a long time, because she got very upset.

Some parents reported marked differences in temperament between their children. Mrs Barker had shared the care of her placid daughter with a childminder, but when John was born he seemed much too delicate and irritable for this to be repeated. Like the Buchans and the Barkers, some parents became very cautious about sharing care because of their child's delicate nature. Others persevered, however. Mary Mitchell had been 'terrible as a child, awake all night. She doesn't settle to change easily.' However, Mary had stayed daily since babyhood with a friend, then a childminder then nursery staff.

It was clear that nearly all the parents showed sensitivity in adapting their patterns of care to the nature of their children, just as it has been found that parent-child interaction in general is responsive and not imposed on the child (Lewis and Rosenblum, 1974). As they grew older, the children could exert influence more directly by verbal expression of their wishes. Many children urged their parents to let them go and stay with relatives or play with friends. On the other hand some resisted staying with carers. Mrs Henderson wanted Douglas to stay and play with friends' children but he had said 'home now' so insistently that she felt obliged to comply and take him away. Likewise on one occasion Mr and Mrs Villiers* had left Simon to stay overnight with friends but when bedtime came he was so adamant about wanting to return home that they were called to collect him in his pyjamas.

Children's shyness and sociability

Children's willingness or otherwise to stay with carers is naturally affected by their more general responses to people

outside the nuclear family. This was not measured precisely
but during the interviews all the parents were asked to
describe their child's personality and to say how he or she
reacted generally with less familiar adults and other children.
Often the child had already been described spontaneously by
respondents as shy, anxious, clingy, friendly or sociable. Using
all this information a global assessment of each child's degree
of social confidence was made. Evidently a child's responses to
other people he or she does not know well vary considerably
according to the person's manner, the context, the child's age,
mood and state of health, and many other factors. Even
specialised psychological studies of temperament have encountered many conceptual and operational difficulties (Hubert *et
al.*, 1982). However, parental descriptions did suggest that
most of the children had a more general disposition to either
shyness or social confidence. Examples of the former include:

Mr Scott*   She's very shy, and she's never spoken at
nursery school since she's been there.
Mrs Taylor*   He's just one of these children that are
clingy. That's an understatement.
Mrs Ritchie* But with her being so clinging – we used
to meet people in the street and she would
just stand beside me – so when she was
three, I thought she needed it (i.e.
playgroup).

The opposite kind of personality might be indicated like this:

Mrs Ferguson* He's pretty friendly with everybody.
Mr Morrison   He's a friendly, wee soul, really.
Mrs Nichols* She's a mixer ( ) She's no strange – it
doesn't matter where you take her.

This twofold classification has to be treated with caution. It
was based on parents' subjective assessments and oversim-
plifies the range and variability of children's temperament.
Bates (1980, 1983) doubts whether parental reports can be
relied upon, but Carey (1982) reviewed evidence which
suggests that parents' observations can be reasonably

accurate. Moreover several pieces of research have shown that many children can be described fairly consistently as either socially inhibited or confident, though sometimes a third category of difficult or non-conforming children is also recognised (Kagan and Moss, 1962; Marcus *et al.*, 1972). The importance of this aspect of children's development is highlighted by the fact that one third of the Milburn and Whitlaw couples mentioned in some way that they had worries about their child's lack of social confidence or clinging behaviour. There is some justification for such concerns. Although shyness has received very little attention compared with aggressive or anti-social behaviour, there is evidence that young children who are inhibited often have adjustment problems when they are older (Kagan, 1982; von Cranach *et al.*, 1976). On the other hand, many children do grow out of or overcome early difficulties (Clarke and Clarke, 1984).

Slightly more than half of the children were classed as broadly friendly or very friendly towards adults. Over one in five (fourteen) appeared to be very shy or anxious. As Batter and Davidson (1979) also found, most were apparently less reserved with other children than they were with adults. Two thirds of parents felt that their child played well with other children and only eleven thought their child had significant difficulties in this respect. That represents a somewhat higher proportion of the sample than the 5 to 10 per cent identified by Asher and Renshaw (1981) as having difficulties with peers at primary school age. Children who were particularly wary about other children were nearly always deficient with adults too ($p < 0.001$). Therefore, the children could be placed in three broad groupings:

Shy-all-round	Shy with adults and children
Shy-with-adults	Shy with adults only
Not-shy	Confident with adults and children

Half of the children who were shy-all-round were to be found in families of intermediate class who made up only one quarter of the sample ($p < 0.02$). A high proportion of shy-all-round children had had sleep difficulties ($p < 0.05$). Longitudinal studies have likewise discovered a distinctive group of children with irregular sleep patterns and poor responsiveness to change (Dunn, 1980a; Thomas and Chess, 1977).

A small study by Simpson and Stevenson-Hinde (1985) found no difference between boys and girls in shyness. This was so for the current sample, too. However, gender was a common element in parents' explanations of differences in children's sociability and reactions to care. There was no consensus about the direction this took, though. Mrs Powell had formed a generalised belief from children she knew that girls are more shy than boys, but Mrs Johnstone had reached the opposite conclusion that girls are more self-reliant and outgoing. Both the Lauries and the Baxters* attributed contrasts in their boy-girl pairs to the fact that the son took after the father and the daughter after the mother. In the first case, the girl was more gregarious, in the second case it was the boy.

It was noted earlier that second born children had fewer friends on average than others. Consistent with that fact, more of them were shy than either first or later borns. Several psychological investigations have reached an opposite conclusion that first borns tend to be less confident and more anxious than other children (Clausen, 1964; McArthur, 1956; Miller and Maryama, 1976). It was also contrary to many parents' birth order explanations of children which suggested that changes in parents' attitudes, sibling interaction and network relationships favoured greater social confidence for second and later borns. Moreover, although second born children tended to be shy, nearly all of the third and fourth children were not shy. Analysis of individual cases showed that it was mostly middle-class parents who had observed that their three-year-old's younger brother or sister appeared to be more confident. Interestingly, Snow et al. (1981) found more first borns to be sociable and assertive than others. Perhaps all that can be concluded from these contradictory results is that sociability is related to fine distinctions of sibling status which interact with other factors.

In this sample shy children were for the most part the ones who had seldom been separated from their mothers; this was true for families in both main social class groupings. All twelve of the children in 'protective' families were shy and so were

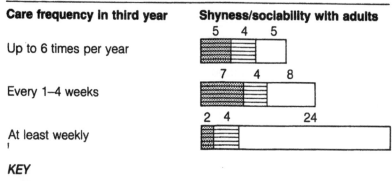

Care frequency in third year   **Shyness/sociability with adults**

Up to 6 times per year — 5 4 5

Every 1–4 weeks — 7 4 8

At least weekly — 2 4 24

KEY

Very shy or anxious with unfamiliar adults

Shy with unfamiliar adults

Not shy; friendly with unfamiliar adults

Figure 7.2 *Shyness-sociability and care frequency*

most of the others in low sharing families. Nearly all children in high sharing families were confident whilst medium sharing families had equal numbers of both shy and not-shy children (p = 0.001; Figure 7.2). In addition only two children from protective families were said to be able to play well with other children (17 per cent) compared with the vast majority in other families (thirty-nine, i.e. 77 per cent). This fits with the conclusion of McCandless *et al.* (1961) that children who are very dependent on adults appear to be inhibited when it comes to getting on with other children. It is noteworthy that Kagan and Moss (1962) also identified maternal protectiveness and encouragement of dependent behaviour before children were aged three as linked to passivity in those children at a later age. The association between shyness and restrictiveness in shared care was further demonstrated by the fact that most of the children with small carer sets were shy-all-round children. Shy children had also usually experienced little or no overnight care (p < 0.01). In addition, those middle-class families with mainly kin carers were significantly more likely to have shy children than other middle-class families (p < 0.05). Clarke-Stewart *et al.* (1980) also observed that frequent interaction and care with relatives went together with lower sociability towards strangers.

Attachment theorists have sometimes generalised from findings about reactions to institutional care and the 'strange situation' experiment to suggest that mother separation is associated with more anxious and less affiliative behaviour in children (Blehar, 1977). It has been feared that this might apply to children with working mothers (Cohen, 1978). In this sample however all the ten mothers who had shared care for work reasons in the first year of the child's life apparently had children who were socially confident ($p < 0.01$). This was also true for all of those currently working outside the home in the daytime. Conversely only one mother with a shy-all-round child had worked in a way which had required care of the children by someone other than the parents. Most of the mothers who were satisfied not working in the daytime had confident children, but a high percentage of the children with mothers who were 'partly-dissatisfied' at home were very anxious or clinging ($p < 0.01$). Gold and Andres (1978a, 1978b) discovered that children of working mothers were better adjusted socially (according to teachers' ratings) than those with non-working mothers.

There are several alternative ways of explaining why most shy children had had much less experience of sharing care with a more restricted range of carers than most friendly children. A social learning explanation would suggest that frequent shared care encourages children to be more sociable. Children who are used to being apart from their parents are thereby encouraged to develop interactive skills without the constant support of parents. Children who are less skilful socially have been shown to be more dependent on parents and less willing to be left (Ferguson, 1970; Light, 1980). Alternatively, frequent sharing care may simply be a sign of greater overall social interaction by families and it is this which assists social confidence. In fact, the positive relationship between care frequency and sociability was found to hold irrespective of the amount of social contact the child had with other adults or other children. Thirdly, parents of constitutionally shy children may respond to their child's sensitivity and so refrain from sharing care (Clarke-Stewart, 1973). A study by Cohen (1979) revealed that parents' confidence or doubts about their children's entry to school was realistically based on the nature of the children in many cases. Fourthly, perhaps genetics plays a part. Reserved parents may give birth to shy children, so that both are reluctant to mix and share care. Twin studies suggest that a fairly stable trait of sociability emerges very early in children's lives. The findings of Scarr (1969) appear to demonstrate that there is a strong genetic component in this but other studies indicate that environmental influences may be important too (Ainslie, 1985; Goldsmith and Gottesmann, 1981; Wilson et al., 1971). In this study the association between care frequency and shyness in the child applied regardless of parents' anxiety levels as measured by MI scores.

Probably several of these mechanisms interact. Many of the shy children in this sample had mothers or both parents who appeared to be diffident as well. They also perceived their children to be too vulnerable to be left with other people except occasionally within the circle of close kin. Lack of social experience apart from parents could then reinforce this. However, this explanation cannot be pushed too far. Quite a few of the low sharing families included older or younger siblings who were described by their parents as being temperamentally more outgoing than the key child. Hence the nature of the family could not by itself be said to determine the shyness of the one child but not the other. Overall, there were only four families of two or more children all of whom appeared to be shy or clinging. Three children who had no brothers or sisters were shy. All seven of these families were low sharers.

At any event, it may be concluded that frequent shared care by mothers in these families did not lead to withdrawn or difficult behaviour as has sometimes been inferred from attachment theory. Given a basic stability of family life, a considerable degree of sharing care and social interaction appeared to foster social confidence. The most inhibited children were more likely to have the kinds of parents who themselves lacked the confidence or ability to create the circumstances for such social experience in their own networks. As a result, many parents of shy children hoped that group care would help their child gain confidence and some thought it had done so.

Children who were deemed to be shy made up a high proportion of those who had been upset when apart from both parents, but this is in part tautologous since assessments of shyness by parents took account of such reactions. Even so, two very shy children had had mainly good reactions to care, for this could also depend on how well they knew the carer and the general context of sharing care. Thus, Kirstie Chalmers* 'does like to cling to us', but had felt 'fine, great' about shared care by her grandparents whom she saw several times a week. Ninety per cent of sociable children were said to be mixing well at group care but over half of the shy children who were attending group care were quiet or played on their own (p < 0.001). Some shy children did settle in quite well, but most of those children who had been very clinging or loath to be left when younger were also unhappy about staying at group care, to begin with anyway.

Somewhat more shy children attended playgroup than nursery schools (p < 0.1). It seemed that parents who believed their own child or children in general were especially sensitive to separations were more liable to seek out a facility with short hours of attendance. This is a more probable explanation than organisational differences for the fact that more children had found it hard to settle in at playgroups than at nursery school. Those with children who were not good mixers were mostly against an early start to group care out of concern that the child would be unhappy, rather than in favour of it in order to assist the child's sociability. This represented an application of the attachment model in that the children were seen as needing to pass through a sensitive period before being ready for major separations of this kind. Parents of shy children were significantly more inclined to perceive an early entry to group care as harmful to children (p = 0.001). Perhaps this was an accurate reflection of their own child's likely reactions.

8 *Discussion and implications*

Traditionally, social policy had been concerned with people who are disadvantaged or exceptional in some way. In contrast this research was designed to respond to commentators who have pointed to the need for greater understanding of the needs, resources and solutions which occur in the everyday life of all kinds of people (Cullen, 1979; Sinfield, 1980; Titmuss, 1976). In doing so it has attempted to apply interpretive sociology to ordinary families. This follows a recent trend illustrated by Backett (1982), Boulton (1983) and Askham (1984). Knowledge about the normal range of experience can provide reference points against which to judge patterns of behaviour and need. It also reveals how most people cope with crises and problems which lead those with fewer material or human resources to seek official help.

Significant details from the research are incorporated in the following discussion, but it may be helpful to recall the main points briefly before broadening our perspective. In the first chapter it was pointed out that non-parental care of young children has conventionally been viewed as 'day care', which embraces services in officially recognised groups together with arrangements made by families with working mothers. Yet children are looked after by people other than parents in a much wider range of ways and for more diverse reasons. This study set out to understand more systematically the totality of particular children's experience of being apart from their parents in the first three years of their lives. It was concerned with the social as well as the emotional consequences of different types and sequences of such shared care. Therefore, interviews were carried out with seventy-three two-parent families living in contrasting areas of Edinburgh. Judged by a number of criteria Milburn was a predominantly 'middle-class' neighbourhood and Whitlaw primarily 'working class'.

It was found that the patterns and processes of shared care were affected both by families' network relationships and parents' beliefs and attitudes. Some aspects of these were in turn strongly influenced by social class. Significantly more middle-class than working-class parents shared care at least weekly. Couples in both classes preferred to use relatives for looking after their children, but many working-class parents were very averse to the idea of sharing care with anyone other than close kin or well-established friends, whereas most middle-class children had stayed frequently with other mothers in nearby streets. In the middle-class area there were quite formalised friendship and shared care networks as well as babysitting groups. These were absent in the working-class area.

Virtually all the families held strong values about avoiding emotional harm to children and encouraging close, continuous relationships between children and parents. However, some people thought this required children to be with their parents particularly the mother for nearly all the time, at least until the age of three. To others the same values were compatible with relatively frequent shared care. The second type of family laid greater emphasis on helping children become independent and on mothers' rights to have breaks from children and to work. Whatever their initial views, most parents tended to feel more comfortable about sharing care more often for second and later children. This was linked to a common experience that minimal shared care could lead to the child having difficulties in adjusting to pre-school groups or school itself.

Even though care patterns and perceptions of children's natures and parents' responsibilities were very diverse, there was a broadly accepted norm that some kind of group experience is very helpful to children from at least the age of three onwards. This rested on a nearly universal view that children have strong social needs and impulses which in a modern urban environment are best met in safe child-centred settings like playgroups and nursery school.

What are the implications of these findings? The short answer is that the wide array of practices and opinions in the sample could be interpreted to fit with any of the main day-care standpoints summarised in chapter 1 – traditional, institutional and radical feminist. Rather than argue simply from one of these perspectives it may be more useful to see how the evidence from this and related research fits with two major linked themes which have been central to social policy thinking over the last decade in relation to the care of dependent people in our society, including not only children but the frail elderly, the handicapped and the mentally ill. One theme concerns the division of responsibilities between the 'state' and the 'community' and the other deals with the similar demarcation between women and men. Many people have argued that 'community care' is preferable to state provision. This approach appeals to a wide spectrum of people for varied reasons. Some hope it will contain public expenditure. Others wish to foster self-help and family responsibility. Community care has also been advocated in order to keep children and adults out of institutions or to transfer power from professionals and bureaucracies to ordinary people (Barclay, 1982; Coote and Hewitt, 1980; Timms, 1983). In practice, care in the community for the under-fives has meant care mainly by mothers, perhaps supplemented by help from social networks and part-time groups after the age of three. From an opposite viewpoint the increasingly prominent body of feminist writings have questioned the fairness and desirability of such patterns since they rely on obligations for women but not men to let domestic responsibilities override their other interests, inclinations and freedoms (Finch and Groves, 1983; New and David, 1985). Exponents of this perspective argue that there is a need for more rather than less public day care provision for the sake of both women and children (Hughes et al., 1980; Mayall and Petrie, 1983).

These issues will now be looked at in turn by consideration of progressively wider frameworks in which shared care occurs. Firstly implications for individuals and relationships within the nuclear family will be suggested. Then the perspective is widened to take account of networks in the 'community'. Finally the role and importance of public provision is discussed in the light of families' needs, networks and resources.

Children, women and men

In our present society child care is mainly carried out by women. Whether this should or must continue is now at the forefront of public and academic debate (Nicholson, 1984; Rossi, 1984). There are powerful and opposing sentiments about this complex issue so that a small-scale study can only hope to elaborate and not resolve some of the arguments. This research provided the unsurprising finding that not only was the primary care of these Edinburgh youngsters carried out by mothers, but non-parental care was mainly performed by women too. Shared care was also mostly arranged by women – even when their husbands were at home. Swop networks and babysitting circles were established and organised by mothers. In many households the man appeared to feel more entitled than his wife to be away from the children even when he was not working.

Whether this unequal division of care responsibility matters or not depends on your viewpoint. From a feminist perspective it provides corroboration of women's insubordination and highlights the need to engage men more substantially in child care. This view predominates in the day care and social policy literature, although there have been voices of dissent (e.g. Leach, 1979; Pringle, 1983). Perhaps constrained by an interview with two men (myself and the husband), few women in the present sample questioned the status quo in any substantial way. Some stoutly defended their conventional role. It would be disrespectful to treat this simply as the product of socialisation and false consciousness. The important issue is no longer to demonstrate that most men and women lead very different lives in which the opportunities for status and power are usually easier for men to take advantage of. What needs doing is to understand people's responses to this situation. This includes examination not only of men's desire to preserve their privileged position, but also of many women's resistance to challenges that they are victims and should act differently (Ungerson, 1983).

A central aspect of course is the special nature and rewards of relationships with children which can obscure or compensate for more negative aspects of women's traditional roles.

Even when there is regret or resentment at the daily grind of meeting children's practical needs many mothers derive an overall sense of satisfaction from bringing up their children (Boulton, 1983; Oakley, 1974b). Some mothers in the present survey described the special joy of watching each detail and stage of a child's development. Fathers too often spoke of the pleasures they experienced with their children but none had apparently concluded that it was necessary to be a full-time carer to derive such satisfaction.

Closely linked to this positive satisfaction was a sense of maternal duty rooted in a mixture of beliefs and values about child development. Although parents' attitudes to sharing care were differentiated according to particular circumstances, there was an underlying negative presumption that it was harmful or risky for children to be away from their mothers unless the set-up was clearly arranged for the child's benefit as in a playgroup. These ideas apparently had deep roots in people's own upbringing. They were embedded and sometimes disguised in the way that people described parenthood, children and sharing care. Statements which embodied value judgments were expressed as if they were matters of fact (e.g. about children's needs). Moral imperatives about responsibilities for children were often stated in a way that appeared to apply to both parents but in practice were largely placed on mothers. Likewise carers referred to as 'family' were mostly grandmothers or aunts. If people spoke with greater honesty this would at least clarify the real position of women's much greater responsibility.

Particularly strong disapproval was expressed by many men *and* women towards working mothers. They assumed that such mothers neglected their children's needs. Such negative epithets may apply in extreme cases but are inappropriate to describe what is normally a careful and conscientious arrangement made by parents. Besides, many mothers took low status jobs for short and perhaps unsocial hours in order to minimise disruption to arrangements for their children. They did so partly because they adhered to the same values and beliefs about children's needs as non-working mothers. This casts doubt on the common inference that the large increase in the number of employed mothers in recent decades really represents a sea-change in social values. The popularity of evening/night work by working-class women while their husbands were responsible for the children also signifies an important divergence from the familiar stereotype of segregated roles. It offers an additional reason besides greater financial strains to explain why a considerably lower proportion of lone mothers than married mothers work part-time (Popay *et al.*, 1983).

Alongside the predominant caution shown about sharing care the study also yielded evidence that a more positive attitude could benefit children and adults. We shall examine in turn the relevant implications for children, women and men. There is no doubt that a child is likely to be very damaged emotionally and socially when *both* separated for an extended period from familiar people and surroundings *and* deprived of consistent loving care. However, there has been an overgeneralisation of this negative extreme of non-family care to apply to much milder forms of non-maternal care. From this sample it was clear that sharing care within social networks was to a greater or lesser extent a normal experience. Average and above average frequencies of shared care did not appear to be harmful and indeed seemed to be advantageous to the children in some respects. All the children had been apart from both parents at some point before they were three and half the children had experienced shared care at least once a week by the time of their third birthday. According to parents' accounts (which may be biased) most children had enjoyed or been little affected by most of their separations from parents. Parental reports supported the view of Greif (1977) that most young children are socio-centric in that they are attracted to interaction with others, especially peers. To be sure many children had been upset by separation at least once and sometimes more often. With a few exceptions, this seemed to have had no lasting effects. Like other forms of transient crying in young children, brief separation protests (though not prolonged distress) may be regarded as a natural part of growing up rather than something to be strenuously avoided.

As there were no independent assessments of the children, any further inferences must be very tentative. Even so it was quite striking that children who were described as clinging, anxious or shy were mainly those who had been with their mothers nearly all the time. Similar conclusions have been reached independently from research in Germany and America (Gudat and Permien, 1980; Thomas and Chess, 1977). Current negative ideas about sharing care may well be self-fulfilling. Anxiety or unfavourable attitudes to shared care may be transmitted to children who therefore perceive being away from their mothers as a rejection rather than a positive gain from someone else. A number of parents in this study had themselves concluded that their strong feelings about not leaving the child had perhaps contributed to lack of beneficial socialising experience. In consequence some decided to share care more freely with second and later children.

It might well benefit young children to get used to operating independently from both parents more than is now the case. It is rare for parents not to have people within their networks willing and able to do this in ways which can be sensitive to the child's capacities and feelings. Good experiences with different carers and settings probably help children to adjust happily on entry to pre-school groups and school itself, as most parents in this study believed. When they have been accustomed to being apart from their mothers they are likely to suffer less should they need to go into hospital alone. Large numbers of children will experience their parents' separation or divorce (Haskey, 1983; Mitchell, 1985). Many may be able to keep in touch with both parents more easily and adjust to having two parental homes better if they have already experienced that other people as well as their mothers can make major contributions to looking after them.

A somewhat more relaxed (though not lax) attitude about sharing care could help women too, by permitting other avenues of fulfilment and assuaging the guilt felt even by mothers who think that high frequency shared care is justified (Ungerson, 1982). There was support for previous findings that it is less crucial to a family whether a mother works or not than whether she is satisfied with whichever of these two options she follows (Hock, 1978, 1980; Yarrow, 1964). Quite a few mothers at home said they were leading satisfied lives though some of these had originally been unsettled or depressed when they began full-time motherhood. A fair number of mothers at home still felt bored or isolated. This appears to be a common consequence of the way in which mothers are expected to assume sole responsibility for infants (Brown *et al.*, 1975; Richman, 1978). One group of women enjoyed having an exclusive relationship with their children but then experienced a strong sense of loss and lack of purpose when they started to go to group care or school. Such people are often keen to fill the gap by looking after other people's children. This leads to the paradox that people who strongly disapprove of sharing care themselves come to rely for their own fulfilment on the fact that other people are willing to have their children minded or even fostered. This contradiction can be a major source of tension (Adamson, 1973; Bryant *et al.*, 1980; Erler, 1980; Rowe *et al.*, 1984).

More involvement in child care by men could be of value and satisfaction to them as well as their wives and children. Moreover, it would help prepare them for the possibility of taking care responsibilities later. More than one in ten of lone parent families are headed by a man (Ferri, 1973; Census, 1981). Children are still sometimes received into care because the mother is absent and the father is unwilling or unable to cope (Grampian, 1978). In old age, many men have to begin for the first time to assume care responsibilities for someone else: 40 per cent of the main carers of elderly infirm people are men, usually husbands looking after their wives (Charlesworth *et al.*, 1984).

No man in this sample had looked after his child as much as his wife. The extent to which fathers looked after their children alone was highly variable. *On average* this occurred about as often as shared care outside the family (excluding group care) but far less than sole care by mothers alone. Many fathers appeared to exercise more selectivity in what tasks, including child care, they carried out. In some cases, even when the father did take charge of his child(ren) the mother had already done or prepared the practical things required. Yet within the overall picture of a sharply uneven role distribution there were some hints of interest in and potential for change. Some men had more experience of young children than their wives and some women had a higher earnings potential than their husbands. Those parents who did voice complaints about their situation (admittedly a minority) often spoke of the excessive demands of the husband's work or insufficient stimulation of the wife's role. In most families it was thought that both parents were equally acceptable to the child as carers and for many couples the father was the main sole carer after the mother.

It does appear that men's involvement in child care may be increasing (Beail and McGuire, 1982) but it clearly remains much less than that of women. A fundamental change is only likely if fathers of young children can spend considerably more time at home. Only then would we approach a situation where couples decided on their particular division of arrangements for work and the family without the presumption that the woman should take the major responsibility for the children. Public policy could encourage this more. A small beginning would be the introduction of parental rather than maternity leave as happens in Sweden (Trost, 1983). Transformations in the nature of work resulting from technological change may or may not assist this process, partly depending on whether there is a will to do so. The sharp distinction between home and work which buttresses the present unequal system of child care may be radically altered in ways which are hard to predict. Theoretically at least, this should give more freedom to both fathers and mothers to determine how, when and where they work and look after their children. This study took place just before the abrupt rise in unemployment. Some people have thought this could weaken conventional role differences but in certain instances it may reinforce them (Binns and Mars, 1984; Fagin and Little, 1984).

Families, networks and exchange relationships

Social science has not given much attention to the ways in which becoming and being a parent alters people's wider social relationships, although some of these consequences may be evident enough to parents themselves. Having children usually causes major changes in social activities and contacts, particularly for women. As we have seen, sharing care can itself play an important part in these alterations. Carers were normally chosen at first from amongst members of parents' prior social networks (especially relatives). The extent to which different kinds of non-relatives were involved in sharing care depended not only on the distance at which close relatives lived but also on parents' differing boundaries of trust and imposition. With experience many couples tested and extended these boundaries so that people who were less close and even strangers became carers. Sharing care was then often a means of making new acquaintanceships or friendships. This particularly involved mothers of similar aged children living close to each other. Parents' influence on children's friendships has been acknowledged (Rubin, 1980) but it has been thought that there is little effect in the opposite direction (Babchuk, 1965). This was not the case in Milburn and to a lesser extent in Whitlaw where having children in general and the interaction of children as individuals often led to a major re-orientation of the parents' friendship networks. Both willingness to share care and the nature of most people's networks were in a greater state of flux and tentativeness with a first child. By the time they had a later child, it was common for people to have become familiar with more people locally and to have lessened their fears about leaving their children.

Looking after children is not simply a very personal aspect of social relationships. It is also in one sense a service performed for parents. That evokes feelings and expectations about doing something in return. Depending on the situation this can involve cash payments, reciprocal child care or a more notional form of 'repayment'. There were four main types of social relationship relevant to sharing care and each was characterised by a distinctive kind of exchange (Table 8.1). Litwak and Szelenyi (1969) provided a classic summary of how services performed within networks tend to take different forms according to the type of relationship involved. They stated that kin are used for major care commitments, neighbours assist with brief or sudden immediate needs and friends provide mainly non-practical help. This picture was broadly confirmed in the present study but it was also seen that neighbours can become friends and then give much day to day practical assistance. In addition kin may live close enough to fulfil most or all network care needs, if the parents wish this.

Writers from diverse backgrounds have pointed out that the

social distance and relative status of the parties engaged in social exchanges affect the implicit rules which govern interaction. In particular, relatives are more likely to engage in unbalanced or delayed exchange than friends and neighbours (La Gaipa, 1981; Leach, 1982; Sahlins, 1965). This was borne out in relation to sharing care. With a few exceptions, parents did not expect to give relatives any direct or equivalent 'repayment', whereas care by non-relatives was usually seen to need more immediate and exact reciprocation. Sometimes parents or their relations vehemently denied any implication that looking after children within the extended family had any exchange connotations. This did not mean that they were irrelevant. The norm of kin giving (Halbertsma, 1968) meant that it was important for relatives to think they were doing something out of selfless family commitment, yet parents themselves were affected by feelings that they should do something in appreciation. Therefore, they often made symbolic or indirect returns. It was 'intercategorical' in the sense that the means of return was different in nature from the original care service (Cook, 1982). Exchange with relatives was also often viewed in an intergenerational context, particularly in working-class extended families. In other words, someone (usually a female) had been looked after as a young child by an older sister, cousin or aunt, then in later years babysat for the children of that relative.

The second main type of exchange relationship concerned neighbours – people living close by, some but not all of whom were also friends. Several observers of the urban scene have doubted whether there is much sense of mutual obligation or support given by people living in the same neighbourhood unless they are related to each other (Abrams, 1978; Fisher, 1975; Stacey, 1969). This is based in part on the idea that most people's social contacts in urban areas do not live in the same district (Clarke, 1982). High rates of movement in and out of an area are seen as particularly inimical to service-giving by neighbours. Following Bott's hypothesis it has been thought that close-knit networks usually consist mainly of kin and are most prevalent in working-class areas. Contrary to all these suppositions, in Milburn a number of self-help social systems of high connectedness had developed amongst un-

Table 8.1 Summary of the patterns of shared care and exchange relationships found in the sample

Type of relationship	Social intimacy and child care	Exchange aspects	Typical working-class variants	Typical middle-class variants
1 Relatives	Socially close on a lifetime basis. Child care often a small element of overall relationship	Unbalanced exchange. If at all, the return given to carers is delayed; of a different kind; often symbolic.	Grandparent care common, but also often other generations with interwoven reciprocity over the years. Sometimes kin carers used exclusively.	Mainly grandparent care. Often combined with non-kin care for other purposes/time of day.
2 Friends/ Neighbours	A Previously close friends commonly used in early stages of parenthood for sharing care.	Balanced giving and receiving of the same kind of practical childcare service.	A Rare or non-existent.	Generalised exchange amongst several or many families. Highly formalised evening care arrangements (babysitting circles).
	B Particularly later on, friendships develop partly as a result of sharing care.		B Exchange between a pair of families primarily for daytime care.	

3 Paid Childcarers	Normally, social distance and status difference is maintained.	Immediate cash payment at market value.	A Use of minders for long hours of work care. B Payment to kin teenagers for evening care.	A Use of minders or au pairs for long hours of work. B Payment to non-kin teenagers for evening care. C Daily helps for occasional care.
4 Group Care Staff	Normally social distance is maintained.	A Indirect cash payment (rates); perceived as free service. B Immediate cash payment at market value or reduced by subsidy.	Use of state nursery schools; or voluntary organisation playgroups.	Use of state nursery schools; or private profit-making playgroups and nursery schools; or self-help playgroups.

related neighbours in a limited locality. This happened even though there was a considerable turnover of population. Exchanges of child care services with friends and neighbours normally involved rough equivalence of giving and receiving. Many shared care arrangements in both areas just entailed pair exchange whereby two mothers looked after each other's children with more or less equal frequency. However, most parents in Milburn belonged to more extended swop networks or circles. These are examples of generalised exchange in which obligations to return are governed by the overall system and not tied to specific individuals. In such multi-family constellations it is not necessary to share care at the same frequency with each partner so long as there is an overall balance within the whole network or group. Amongst the benefits of generalised exchange are easier matching of the supply and demand of care services, diffusion of the sense of personal indebtedness to individual carers and opportunities for making friends and developing joint social activities.

A third form of reciprocity was based on complementarity rather than kinship or symmetry. For teenagers and sometimes for strangers the balance of exchange was preserved not by equivalent services but by cash payment. This was normally seen as incompatible with friendship which is a relationship of equals, so that friends were hardly ever paid for sharing care. Conversely, paid childcarers did not become friends.

Can any helpful inferences be drawn about the wider applicability of such kinds of service-giving? With regard to child care, it would seem that some isolated parents who lack close kin support nearby might benefit from being carefully introduced by community leaders or professionals to either existing or artificially created local networks. This would need sensitivity to people's concerns about stranger care. In theory it is possible to envisage caring networks which included other kinds of dependent people beside children such as the handicapped or infirm elderly. However, this did not happen in practice. As Weitman (1978) has pointed out, helping networks have limitations in that they exclude as well as include people. Circles and swop networks included only people at a similar life-cycle stage so that there were common interests and equivalence of exchange implications. Even single parents find it difficult to comply with the need for reciprocity since they have nobody at home to free them to go out and babysit as couples do. Some networks did seek to adjust to this factor. On the whole it seems more promising to encourage separate self-help and relief care networks for the carers of different kinds of dependent person. The Equal Opportunities Commission (1982a, 1982b) has documented the many strains which can be experienced by those looking after elderly or handicapped people. Besides officially sponsored relief schemes, some form of swop care by people in the same position and modelled on babysitting circle principles could ease the burdens and perhaps also provide social benefits. Indeed this is already happening in small ways (Rossiter and Wicks, 1982; Walker, 1982). The idea of paying teenagers and others to act as carers may also have wider applicability, but caution would be needed because of common misgivings about young people's competence and trustworthiness.

Much of our theoretical understanding of exchange derives from the analyses about the motives and interests of the giver. The present study showed how the feelings of *recipients* about an actual or potential child care service were also crucial in determining whether it might start or persist. This finding fits with our growing understanding about aid to needy old people (Abrams, 1980; Leat, 1982, 1983; Sundstrom, 1983). One consequence is that those wishing to help others may do well to provide opportunities for the receiver of help to give something back, even if this is done in a symbolic, non-equivalent way. Otherwise the helping relationship may be curtailed by the recipient in order to preserve pride or feelings of autonomy. As Emerson (1976) has argued, ideas about exchange drawn from economics and psychology which emphasise self-interest and reward may need modification when applied to ongoing social relationships. In this study, people felt most at ease with arrangements which were co-operative and mutual in some way. Pinker (1979) postulated that people's willingness *to give* to others diminishes through concentric circles of people of decreasing closeness and identification. Most of the couples interviewed also had concentric 'we-groups' in relation to *receiving help* with their children. Relatives and close friends normally but not invariably formed the inner circle, beyond which willingness to venture for sharing care varied greatly.

Class, networks and exchange

For a long time now both social scientists and lay people have looked upon social class as a major determinant of differences in family life. In recent times there have been suggestions that these contrasts have lessened as a result of the 'embourgeoisement' of working-class families, a 'downward' diffusion of values or convergence of life-styles (Buttimer, 1972; Goldthorpe and Lockwood, 1963; Young and Willmott, 1973). In this sample there were important characteristics which appeared to be largely independent of class such as 'protectiveness' in sharing care, the range of hours that mothers worked, and the desire for group care at the age of three. Nevertheless, striking class contrasts in social relationships and care patterns were still apparent in these two areas of Edinburgh in the early 1980s (Table 8.1). This had a big influence on the degree and manner of involvement in a child's early development of kin and non-kin, men and women, teenagers and peers.

In both classes a spectrum of care sequences was to be found but there was a definite trend for most working-class parents to share care less often than most middle-class parents. By and large they were reluctant to trust or impose on people they had not known for a long time. This was linked to an ideal of neighbouring which valued peaceful non-interference rather than personal intimacy or mutual service-giving. The main exceptions to this occurred when a pair of families living next door formed a close bond. Relatives were frequently involved in working-class families' home life and child care, but parents' friends were often seen outside the home away from the children in the evenings (cf. Allan, 1979). The working-class couples' reluctance to accept help *with child care* and *inside the home* from outside the kin network may have wider significance. For example, in the fields of educational enrichment and social work prevention much emphasis is not put on professionals or volunteers facilitating change by intervention in the home. Some are undoubtedly successful (van der

Eycken, 1982), but others may founder unless they are sensitive to people's boundary maintaining mechanisms.

In contrast most middle-class couples expected to develop close relationships with other families living round about. They hoped and planned that this would provide playmates and play activities for the children and also facilitate their own ability to carry on an active social life. This had resulted in quite elaborate and formalised systems of reciprocal shared care. There was not the same necessity for close personalised links before someone became a carer and sometimes the relationships with other local parents were largely confined to practical help. Whereas some working-class parents were outraged at the thought of sharing care outside the kin network, some middle-class parents preferred the clear 'contract' they associated with care by non-relatives in contrast to the emotional complications which they felt arose with relatives as carers. On the other hand many couples had formed social ties of considerable strength and personal importance with other parents living nearby. Sharing care was often a vital element in initiating or extending these relationships.

It would be necessary to compare people in other areas before it can be concluded that these differences represent wider social class characteristics rather than local variations. A few interviews carried out in other districts showed that they at least had a wider generality within Edinburgh. In addition, the patterns are consistent with earlier analyses of social relationships, class and community (Seabrook, 1967; Willmott and Young, 1960). The class differences in boundaries of trust and imposition which applied to sharing care also resemble contrasts in the structuring of communication and authority discerned by other writers. Bernstein's theory of linguistic codes suggested that middle-class children learn from their parents to express themselves in flexible and individualistic ways. Working-class children are more inclined to converse without making clear the contexts of what they are talking about (Bernstein, 1971, 1977). The working-class children in the present study usually spent more of their time with close relatives who were very familiar and understood their situation very well so that there would be less need to explain everything to them. Middle-class children were more likely to have graduated opportunities to meet varied people outside the family which may call for more adaptable modes of communication. Likewise Kohn (1969) identified somewhat similar dispositions for working-class parents to encourage conformity and traditionalism in their children, whereas middle-class parents were seen to favour autonomy and self-control for their offspring. Thus both Kohn and Bernstein were implicitly discussing the closeness and fixity of boundaries around the family.

Kohn attributed these differences to features of men's work settings. He argued that fathers repeat at home the kinds of communication and thinking required for their jobs. Similarly, both parents may foster the qualities in their children which may suit them in the kinds of work for which they are likely to be destined. Manual jobs usually require obedience to routines whilst non-manual jobs give opportunities for greater independence of action and rely on more internalised responsibility for carrying out tasks. Without denying the importance of fathers' work situations for family life, it is at least as plausible that women's educational and work experience will be very important in affecting parental values, given that most child care is done by mothers. Many middle-class mothers in this sample and more generally have had education which builds up an expectation of some kind of career and therefore a future orientation. Often the specific kind of work done before parenthood embodies ideas about children and play since many have worked as nurses, teachers, doctors, social workers, etc. It seems quite likely that theories and practices which emphasise the social and intellectual importance of the pre-school period have been transmitted through middle-class mothers' networks which therefore emphasise opportunities for play, learning and mixing. Many working-class mothers have done clerical or manual work which does not encourage an active role nor provide guidance about child care. 'Learning' is highly valued as a means of providing their own children with better life-chances but their own experience has often given them little of the knowledge or confidence to believe that they can contribute much to this themselves. Therefore it is best left to teachers in formal pre-school groups.

The working-class pattern of near exclusive care by relatives is a more universal one since kin care predominates in most non-Westernised societies. One obvious explanation of the greater middle-class openness to care by non-relatives is mobility but this is coupled with resocialisation processes. In this research and in the wider survey by Goldthorpe *et al.* (1980) it appeared that social status and mobility were less important than geographical mobility. When middle-class couples lived near kin they normally shared care at least as often with them as working-class couples. More crucial than the fact in itself of having moved from one's area of origin was the distance from close relatives, who often though not always remained in the original locality. Most respondents in both areas now lived away from the district they had grown up in, but a far higher proportion of middle-class parents had moved beyond the easy reach of close relatives. Moreover the influence of distance from kin operated at a social as well as an individual level. In Whitlaw the majority of families felt they could meet their routine care needs within the kin network. This meant that the minority of families lacking nearby kin support did not encounter other people nearby who also wanted to share care with unrelated local people. In Milburn the majority of middle-class families had to look outside the kin network if they were to share care routinely. That common need prompted reciprocal arrangements. The substantial minority who had regular kin carers in Edinburgh became involved with the street care networks around them in order to meet with tacit requirements of social exchange. It was difficult to become friends without being prepared to look after someone else's child. It was hard to do that unless you also allowed the other person to look after your child, even if you already had relatives already willing and available. This illustrates how the form and composition of people's social networks can both create opportunities and may apply pressures to conform (Marsden and Lin, 1982). Membership of street care networks was not always immediate or automatic. Both native and incomer couples described how they had only gradually accepted the idea of using people outside 'the family' and perhaps eventually strangers. A process of persuasion and desensitisation of anxieties about stranger care led them to relax their boundaries of trust step by step. The few working-

class couples living in Milburn appeared to be excluded from
such processes partly out of feelings of status distance from
the majority of people around them.

What are the implications of these differences? It must be
emphasised that there is no desire to establish new stereo-
types. There were exceptions to all the generalisations and
families differed for many reasons other than class. Even so
some conventional ideas may need modifying. It is commonly
thought that working-class parents encourage more street
interaction with peers and encourage their children to be independent (Donachy, 1979; Lewis *et al.*, 1975). The evidence from
this research is that *at the pre-school stage* those children who
mixed little with other children nearby were mainly working
class whereas many middle-class children had very active
social lives with street friends. Similarly the idea that old
established working-class areas have intimate communities
is contradicted by the situation in Whitlaw. The persisting
predominance of manual workers in an inner city area may
disguise the fact that the majority are newcomers and there
is no common occupation to act as a focus for integration.

Networks, group care and collective responsibility

A family's network contacts can influence attitudes about
group care and reactions to it in a number of ways. Parents'
preparedness to make use of facilities and their perception of
them as 'a good thing' were often instigated and confirmed by
observing or holding detailed discussions with neighbours or
friends who had made use of them. In just a few cases normative pressures led some people to use group care when they
preferred not to. These correspond to the child-centred mothers
identified in other research as being non-users of group care
(Blomart, 1963; Shinman, 1981). Social networks rather than
professionals, educationalists or local authorities were the
prime source of information and evaluation about group care.
For the most part such informal communication was effective
and satisfactory, but some people who did not have contacts
with existing users wanted more official information about
pre-school facilities. This is likely to apply even more to
newcomers to an area who were not present in this sample.

The nature of network interactions also influence children's and parents' responses to group care through their effects on social and emotional development. This was in turn mediated by differences in parental attitudes and social class. Either by design or as a by-product of other values, some parents had given their children plenty of practice in dealing with separations whereas others had not. Many middle-class mothers deliberately set out to prepare their children for playgroup or nursery school by means of mini-groups and regular peer play. The playgroup movement has been explained by reference to middle-class mothers' skills in organising their children's experiences. These were here seen in operation *prior* to attendance at pre-school groups. This meant that middle-class children usually started at playgroup or nursery school with at least one familiar companion. That was true for far fewer of the working-class children. That is perhaps offset by the fact that they were more closely integrated into a stable set of familiar people whose relationships extended back far longer in time. This often included more contact with men, older people and teenagers than was the case for many middle-class children.

Group care experience also had feedback effects on network interaction. As Warren and Rothman (1981) have argued, public and voluntary services do not necessarily undermine network support systems. They may even assist their development. Particularly in Milburn, pre-school groups were places where some mothers initiated and elaborated local acquaintanceships. Most working-class mothers appeared to lack the shared expectations and necessary confidence to do this unless there was some formalised opportunity to mix at the group itself. That is something which is encouraged at most playgroups but arranged less frequently at nursery schools, yet these are the main kinds of group in working-class areas.

Some experts have characterised entry to playgroups, nurseries and nursery schools as children's first major step outside the nuclear family or at least as their first experience of an organised group (e.g. Blatchford *et al.*, 1982:1–2; Bruner, 1980). In fact, all the children in the present sample had been previously looked after by someone other than their parents and for many this had occurred at least once a week. Over half had prior experience in some other kind of group (such as toddler groups, church and sports creches, ballet classes). More than one in three had stayed in a group without a parent being there. There seems to be a need to pay more attention to the significance of these miscellaneous groups. Some had been fine but others appeared to lack adequate facilities or supervision.

To what extent did group care duplicate network care or provide a distinctive alternative? Networks did meet many couples' wishes for alternative child care in day to day living. Potential crises such as the hospitalisation of the mother for childbirth were coped with informally – usually by means of care by grandmothers and fathers. There were limitations, though. Only rarely did people's prior social networks sustain any need or wish for prolonged daily care whether this be to permit both parents to work at the same time or to cater for children's perceived socio-educational needs. This is because of carers' other commitments, parents' concern not to impose and requirements of reciprocity in relation to friends and neighbours (see also Allan, 1983).

All but a few of the families had several network members willing and able to share care. Nevertheless, nearly everyone thought that attendance at a playgroup or a nursery school was an essential supplement to what they and their networks offered to their children. Similarly, the vast majority were highly satisfied with what such groups provided. The rate of attendance was exceptionally high in comparison with other survey results for children before their fourth birthday. This seems only partly explicable by the fact that the sample was confined to two parent families who had lived in the same area for some time. It is also improbable that these areas represent exceptional needs since they are located in a comparatively prosperous city. Two major factors seem to account for the high take-up of places. One is the relatively large number of facilities which itself means that demand which is hypothetical elsewhere can be actualised here. Just as important was that informal communications had established traditions such that arranging for one's child to go to group care had mostly come to be taken for granted. It was seen as a natural and appropriate response to the needs and capacities of children at the age of three in a modern urban environment. Almost universal agreement about the multiple benefits of group care for children was to be found amongst families with high and low incomes, spacious and cramped accommodation, good and poor access to play space. Similar values about group care applied regardless of sharply contrasting attitudes to other forms of sharing care.

Contrary to some opinions, it was clear that group care was not used for parental convenience but co-existed with strong values about maternal duty. When mothers worked they had nearly always begun to do so well before the child went to a playgroup or nursery school. The wish to place their child in a group did not derive from their own motivation to work. Looked at from a different angle this simply means that on the whole children with working mothers started at group care at similar times and for similar reasons as those with non-working mothers. This explains the situation, which puzzled Halsey and Smith (1976), that far more mothers work while their child is at a group than give work as a reason for using that group. Group care was seen by nearly every parent to offer opportunities for play, social interaction and professional stimulation which mothers could not provide in their own homes or with the help of their social networks. In many cases, a child's own enthusiasm to attend was an important factor too. Thus the case for provision of group care on demand does not need to rest on the needs of working mothers or special categories of children. It can give all children access to peers and learning opportunities in a child-centred setting which is otherwise difficult to achieve in an environment largely designed with adults and traffic in mind.

Only a decade ago, these findings would have fitted happily with an admittedly brief acceptance by policy-makers that it was desirable to provide pre-school facilities for all parents who want a place (Plowden, 1967; White Paper, 1972a, 1972b). Since then Lady Plowden has changed her mind about the desirability of public pre-school education (Finch, 1982; Granada, 1985). Expansion of nursery education has also ceased to be a government priority. This study has shown that the demand has not gone away and is more widespread than is commonly assumed. Even in this relatively trouble-free sample a fair number of mothers indicated that they or their children had or would have had considerable frustration or tensions without group care. This applied particularly to mothers who were somewhat isolated from street networks, had very active two-year-olds or twins, or spoke English as a second language. Although ambivalence about the value of pre-school care has always made it vulnerable at times of recession, it is also true that falling school rolls have meant that parts of educational buildings may now be under-used. There are also unemployed teachers needing work. These resources could be put to work for the benefit of the under-fives.

Of course pre-school groups do not all need to be provided directly by the state, though much of the voluntary sector receives subsidies from local government (Lothian, 1984). Some parents like to have a choice and the opportunity to shop around. However, there are problems resulting from the fragmentation and diversity of pre-school daytime facilities (Watt, 1976; Dicks, 1983). This has contributed to the pleas for publicly provided combined centres which might cater for all needs under one roof (Hughes *et al.*, 1980; Sheffield, 1986). That idea received some support from the present findings. Parents used playgroups and nursery schooling for the same reasons and evaluated them with comparable criteria, so that in most respects it seems legitimate to regard them as similar services. A majority of parents preferred local authority provision to others and the main deficit identified was in the need which was expressed but not fully met in the middle-class area for more nursery education places. Three quarters of all the parents in the sample wanted their child to attend a state nursery school by the age of four. On the other hand, a significant minority preferred the intimacy and informality of a playgroup; this would be hard to maintain within a larger unit. There seems to be a continuing need for playgroup-type settings, although perhaps as much to provide a preparation for nursery school as an alternative.

Contrary to much professional opinion, issues of involvement in group care were not prominent for many mothers. Most welcomed social and fund-raising activities but only a minority in both classes liked the idea of helping to run a group. There were many instances where there was a mismatch between desired and actual involvement. In the day care field, there has been much discussion about the desirability and practicability of extending 'middle-class' arrangements such as participative playgroups to working-class areas. A section of hard-pressed working-class families find the idea of playgroups irrelevant or difficult to make use of, because of life-style factors, women's work patterns and lack of organising skills or connections (Finch, 1983, 1984). Most working-class parents in this study had strong doubts about the suitability of other untrained parents taking responsibility for their children but several happily made use of professionally run playgroups and others were attracted by this format. Preferences for playgroups and mothers' participation were not so much related to social class as to a high valuation of a particularly close mother-child relationship.

Professionals impinge on shared care in two ways – as advisers and as group carers. In certain cases health visitors had clearly given very useful advice to parents but there remains a need for a ensuring that all parents have adequate knowledge about local provision for their young children. Conversely, playgroup leaders and nursery school staff often know little about children before they come. This avoids potential dangers of intrusiveness and stereotyping but group carers might be in a better position to help children adapt to the new setting if they knew more about a child's prior sequence of care and previous reactions to shared care. Other relevant considerations would be a child's general sociability and experience with peers. It may also be helpful if staff and parents communicate with each other more openly about their respective views on the best ways to help children settle in. Group carers are naturally very busy with the children in their charge but some also pay attention to the social functions of group care for parents. It would be beneficial if all groups gave conscious attention to opportunities for mothers to mix, should they want to, by means of coffee rooms, social events or meetings. This could be especially useful to first-time mothers and those not linked to street networks. A number of fathers are free in the daytime too though some may be inhibited about participating in what may be looked upon as a 'woman's place' (Mr Robertson*). Evening events can help overcome this.

Conclusions

This study has hopefully shown the richness of examining the interaction between children's development and their social milieux which are often investigated separately. There were limitations of scale so that it would be useful to test the applicability of the findings in other areas and with different kinds of families such as one parent households or those with two unemployed parents. A longitudinal project would be valuable to see the subtle interplay of parents' and children's social relationships, of parental and non-parental care, as they affect each other over time.

Secure continuing relationships with a limited number of adults appears to be vital for children's satisfactory development (Smith, 1979). However, there is now a considerable body of evidence to show that this generalisation has been interpreted too narrowly by many 'experts' and parents. Children's needs are compatible with a considerable range of carers and care experiences. Indeed excessive concentration on the mother-child bond may hamper children's adaptability and eventual independence. Some of the undoubted constraints and stresses of parenthood could be relieved by more positive attitudes to sharing care. Provided that the carers are or become familiar and trusted, this should not harm the children and may benefit them. This means that there is scope for a fairer distribution of responsibilities for child care amongst mothers, fathers, network members and organised group arrangements.

Appendix

Research questionnaire
Please note that questions were asked in the context of a semi-structured interview, so that the order and wording were not precisely as stated here but adjusted to the course of the conversation in each interview.

In each family, just one three-year-old child was the focus of the interview and is referred to as C in the questionnaire. M denotes the mother and F the father. Some questions were put using written forms and these are included at the end of the questionnaire (Forms A–G). Form H gives an outline of the diary which recorded children's carers and activities for a two week period.

Interview details

Date, time and length of interview
People present at interview

Basic family data

C's date of birth
C's sex
C's birth order
Ages and sexes of C's siblings
Is family complete or not?

Non-group care

First year   Who looked after C, when, how often, for how long, where and for what reason? Who took the initiative and how was it arranged? How did the child react to care? Where did the care take place and what travel arrangements were involved?

Second year   As first year

Third year   As first year
Has C ever asked to stay with other people? In what circumstances?
Have the parents looked after the carers' children?
What difference does it make to C if care is at home or away?
Who is the current main daytime carer?
Who is the current second daytime carer?
Who is the current main evening carer
Who is the current second evening carer?
How often do you use an evening babysitter?
Have you ever used a paid babysitter? In what circumstances?
Do you have any reciprocal care arrangements?
Do you belong to a babysitting circle or group?
If not, what do you think about them?
If yes, how many members are there? How is it organised? How did it develop? How far are fathers involved in the circle? How did you come to join the circle?

Group care

Did C go to a mother and toddler group?
If yes, what was the experience like?
Has C been to any form of group?
In the case of a group other than a playgroup or nursery school, what kind of place was this, how did C react and what was the purpose of the arrangement?
At what age did C start at playgroup or nursery school?
At what age did C change group, if at all?
What is the group currently attended? Where is it?
How many children and staff are there at the group?
What are the days and hours of attendance?
Who takes and collects C? How do they get there?
How did C react when he/she first started?
How have C's reactions changed?

Before C started, how did you think he/she would react?

What do you think is the best way to help children settle in a group?

What changes in C's behaviour have you noticed?

What worries, if any, did you have about C going?

How many children did C know at the group before starting?

How have the other children there affected C?

Why did you decide that C should go to playgroup or nursery school?

Why did you choose that particular group?

Why did you choose that age for starting? What difference would it have made if C had started earlier or later?

How did you first learn about the group?

Have you received any advice from a professional person?

What benefits have there been for C?

What benefits have there been for M?

What benefits have there been for F?

What disadvantages have there been for C?

What disadvantages have there been for M?

What disadvantages have there been for F?

What are your views about the staff?

What are your views of the facilities?

What, if any, improvements would you like to see in the group?

What, if any, improvement would you like to see in the general provision for pre-school children round here?

What kind of involvement does M have with the group?

What kind of involvement would M like with the group?

What kind of contact does F have with the group?

How much interaction do M and F have with other parents?

Costs of care

Weekly costs of group care?

Weekly costs of non-group care?

Cost per hour or evening of babysitter?

Future plans

Do you expect C to change playgroup or nursery before starting school?

If so, what would the change be?

Do you envisage any changes in the days and hours of attendance for C before starting school?

Do you foresee any changes in your babysitting arrangements?

Non-users of group care

Do you expect C to go to a playgroup or nursery school?

Is C booked into a playgroup or nursery school?

When do you think C will start?

Why would you like C to go?

Why did you choose that particular group?

What hours and days do you expect C to attend for?

What kind of involvement would M like?

How did you first learn about the group you expect C to go to?

Have you been given advice by a professional person?

What difference would it have made if C could have started earlier?

How do you think C will react?

C's siblings and care

From what age(s) did C's older sibling(s) attend a group?

How did they get on?

How did this affect arrangements for C?

How, if at all, do you think you may change arrangements for a younger sibling, based on your experience with C?

Network relationships

Could you please tell me which relatives C has seen in the last year? For each one, where do they live and how often has face to face contact occurred? Are they working? Do they have a car? (See Form A)

How old are C's grandparents?

If a grandparent is dead, how long ago did he or she die?

What does C call his/her grandparents?

Do the grandparents have any health problems?

Did F's and M's relatives know each other, before M and F met? If so, how well?

Do the two sides of the family meet each other?

Do your family know your friends?

Which relatives, if any, have you been away on holiday with since C was born?

How many cousins under five does C have?

What kind of contact does C have with his/her cousins?

Could you tell me about your friends who are important to C? (See Form B) Where do they live? How often does C meet them? Which ones are single? If they have children, how old are they?

How did you come to know them?

Have you made any friends through C? If so, how?

Have there been friends you have less contact with as a result of having children? If so, which ones and why?

Do your friends mostly know each other or not?

How do you get on with people in the street?

How do you get on with the people next door?

How many people in the street have become friends?

How many young children are there in the street?

Does C play with children in the street?

How many friends does C have in the street?

The child's attachments (See Form C)

(a) Adults
Ranking of parents – equal, M first or F first
Description of people who are ranked first, second and third
Total number of people in the list
Number of kin
Number of parents' friends
Number of care staff
Number of females

(b) Children
Total number in the list
Number who are relatives
Number who are female
Number who do not live locally
Number at each age

Details of anyone C does not like

The child's development

Was the birth straightforward? If not, what complications were there?

Was F present at birth?

How well prepared for parenthood did M feel?

How well prepared for parenthood did F feel?

What worries have you had as parents?

Has C's development been normal?

Has C had any serious illnesses? If so, what and when?

Details of any time C has been in hospital overnight – duration, reasons, age

Details of any time C has been apart from parents overnight – carer, duration, reasons, age, home or away

How did C react to these separations?

Who would be the first choice person for an overnight stay now?

What arrangements would the family make if M had to go into hospital (a) for a few nights (b) for an extended period?

How would you describe C's personality?

What kind of things does C enjoy doing most?

How does C get on with other children?

How does C get on with adults he/she does not know so well?

Parents' personal data

Note The same questions were asked of both F and M in turn

Date of birth

Area where brought up

Occupations of parents (i.e. the child's grandparents)

How old were you when your mother went back to work after having children (a) part-time (b) full-time?

Number of siblings and birth order

Did you attend any form of group before you were five?

Who would have been the main person who babysat for you when you were a child?

What experience of young children did you have before you were married?

Did you ever act as a babysitter?

Did you have any major separations from your parents as a child? If so, give details

Did anyone close to you die, when you were a child? If so, who was it and how old were you?

What type of secondary school did you attend?

What has been your highest qualification?

How do you think your childhood experiences have affected your views of care of children and babysitting, the kinds of thing we have been talking about?

F's work

Note Non-working fathers were asked about their last job and how long ago they became unemployed

What is your job (and position)?

Where do you work?

How do you travel to work?

How long does it take to get there?

What are your normal hours of work?

How long have you been with your present employer?

What are the good things about your job?

What are the things which are not so good about your job?

How much contact does C have with your workplace?

How much contact does C have with the people you work with?

M's work

(a) All mothers

Did you work until you were married or until you had children?

What was your job, then?

When you stopped work, when did you think you would go back to work?

What did you miss about work?

What were you glad to have given up?

What work have you done since C was born? Give details

Did you work in between children? Give details

(b) Mothers currently working

What is your current job (and position)?
Where do you work?
How do you travel there?
How long does it take?
What are your normal working hours?
How long have you been with your present employer?
What are the good things about your job?
What things are not so good?
Why did you go back to work?
What effects do you think your working has had on C?
How much contact does C have with your workplace?
How much contact does C have with the people you work with?
What are F's views about M's return to work?
What are M's and F's views about working mothers in general?

(c) Mothers not currently working

What are the benefits of being at home?
What disadvantages are there?
What are M's and F's views about working mothers?
Would you consider working at a time when F could look after
    the children?
When does M expect to return to work?

Income

F's net weekly take home pay
M's net weekly take home pay

Parents' opinions about care and children

Answers to attitude questions on Forms D, E, F
What do you think has most effect on a child's personality?
What age, if any, do you think is most important for affecting
    a child's personality?
What has influenced your attitudes about care of young
    children?
It seems that many more children now go to some kind of
    playgroup or nursery school than in the past. What do you
    think of this change?

What do you think about the differences between playgroups and nursery schools?

At what age have you found C most enjoyable?

At what age has C been most difficult?

Family life and parental roles

How long have you been married?

How long did you know each other before that?

What do you think helps most to make a happy family?

Is there anything which gets in the way of happiness for your family?

Answers to the questions about housework and care of children from Form E

In your family, who does what in the following activities?

Shopping

Cleaning the house

Cooking

Washing up

Washing clothes

Bathing the children

Nappy changing (when C was younger)

Does the pattern for housework differ from before you had children?

How often, and for what reason, does F look after C while M is not there?

How often do you go out together in the evenings?

How often do you go out separately?

What are F's main interests?

What are M's main interests?

Where have you been for your main holiday each year since C was born?

Class

What social class would you say you belong to?

What does class mean to you?

What other classes are there?

Stress

Malaise inventory scores from Form G
What pressures do you have as parents?
How do these compare with other pressures on you?

Housing and mobility

How long have you lived at the present address?
How long have you lived in the present area?
Why are you living in Edinburgh?
Why did you come to this part of Edinburgh?
Housing tenure
Does C have his/her own bedroom?
What kind of garden do you have?
What is the area round here like for playspace?
Do you use the playspace much?
Do you own a car?
Who drives in the family?
Does M have access to a car in the daytime?
If you have a car, what difference has this made to care arrangements for C?
If you do not have a car, what difference might it have made, if you had had one?

Neighbourhood

What is the name of this area?
What do you think of it as an area for bringing up children?
What advantages are there for children in this area?
What disadvantages are there for children in this area?
What do you think of this area for adults?
What are the advantages for adults?
What are the disadvantages for adults?
Would you like to move anywhere else? If so, where?
Would you say you are similar to other people round here?

II Research forms

Form A

Contacts with relatives
The following information was obtained about each relative, who had been seen by the child at least once in the last year:
Relationship to child
Area of residence
Approximate frequency and duration of contacts with the child
Working or not
Has a car or not

Form B

Contacts with non-kin
The following information was obtained about friends or neighbours who were considered by the parents to be important to the child:
Nature of relationship to parents
Marital status
Area of residence
Approximate frequency and duration of contact with the child
Ages of children

Form C

The child's attachments
A list was made of the adults C was thought to be most fond of, in order. The person's relationship to the child was noted. A similar list was made of the children C was said to be most fond of, with their age and relationship to C. A note was also made of any person the child was thought to dislike.

Form D

Parents' views about sharing care at different ages
Parents were asked to indicate at which age they thought it
was all right for a child to be away from his or her parents in
the following circumstances:

1 With relatives or friends
For brief periods
Regularly for part of the day
Regularly for the whole day

2 In a playgroup or nursery centre or nursery school
For brief periods
Regularly for part of the day
Regularly for the whole day
In each case, parents were asked to indicate an age at half
yearly intervals from six months to five years.

Form E

Views about care of young children
Parents were asked to respond to a number of statements with
one of the following:
  1 Disagree
  2 Strongly disagree
  3 Agree
  4 Strongly agree
  5 Feel neutral about
  6 Have mixed feelings about
These were the statements:
  1 Care of young children should be the equal responsibility
    of both parents.
  2 Children under five should not normally attend any form
    of day care for the whole day.
  3 It should be made easier for fathers of young children to
    work for shorter hours.
  4 There should be a money allowance to encourage
    mothers of young children to stay home.

5 It benefits the family if the mother works at least part-time.

6 Mothers of young children should not normally work at all during the day.

7 Boys and girls need to be treated differently by their parents.

8 It helps children to have experience outside the home for a full day from three to five.

9 Children under five are harmed if both parents work full-time.

10 Part-time experience outside the home is good for children under three.

11 Day care centres should be used only by families with special needs.

12 Any parents who wish to do so should be able to use a day care centre.

13 Children should be encouraged to be independent from their parents.

14 Housework should be mainly a woman's responsibility.

In addition, parents were asked to complete the following sentence:

What I feel most strongly about in relation to the care of young children is . . .

Form F

Views about types of care

Parents were asked to note which care arrangements from the following list they thought to be the two which were most helpful to families, and the two which were least helpful.

1 Corporation day nursery

2 Private day nursery

3 Nursery school or class

4 Private school or kindergarten

5 Playgroup run by mothers

6 Playgroup run by trained staff

7 Workplace creche or nursery

8 Childminder

9 Mother and children's group

Form G

Malaise inventory
NB The original inventory was used in the Isle of Wight and
CHES studies (Osborn *et al.*, 1984; Rutter *et al.*, 1970). As a
result of an unfortunate error, one question was inadvertently
omitted in copying this. That did not significantly affect the
variations within the sample but must have reduced score
levels slightly in comparison with other samples.

Parents were asked to state how many of the following questions they answered 'Yes' to.

1 Do you often have backache?
2 Do you feel tired most of the time?
3 Do you often feel miserable or depressed?
4 Do you often have bad headaches?
5 Do you usually have great difficulty in falling asleep or
staying asleep?
6 Do you usually wake unnecessarily early in the
morning?
7 Do you wear yourself out worrying about your health?
8 Do you often get into a violent rage?
9 Do people often annoy or irritate you?
10 Have you at times had a twitching of face, head or
shoulders?
11 Do you often suddenly become scared for no good reason?
12 Are you scared to be alone when there are no friends
near?
13 Are you easily upset or irritated?
14 Are you frightened of going out alone or of meeting
people?
15 Are you constantly keyed up or jittery?
16 Do you suffer from indigestion?
17 Do you often suffer from upset stomach?
18 Is your appetite poor?
19 Does every little thing get on your nerves and wear you
out?
20 Does your heart often race like mad?

21 Do you often have bad pains in your eyes?
22 Are you troubled with rheumatism or fibrositis?
23 Have you ever had a nervous breakdown?

Form H

Daily record
Parents were asked to complete a daily record for two weeks.
They showed on the form how the child spent each of five
sessions – breakfast, morning, lunch, afternoon and evening.
For each session, the following were recorded:
  Place where child is
  Person(s) in charge
  Other adults and children present
  Main activities
  Incidents or meetings with others
  Any other comments
Parents were requested to describe any person mentioned if it
was not clear and to record the ages of individual children
present, except when the child was at group care.

Bibliography

Several references in the text to works issued by organisations have been given their initials only. These are listed here together with the full title of the organisation so that the full reference can be traced in the bibliography.

CPRS   Central Policy Review Staff
EOC   Equal Opportunities Commission
GHS   General Household Survey
OECD   Organisation for Economic Co-operation and Development
OPCS   Office of Population, Censuses and Surveys
SED   Scottish Education Department
SWSG   Social Work Services Group
TUC   Trades Union Congress

ABRAMS, P. (1978), 'Community care: some research problems and priorities', in J. Barnes and N. Connelly (eds), *Social Care Research*, London, Bedford Square Press.

ABRAMS, P. (1980), 'Altruism and reciprocity: altruism as reciprocity', University of Durham, Rowntree Research Unit Working Paper No. 10.

ADAMSON, G. (1973), *The Care-Takers*, London, Bookstall Publications.

AINSLIE, R. C. (1985), *The Psychology of Twinship*, Lincoln, Nebraska, University of Nebraska Press.

AINSWORTH, M. D. S. (1962), 'The effects of maternal deprivation: a review of findings and the controversy of research strategy', in World Health Organisation, *Deprivation of Maternal Care: A Reassessment of its Effects*, Geneva, WHO.

AINSWORTH, M. D. S. (1965), 'Further research into the adverse effects of maternal deprivation', in J. Bowlby, *Child Care and the Growth of Love* (2nd edition), Harmondsworth, Penguin.

ALBRECHT, R. (1954), 'The parental responsibilities of grandparents', *Marriage and Family Living*, pp. 201–4.

ALDOUS, J., OSMOND, M. W. and HICKS, M. W. (1979), 'Men's work and men's families', in W. R. Burr, R. Hill, F. I. Nye and I. L. Reiss (eds), *Contemporary Theories about the Family*, volume 1 – Research-Based Theories, New York, The Free Press.

ALLAN, G. (1979), *A Sociology of Friendship and Kinship*, London, George Allen and Unwin.

ALLAN, G. (1983), 'Informal networks of care: Issues raised by Barclay', *British Journal of Social Work*, vol. 13, pp. 417–433.

ALLBESON, J. and DOUGLAS, J. (1982), *National Welfare Benefits Handbook 1982/3*, London, Child Poverty Action Group.

ALLEN, V. L. (1981), 'Self, social group and social structure: surmises about the study of children's friendships', in S. R. Asher and J. M. Gottman (eds), *The Development of Children's Friendships*, Cambridge, Cambridge University Press.

ANESHENSEL, C. S., FRERICHS, R. R. and CLARK, V. A. (1981), 'Family roles and sex differences in depression', *Journal of Health and Social Behaviour*, vol. 22, pp. 379–393.

ANTONUCCI, T. (1976), 'Attachment: A life-span concept', *Human Development*, pp. 135–142.

APPLE, D. (1956), 'The social structure of grandparenthood', *American Anthropologist*, vol. 58, pp. 656–663.

ARIES, P. (1971), *Histoires des Populations Françaises*, Paris, Editions du Seuil.

ASHER, S. R. and RENSHAW, P. D. (1981), 'Children without friends; social knowledge and social skill training', in S. R. Asher and J. M. Gottman (eds), *The Development of Children's Friendships*, Cambridge, Cambridge University Press.

ASKHAM, J. (1984), *Identity and Stability in Marriage*, Cambridge, Cambridge University Press.

BABCHUK, N. (1965), 'Primary friends and kin: a study of the associations of middle class couples', *Social Forces*, vol. 43, pp. 482–493.

BACKETT, K. C. (1977), 'The Negotiation of Parenthood', University of Edinburgh, PhD Thesis.

BACKETT, K. C. (1980), 'Images of parenthood', in M. Anderson (ed), *The Sociology of the Family* (2nd edition), Harmondsworth, Penguin Books.

BACKETT, K. C. (1982), *Mothers and Fathers*, London, The Macmillan Press Ltd.

BAERS, M. (1954), 'Women workers and home responsibilities', *International Labour Review*, vol. 69, pp. 338–354.

BALDWIN, D. A. (1978), 'Power and social exchange', *The American Political Science Review*, vol. 72, pp. 1229–1242.

BARCLAY, P. (1982), *Social Workers: Their Role and Tasks*, London, Bedford Square Press.

BARNES, F. (1975), 'Accidents in the first three years of life', *Child: care, health and development*, vol. 1, pp. 421–433.

BARNES, J. and CONNELLY, N. (eds) (1978), *Social Care Research*, London, Bedford Square Press.

BARRY, III, H. and PAXSON, L. M. (1971), 'Infancy and Early Childhood', *Ethnology*, vol. 10, pp. 466–508.

BATES, J. E. (1980), 'The concept of difficult temperament', *Merrill-Palmer Quarterly*, vol. 26, no. 4, pp. 299–319.

BATES, J. E. (1983), 'Issues in assessment of difficult temperament: A reply to Thomas, Chess and Korn', *Merrill-Palmer Quarterly*, vol. 29, no. 1, pp. 89–97.

BATTER, B. B. and DAVIDSON, C. V. (1979), 'Wariness of strangers: reality or artifact?', *Journal of Child Psychology and Psychiatry*, vol. 20, pp. 93–109.

BEAIL, N. and McGUIRE, J. (1982), *Fathers – Psychological Perspectives*, London, Junction Books.

BECKER, G. S. (1965), 'A theory of the allocation of time', *The Economic Journal*, vol. 75, pp. 493–517.

BECKER, J. M. T. (1977), 'A learning analysis of the development of peer-oriented behaviour in nine month old infants', *Developmental Psychology*, vol. 13, no. 5, pp. 481–491.

BEFU, H. (1977), 'Social exchange', *American Review of Anthropology*, vol. 6, pp. 255–281.

BELL, C. (1968), *Middle Class Families*, London, Routledge and Kegan Paul.

BELL, C., McKEE, L. and PRIESTLEY, K. (1983), *Fathers, Childbirth and Work*, Manchester, Equal Opportunities Commission.

BELL, C. and NEWBY, H. (1977), 'Introduction: The age of methodological pluralism', in C. Bell and H. Newby (eds), *Doing Sociological Research*, London, Allen Unwin.

BELL, W. and BOAT, M. D. (1957), 'Urban neighbourhood and informal social relations', *American Journal of Sociology*, pp. 391–398.

BELSKY, J. and STEINBERG, L. D. (1978), 'The effects of day care:

A critical review', *Child Development*, vol. 49, pp. 929–949.

BERGER, P. and BERGER, B. L. (1983), *The War over the Family – Capturing the Middle Ground*, London, Hutchinson.

BERGER, P. and KELLNER, H. (1965), 'Marriage and the construction of reality', *Diogenes*, vol. 46, pp. 1–24.

BERGER, P. and LUCKMANN, T. (1971), *The Social Construction of Reality*, Harmondsworth, Penguin University Books.

BERNAL, J. F. (1973), 'Night waking in infants during the first 14 months', *Developmental, Medicine and Child Neurology*, vol. 15, pp. 760–769.

BERNSTEIN, B. (1971), *Class, Codes and Control*, vol. 1, London, Routledge and Kegan Paul.

BERNSTEIN, B. (1977), *Class, Codes and Control*, vol. 3 – *Towards a Theory of Educational Transitions*, London, Routledge and Kegan Paul.

BIGELOW, B. J. and LA GAIPA, J. J. (1980), 'The development of friendship values and choice', in H. C. Foot, A. C. Chapman, and J. R. Smith (1980), *Friendship and Social Relations in Children*, New York, J. Wiley and Sons.

BINNS, D. and MARS, G. (1984), 'Family, community and unemployment: A study in change', *Sociological Review*, vol. 32, pp. 662–95.

BLACKSTONE, T. (1971), *A Fair Start: The Provision of Pre-school Education*, London, Allen Lane – The Penguin Press.

BLATCHFORD, P., BATTLE, S. and MAYS, J. (1982), *The First Transition – Home to Pre-school*, Windsor, Berks, NFER-Nelson.

BLAU, P. (1964), *Exchange and Power in Social Life*, New York, J. Wiley and Sons.

BLAU, P. M. and DUNCAN, O. D. (1975), 'Measuring the status of occupations', in A. P. M. Coxon and C. L. Jones (eds), *Social Mobility*, Harmondsworth, Penguin.

BLAXTER, M. and PATERSON, E. (1982), *Mothers and Daughters*, London, Heinemann.

BLEHAR, M. C. (1977), 'Mother-child interaction in day-care and home-reared children', in R. A. Webb (ed.), *Social Development in Childhood: Day-care programs and research*, Baltimore, Johns Hopkins University Press.

BLOCK, J. H. (1976), 'Issues, problems and pitfalls in assessing sex differences: A critical review of the psychology of sex differences', *Merrill-Palmer Quarterly*, vol. 22, no. 4, pp. 283–308.

BLOMART, J. (1963), 'Attitudes maternelles et réactions à l'entrée au jardin d'enfants', *Acta Psychologica*, vol. 21, pp. 75–99.

BLURTON-JONES, N. (1974), 'Ethology and socialisation', in
M. P. M. Richards (ed.), *The Integration of a Child into a
Social World*, Cambridge, Cambridge University Press.

BLURTON-JONES, N., ROSETTIE FERRIERA, M. C., FARQUAR
BROWN, M. and MACDONALD, L. (1978), 'The association
between perinatal factors and later night waking', *Developmental Medicine and Child Neurology*, vol. 20, pp. 427–34.

BOARD OF EDUCATION (1933), *Infant and Nursery Schools* (The
Hadow Report), London, HMSO.

BOISSEVAIN, J. (1974), *Friends of Friends*, Oxford, Basil
Blackwell.

BONE, M. (1977), *Pre-school Children and the Need for Day-
care*, London, HMSO.

BOTT, E. (1957), *Family and Social Network*, London, Tavistock
Publications.

BOTT, E. (1971), *Family and Social Network* (2nd edition),
London, Tavistock Publications.

BOULTON, M. G. (1983), *On Being A Mother*, London, Tavistock.

BOWERMAN, C. E. and DOBASH, R. M. (1974), 'Structural variations in inter-sibling affect', *Journal of Marriage and the
Family*, vol. 36, pp. 48–54.

BOWLBY, J. (1965), *Child Care and the Growth of Love* (2nd
edition), Harmondsworth, Penguin.

BOWLBY, J. (1969), *Attachment*, Harmondsworth, Penguin.

BOWLBY, J. (1973), *Separation: Anxiety and Anger*, Harmondsworth, Penguin.

BRONFENBRENNER, U. (1975), 'Is early intervention effective?',
in U. Bronfenbrenner and M. A. Mahoney (eds), *Influences
on Human Behaviour*, Hinsdale, Illinois, The Dryden Press.

BRONFENBRENNER, U. (1977), 'Towards an experimental
ecology of human development', *American Psychologist*,
vol. 32, pp. 513–31.

BRONFENBRENNER, U. (1979), *The Ecology of Human Development*, Cambridge, Mass., Harvard University Press.

BROWN, G. W., NI BHROLCHAIN, M. and HARRIS, T. (1975),
'Social class and psychiatric disturbance among women in
an urban population', *Sociology*, pp. 225–54.

BROWN, G. W. and HARRIS, T. (1978), *Social Origins of
Depression*, London, Tavistock Publications.

BRUNER, J. (1980), *Under Five in Britain*, London, Grant
McIntyre.

BRYANT, B., HARRIS, M. and NEWTON, D. (1980), *Children and
Minders*, London, Grant McIntyre.

BURGESS, R. L. (1981), 'Relationships in marriage and the family', in S. Duck and R. Gilmour (eds), *Personal Relationships*, volume 1 – *Studying Personal Relationships*, London, Academic Press.

BURGESS, R. L. and NIELSEN, J. M. (1974), 'An experimental analysis of some structural determinants of equitable and inequitable exchange relations', *American Sociological Review*, pp. 427–443.

BURLINGHAM, D. and FREUD, A. (1943), *Infants with no Families*, London, George Allen and Unwin.

BUSFIELD, J. (1974), 'Family ideology and family pathology', in N. Armistead (ed.), *Reconstructing Social Psychology*, Harmondsworth, Penguin Books.

BUTTIMER, A. (1972), 'Community', in Stewart (ed.), *The City*, Harmondsworth, Penguin.

CALDWELL, B. M. (1973), 'Infant day care – the outcast gains respectability', in P. Roby (ed.), *Child Care – Who Cares?*, New York, Basic Books.

CAREY, W. B. (1970), 'A simplified method for measuring infant temperament', *The Journal of Paediatrics*, vol. 77, no. 2, pp. 188–194.

CAREY, W. (1982), 'Validity of parental assessments of development and behaviour', *American Journal of Dis. Child*, vol. 136, pp. 97–99.

CENSUS (1971), *County Report – Edinburgh City*, Edinburgh, HMSO.

CENSUS (1981), London, HMSO.

CENTRAL ADVISORY COMMITTEE FOR EDUCATION (England) (1967), *Children and their Primary Schools* (The Plowden Report), London, HMSO.

CENTRAL POLICY REVIEW STAFF (1978), *Services for Young Children with Working Mothers*, London, HMSO.

CHALLIS, L. (1974), 'Day care needs of the under fives', *Greater London Intelligence Quarterly*, pp. 53–58.

CHALLIS, L. (1980), *The Great Under-fives Muddle*, University of Bath, Bath Social Policy Papers.

CHALLMAN, R. C. (1932), 'Factors influencing friendships among preschool children', *Child Development*, vol. 3, pp. 146–158.

CHAPLIN, J. B. (1975), 'The social worker's role in day care', *Royal Society of Health Journal*, vol. 95, pp. 229–232.

CHARLESWORTH, A., WILKIN, D. and DURIE, A. (1984), *Carers and Services*, Manchester, Equal Opportunities Commission.

CHAZAN, M. (ed.) (1973), *Education in the Early Years*, University of Swansea, Faculty of Education.

CLARK, B. R. (1956), 'Organisational adaptation and precarious values: A case study', *American Sociological Review*, vol. 21, pp. 327–336.

CLARK, D. H. (1967), *The Psychology of Education*, New York, The Free Press.

CLARK, M. M. (1978), 'Developments in pre-school education and the role of research', in M. M. Clark and W. M. Cheyne (eds), *Studies in Pre-school Education*, London, Hodder and Stoughton.

CLARKE, A. M. and CLARKE, A. (1976), *Early Experience: Myths and Evidence*, London, Open Books.

CLARKE, A. and CLARKE, A. M. (1984), 'Constancy and change in the growth of human characteristics', *Journal of Child Psychology and Psychiatry*, vol. 25, no. 2, pp. 191–210.

CLARKE, M. (1982), 'Where is the community which cares?', *British Journal of Social Work*, vol. 12, pp. 453–469.

CLARKE-STEWART, A. (1973) *Interaction between Mothers and their Young Children: Characteristics and Consequences*, Monographs of the Society for Research in Child Development, vol. 38, nos 6–7, Chicago, University of Chicago Press.

CLARKE-STEWART, ALISON (1980), 'The father's contribution to children's cognitive and social development in early childhood', in F. A. Pedersen (ed.), *The Father-Infant Relationship*, New York, Praeger.

CLARKE-STEWART, A. (1982), *Day Care*, Glasgow, Fontana.

CLARKE-STEWART, K. A., UMETT, B. J., SNOW, M. E. and PEDERSEN, J. A. (1980), 'Development and prediction of children's sociability from 1 to 2½ years', *Developmental Psychology*, pp. 290–302.

CLAUSEN, J. A. (1964), 'Family structure, socialisation and personality', in L. W. Hoffman and M. L. Hoffman (eds), *Review of Child Development Research*, New York, Russell Sage Foundation.

COHEN, J. (1979), 'Patterns of parental help', *Educational Research*, vol. 21, no. 3, pp. 186–193.

COHEN, S. E. (1978), 'Maternal employment and mother-child interaction', *Merrill-Palmer Quarterly*, vol. 24, pp. 189–197.

COOK, D. (1982), 'Network structures from an exchange perspective', in P. V. Marsden and N. Lin (eds) (1982), *Social Structure and Network Analysis*, Beverly Hills, Sage.

COOTE, A. and HEWITT, P. (1980), 'The stance of Britain's major parties and interest groups', in P. Moss and N. Fonda (eds), *Work and the Family*, London, Temple Smith.

CORNELIUS, S. W. and DENNEY, N. W. (1975), 'Dependency in day-care and home-reared children', *Developmental Psychology*, vol. 11, no. 5, pp. 575–582.

CORSARO, W. (1981), 'Friendship in nursery school: social organization in a peer environment', in S. R. Asher and J. M. Gottman (eds), *The Development of Children's Friendships*, Cambridge, Cambridge University Press.

COX, M. V. (ed.) (1980), *Are Young Children Egocentric?*, London, Batsford.

COX, T. (1983), *Stress*, London, Macmillan.

CRAWFORD, M. (1981), 'Not disengaged: Grandparents in literature and reality, an empirical study in role satisfaction', *Sociological Review*, vol. 29, pp. 499–519.

CROWE, B. (1973), *The Playgroup Movement*, London, George Allen and Unwin.

CUBITT, T. (1973), 'Network density among urban families', in J. Boissevain and J. C. Mitchell (eds), *Network Analysis in Human Interaction*, The Hague, Mouton.

CULLEN, I. (1979), 'Urban social policy and the problems of family life', in C. Harris (ed.), *The Sociology of the Family: New Directions for Britain*, University of Keele, Sociological Review Monograph, no. 28.

CUNNINGHAM-BURLEY, S. J. (1983), *The Meaning and Significance of Grandparenthood*, University of Aberdeen, PhD thesis.

CUNNINGHAM-BURLEY, S. (1984), ' "We don't talk about it . . ." – Issues of gender and method in the portrayal of grandfatherhood', *Sociology*, vol. 18, no. 3, pp. 325–337.

CUNNINGHAM-BURLEY, S. (1986), 'Becoming a grandparent', *New Society*, vol. 75, no. 1206, pp. 229–230.

DAHLBERG, F. (ed.) (1981), *Woman the Gatherer*, New Haven, Yale University Press.

DANIEL, W. W. (1981), 'Maternity rights: the symbol and the power', *New Society*, vol. 58, pp. 147–148.

DANZIGER, K. (1970), *Socialization*, Harmondsworth, Penguin.

DANZIGER, K. (ed.) (1971), *Readings in Child Socialization*, London, Pergamon Press.

DAVIDSON, F. (1970), 'Day care centers in Paris and its suburbs', in A. Kadushin (ed.), *Child Welfare Services*, New York, Macmillan.

DAVIE, R., BUTLER, N. and GOLDSTEIN, H. (1972), *From Birth to Seven*, London, Longmans.

DAY, C. (1975), *Company Day Nurseries*, London, Institute of Personnel Management.

DENZIN, N. K. (1977), *Childhood Socialisation*, London, Jossey-Bass.

DICKENS, W. C. and PERLMAN, D. (1981), 'Friendship over the life-span', in S. Duck and R. Gilmour, *Personal Relationships*, volume 2 – *Developing Personal Relationships*, London, Academic Press.

DICKS, E. (1983), 'A family perspective in policies for the under-fives', in A. W. Franklin (ed.), *Family Matters*, Oxford, Pergamon.

DOMINIAN, J. (1982), *Depression*, Glasgow, Fontana.

DONACHY, W. (1979), 'Parental participation in pre-school education', in M. M. Clark and W. M. Cheyne (eds), *Studies in Pre-School Education*, London, Hodder and Stoughton.

DOUGLAS, J. W. B. (1975), 'Early hospital admissions and later disturbances of behaviour and learning' *Developmental Medicine and Child Neurology*, vol. 17, pp. 456–480.

DOUGLAS, J. W. B. and BLOMFIELD, J. M. (1958), *Children under Five*, London, George Allen and Unwin.

DREITZEL, P. (ed.) (1973), *Childhood and Socialization*, London, Macmillan.

DUCK, S. and GILMOUR, R. (eds) (1981), *Personal Relationships*, volumes 1–3, London, Academic Press.

DUNN, J. (1977), *Distress and Comfort*, London, Open Books.

DUNN, J. (1980a), 'Individual differences in temperament', in M. Rutter (ed.), *Scientific Foundations of Psychiatry*, London, Heinemann.

DUNN, J. (1980b), 'Feeding and sleeping', in M. Rutter (ed.), *Scientific Foundations of Psychiatry*, London, Heinemann.

DUNN, J. (1983), 'Sibling relationships in early childhood', *Child Development*, vol. 54, pp. 787–811.

DUNN, J. and KENDRICK, C. (1979), 'Interaction between young siblings in the context of family relationships', in M. Lewis and L. Rosenblum (eds), *The Child and its Family*, New York, Plenum Press.

DUNN, J. and KENDRICK, C. (1980) 'The arrival of a sibling: changes in the patterns of interaction between mother and first-born child', *Journal of Child Psychology and Psychiatry*, vol. 21, pp. 119–132.

DUNN, J. and KENDRICK, C. (1982), *Siblings: Love, Envy and Understanding*, London, Grant McIntyre.

EDGELL, S. (1980), *Middle Class Couples*, London, George Allen and Unwin.

EKEH, P. P. (1974), *Social Exchange Theory – The Two Traditions*, London, Heinemann.

ELIAS, P. (1980), 'Employment prospects and equal opportunity', in P. Moss and N. Fonda (eds), *Work and the Family*, London, Temple Smith.

EMERSON, R. M. (1976), 'Social exchange theory', *Annual Review of Sociology*, vol. 2, pp. 235–262.

EMLEN, A. C. (1973), 'Slogans, slots and slander: The myth of day care need', *American Journal of Orthopsychiatry*, vol. 43, no. 1, pp. 23–36.

EQUAL OPPORTUNITIES COMMISSION (1978), *I Want To Work . . . But What About The Children?*, Manchester, EOC.

EQUAL OPPORTUNITIES COMMISSION (1979), *With All My Worldly Goods I Thee Endow . . . Except My Tax Allowances*, Manchester, EOC.

EQUAL OPPORTUNITIES COMMISSION (1982a), *Caring for the Elderly and Handicapped*, Manchester, EOC.

EQUAL OPPORTUNITIES COMMISSION (1982b), *Who Cares for the Carers?*, Manchester, EOC.

ERIKSON, E. H. (1965), *Childhood and Society*, Harmondsworth, Penguin.

ERLER, G. (1980), 'Tagesmutter und Eltern – ein Feld mit Stoppersteinen', in Bundesminister fur Jugend, Familie und Gesundheit (1980), *Das Modellprojekt Tagesmutter – Abschlussbericht der wissenschaftlichen Begleitung*, Stuttgart, Verlag W. Kochhammer.

ETAUGH, C. (1974), 'Effects of maternal employment on children: A review of recent research', *Merrill-Palmer Quarterly*, vol. 20, no. 2, pp. 71–98.

FAGIN, L. and LITTLE, M. (1984), *The Forsaken Families*, Harmondsworth, Penguin.

FEIN, G. G. and CLARKE-STEWART, A. (1973), *Day Care in Context*, New York, J. Wiley & Sons.

FERGUSON, L. R. (1970), 'Dependency motivation and socialization', in R. A. Hoppe, G. A. Milton and E. C. Simmel (eds), *Early Experiences and the Process of Socialization*, London, Academic Press.

FERGUSON, S. M. and FITZGERALD, H. (1954), *Studies in the*

Social Services, part of the *History of the Second World War*, London, Longmans.

FERRI, E. (1973), 'Characteristics of motherless families', *British Journal of Social Work*, vol. 3, no. 1, pp. 91–100.

FERRI, E. (1978), 'Integrating services for the under-fives', *Concern*, no. 27, pp. 20–24.

FERRI, E., BIRCHALL, D., GINGELL, V. and GIPPS, C. (1981), *Combined Nursery Centres*, London, Macmillan.

FERRI, E., BIRCHALL, D., GINGELL, V. and GIPPS, C. (1982), 'Combined nursery centres: A reply to J. Oates' review', *Early Childhood*, vol. 2, no. 4, pp. 18–21.

FINCH, J. (1982), 'Plowden's reversal: playgroups not nursery education', *Early Childhood*, vol. 2, no. 9, pp. 30–31.

FINCH, J. (1983), 'Can skills be shared? Pre-school playgroups in "disadvantaged" areas', *Community Development*, vol. 18, no. 3, pp. 251–256.

FINCH, J. (1984), 'A first class environment? Working-class playgroups as pre-school experience', *British Educational Research Journal*, vol. 10, no. 1, pp. 3–17.

FINCH, J. and GROVES, D. (1980), 'Community care and the family: A case for equal opportunities', *Journal of Social Policy*, vol. 9, no. 4, pp. 487–511.

FINCH, J. and GROVES, D. (1983), *A Labour of Love*, London, Routledge and Kegan Paul.

FISHBEIN, M. and RAVEN, B. H. (1967), 'Beliefs and attitudes', in M. Fishbein (ed.), *Readings in Attitude Theory and Measurement*, New York, J. Wiley and Sons.

FISHER, C. S. (1975), 'The study of urban community and personality', *Annual Review of Sociology*, vol. 1, pp. 67–89.

FISHER, C. S. (1981), 'The public and private worlds of city life', *American Sociological Review*, vol. 46, pp. 306–316.

FLETCHER, R. (1973), *The Family and Marriage in Britain* (3rd edition), Harmondsworth, Penguin.

FONDA, N. (1976), 'Current entitlements and provisions: a critical review', in N. Fonda and P. Moss (eds), *Mothers in Employment*, London, Brunel University.

FOX, R. (ed.) (1975), *Biosocial Anthropology*, London, Malaby Press.

FURSTENBERG, F. F. Jr (1985), 'Sociological ventures in child development', *Child Development*, vol. 56, pp. 281–288.

GARDINER, J. (1975), 'Women's domestic labour', *New Left Review*, vol. 83, pp. 47–58.

GARVEY, A. (1974), 'The Children's Community Centre', *Where*, no. 98, pp. 328–331.

GAVRON, H. (1966), *The Captive Wife*, London, Routledge and Kegan Paul.

GENERAL HOUSEHOLD SURVEY (1979), *Day Care of Children Under Five*, London, HMSO.

GESELL, A. (1951), *The First Five Years of Life*, London, Methuen.

GEWIRTZ, J. L. (1976), 'The attachment acquisition process as evidenced in the maternal conditioning of cued infant responding (particularly crying)', *Human Relations*, pp. 143–155.

GIDDENS, A. (1976), *New Rules of Sociological Method*, London, Hutchinson.

GINSBERG, S. (1976), 'Women, work and conflict', in N. Fonda and P. Moss (eds), *Mothers in Employment*, London, Brunel University.

GITTINS, D. (1985), *The Family in Question*, London, Macmillan.

GLASS, N. (1947), 'Eating, sleeping and elimination habits in children attending day nurseries and children cared for at home by mothers', *American Journal of Orthopsychiatry*, vol. 59, pp. 697–711.

GOLD, D. and ANDRES, D. (1978a), 'Relations between maternal employment and development of nursery school children', *Canadian Journal of Behavioural Science*, vol. 10, no. 2, pp. 116–129.

GOLD, D. and ANDRES, D. (1978b), 'Comparisons of adolescent children with employed and unemployed mothers', *Merrill-Palmer Quarterly*, vol. 24, no. 4, pp. 243–254.

GOLDSMITH, H. H. and GOTTESMANN, I. I. (1981), 'Origins of variation in behavioural style: a longitudinal study of temperament in young twins', *Child Development*, vol. 52, pp. 91–103.

GOLDTHORPE, J. H. and HOPE, K. (1974), *The Social Grading of Occupations: A New Approach and a Scale*, Oxford, Clarendon Press.

GOLDTHORPE, J. H. and LLEWELLYN, C. (1977), 'Class mobility: Intergenerational and work life patterns', *British Journal of Sociology*, vol. 28, no. 3, pp. 269–302.

GOLDTHORPE, J., LLEWELLYN, C. and PAYNE, C. (1980), *Social Mobility and Class Structure in Modern Britain*, Oxford, Clarendon Press.

GOLDTHORPE, J. H. and LOCKWOOD, D. (1963), 'Affluence and the British class structure', *Sociological Review*, vol. 11, pp. 133–163.

GOLDTHORPE, J. H., LOCKWOOD, D., BECHHOFFER, F. and PLATT, J. (1969), *The Affluent Worker in the Class Structure*, Cambridge, Cambridge University Press.

GOODY, J. (1962), 'On nannas and nannies', *Man*, vol. 62, pp. 179–184.

GOUDER, J. C. (1975), 'A note on the declining relation between subjective and objective class measures', *British Journal of Sociology*, vol. 26, pp. 102–109.

GOULDNER, A. W. (1960), 'The norm of reciprocity: A preliminary statement', *American Sociological Review*, vol. 25, no. 2, pp. 161–178.

GOVE, W. R. (1972), 'The relationship between sex roles, marital status and mental illness', *Social Forces*, vol. 51, no. 4, pp. 34–44.

GRAMPIAN REGIONAL COUNCIL (1978), *Study of Admissions to Care*, Aberdeen, Grampian Regional Council Social Work Department.

GRANADA TELEVISION (1985), *The Under-fives*, Manchester, Granada.

GREEN, E. H. (1933), 'Friendships and quarrels among preschool children', *Child Development*, vol. 4, pp. 237–252.

GREIF, E. B. (1977), 'Peer interactions in pre-school children', in R. A. Webb (ed.), *Social Development in Childhood: Day-care programs and research*, Baltimore, J. Hopkins University Press.

GUDAT, U. and PERMIEN, H. (1980), 'Die kinderpsychologischen Untersuchungen im Tagesmutter Projekt', in Bundesminister fur Jugend, Familie und Gesundheit (1980), *Das Modellprojekt Tagesmutter – Abschlussbericht der wissenschaftlichen Begleitung*, Stuttgart, Verlag W. Kochhammer.

HADOW REPORT (1933), see Board of Education.

HAGEN, E. (1973), 'Child care and women's liberation', in P. Roby (ed.), *Child Care – Who Cares?*, New York, Basic Books.

HALBERTSMA, H. A. (1968), *Informal Systems of Mutual Assistance among Kin and Neighbours in Case of Illness and Death*, Aberdeen, Paper to the First International Conference on Social Science and Medicine.

HALSEY, A. H. (1980), 'Education can compensate', *New Society*, vol. 52, pp. 172–173.

HALSEY, A. H. and SMITH, T. (1976), *Pre-school Expansion: Its Impact on Parental Involvement and on the Structure of Provision*, London, Social Science Research Council, Final Report, Grant Number HR 2915/2.

HANNON, P. (1978), 'Minders of our future', *New Society*, vol. 44, pp. 304–305.

HARDYMENT, C. (1983), *Dream Babies*, London, Jonathan Cape.

HARPER, C. L. (1978), 'New evidence on the impact of day-care centres on children's psycho-social development', *Child Welfare*, vol. 57, pp. 527–531.

HASKEY, J. (1983), 'Children of divorcing couples', *Population Trends*, no. 31, pp. 20–26.

HASSENSTEIN, B. (1974), 'Kritik der wissenschaftliche Begrundung des Tagesmutterprojekts', *Zeitschrift fur Padagogik*, vol. 20, pp. 929 et seq.

HAYES, D. S., CHEMELSKI, B. E. and PALMER, M. (1982), 'Nursery rhymes and prose passages: Pre-schoolers' liking and short-term retention of story events', *Developmental Psychology*, vol. 18, pp. 49–56.

HAYSTEAD, J., HOWARTH, V. and STRACHAN, A. (1980), *Pre-school Education and Care*, Edinburgh, Hodder and Stoughton.

HENDRIX, L. (1979), 'Kinship, social class and migration', *Journal of Marriage and the Family*, vol. 41, pp. 399–407.

HERBST, P. G. (1960), 'Task differentiation of husband and wife in family activities', in N. W. Bell and E. F. Vogel (eds), *A Modern Introduction to the Family*, New York, The Free Press of Glencoe.

HERMANN, A. and KOMLOSI, S. (1972), *Early Child Care in Hungary*, London, Gordon and Breach.

HILL, M. (1984), *Sharing Care of Young Children*, Edinburgh University, PhD thesis.

HILL, R., FOOTE, N., ALDOUS, J., CARSON, R. and MACDONAL, R. (1970), *Family Developments in Three Generations*, Cambridge, Mass., Schenkman Publishing Company.

HOCK, E. (1978), 'Working and non-working mothers with infants: perceptions of their careers, their infants' needs and satisfaction with mothering', *Developmental Psychology*, vol. 14, no. 1, pp. 37–43.

HOCK, E. (1980), 'Working and non-working mothers and their infants', *Merrill-Palmer Quarterly*, vol. 26, pp. 79–101.

HOFFMAN, L. W. (1979), 'Maternal employment, 1979', *American Psychologist*, vol. 34, no. 10, pp. 859–865.

HOFFMAN, L. W. and MANIS, J. D. (1978), 'Influences of children on marital interaction and parental satisfactions and dissatisfactions', in R. M. Lerner and G. B. Spanier (eds), *Child Influences on Marital and Family Interaction: A Lifespan Perspective*, London, Academic Press.

HOGGART, R. (1973), 'Changes in working-class life', in M. A. Smith, S. Parker and C. S. Smith (eds), *Leisure and Society in Britain*, London, Allen Lane.

HOLMAN, R. (1980), 'Exclusive and inclusive concepts of fostering', in J. Triseliotis (ed.), *New Developments in Fostering and Adoption*, London, Routledge and Kegan Paul.

HONEY, M. (1973), 'Day care and play for under fives in Greenwich', *Bulletin of the Greater London Research and Intelligence Unit*, pp. 72–80.

HUBERT, J. (1965), 'Kinship and geographical mobility in a sample from a London middle-class area', *The International Journal of Comparative Sociology*, vol. 6, pp. 61–80.

HUBERT, N. C., WACHS, T. D., PETERS-MARTIN, P. and GANDOUR, M. J. (1982), 'The study of early temperament: measurement and conceptual issues', *Child Development*, vol. 53, pp. 571–600.

HUGHES, M., MAYALL, B., MOSS, P., PERRY, J. and PETRIE, P. (1980), *Nurseries Now*, Harmondsworth, Penguin.

HUNT, A. (1968), *A Survey of Women's Employment*, London, Government Social Survey.

HUNT, D. (1970), *Parents and Children in History*, New York, Basic Books.

HUTT, C. (1972), *Males and Females*, Harmondsworth, Penguin.

HUTTON, G. (1975), *Social Environment in Suburban Edinburgh*, York, Joseph Rowntree Memorial Trust.

INEICHEN, B. (1981), 'The housing decisions of young people', *British Journal of Sociology*, vol. 32, no. 2, pp. 252–258.

IRISH, D. P. (1964), 'Sibling interaction: A neglected aspect in family life research', *Social Forces*, vol. 42, no. 3, pp. 279–288.

IRVING, H. W. (1977), 'Social networks in the modern city', *Social Forces*, vol. 55, no. 4, pp. 867–880.

JACKSON, B. and JACKSON, S. (1979), *Childminder: A Study in Action Research*, London, Routledge and Kegan Paul.

JACKSON, S. (1971), *The Illegal Childminders*, Cambridge, Cambridge Educational Development Trust.

JACKSON, S. (1975), 'A new policy for childminders', *New Society*, vol. 8, no. 13, pp. 19–20.

JENKINS, S., BAX, M. and HART, H. (1980), 'Behaviour problems in pre-school children', *Journal of Child Psychology and Psychiatry*, vol. 21, pp. 5–17.

JENKS, C. (ed.) (1982), *The Sociology of Childhood*, London, Batsford.

JOHNSEN, K. P. and LESLIE, G. R. (1965), 'Methodological notes on research in childrearing and social class', *Merrill-Palmer Quarterly*, vol. 11, pp. 345–358.

KADUSHIN, A. (1970), *Adopting Older Children*, Harvard, Mass., The Harvard Common Press.

KAGAN, J. (1979), *The Growth of the Child*, London, Methuen.

KAGAN, J. (1982), 'The construct of difficult temperament: a reply to Thomas, Chess and Korn', *Merrill-Palmer Quarterly*, vol. 28, no. 1, 21–24.

KAGAN, J. and MOSS, H. A. (1962), *Birth to Maturity*, New York, John Wiley and Sons.

KAHANA, B. and KAHANA, E. (1970), 'Grandparenthood from the perspective of the developing child', *Developmental Psychology*, vol. 3, no. 1, pp. 98–105.

KAHANA, E. and KAHANA, B. (1971), 'Theoretical and research perspectives on grandparenthood', *Aging and Human Development*, vol. 2, pp. 261–268.

KAMMEYER, K. (1967), 'Birth order as a research variable', *Social Forces*, vol. 46, pp. 71–80.

KARRE, M. (1973), 'Social rights in Sweden before school starts', in P. Roby (ed.), *Child Care – Who Cares?*, New York, Basic Books.

KELLERMAN, J. and KATZ, E. P. (1978), 'Attitudes towards the division of child-rearing responsibility', *Sex Roles*, vol. 4, pp. 505–517.

KESSEN, W. (1975), *Childhood in China*, New Haven, Yale University Press.

KLEIN, J. (1965), *Samples from English Cultures*, London, Routledge and Kegan Paul.

KLUCKHOHN, F. R. and STRODTBECK, F. L. (1961), *Variations in Value Orientations*, Evanston, Illinois, Row, Peterson and Co.

KOHN, M. (1963), 'Social class and parent-child relationships – An interpretation', *American Journal of Sociology*, vol. 68, no. 4, pp. 471–480.

KOHN, M. L. (1969), *Class and Conformity*, Homewood, Illinois, The Dorsey Press.

KONNER, M. (1975), 'Relations among infants and juveniles in comparative perspective', in M. Lewis and L. Rosenblum (eds), *Friendship and Peer Relations*, New York, J. Wiley and Sons.

KORNER, A. F. (1974), 'The effect of the infants' state on the caregiver', in M. Lewis and L. Rosenblum, (eds), *The Effects of the Infant on its Caregiver*, New York, J. Wiley and Sons.

KRAUSZ, E. (1969), *Sociology in Britain*, London, Batsford.

LA GAIPA, J. J. (1981), 'A systems approach to personal relationships', in S. Duck and R. Gilmour (eds), *Personal Relationships*, volume 1 – *Studying Personal Relationships*, London, Academic Press.

LAMB, M. (ed.) (1976), *The Role of the Father in Child Development*, New York, John Wiley and Sons.

LAND, H. (1978), 'Who cares for the family?', *Journal of Social Issues*, vol. 7, pp. 257–284.

LAND, H. (1981), *Parity Begins At Home: Women's And Men's Work And Its Effects On Their Paid Employment*, Manchester, Equal Opportunities Commission.

LAND, H. and PARKER, R. (1978), 'Family policies in Britain: The hidden dimensions', in S. B. Kamerman and A. J. Kahn (eds), *Family Policy: Government and Policy in Fourteen Countries*, New York, Columbia University Press.

LA ROSSA, R. and LA ROSSA, M. M. (1981), *Transition to Parenthood*, Beverly Hills, Sage.

LA ROSSA, R. and WOLF, J. H. (1985), 'On qualitative family research', *Journal of Marriage and the Family*, vol. 47, no. 3, pp. 531–541.

LASCH, C. (1977), *Haven in a Heartless World*, New York, Basic Books.

LASKO, J. K. (1954), 'Parent behaviour towards first and second children', *Genetic Psychology Monographs*, vol. 49, pp. 97–134.

LEACH, E. (1982), *Social Anthropology*, London, Fontana.

LEACH, P. (1974), *Babyhood*, Harmondsworth, Penguin.

LEACH, P. (1979), *Who Cares?*, Harmondsworth, Penguin.

LEAT, D. (1982), *Analysing Reciprocity*, London, unpublished paper, Policy Studies Institute.

LEAT, D. (1983), *Getting To Know The Neighbours*, London, research paper no. 83–2, Policy Studies Institute.

LECOULTRE, D. (1976), 'Family, employment and the allocation of time', in N. Fonda and P. Moss (eds), *Mothers in Employment*, London, Brunel University.

LEE, G. R. (1979), 'Effect of social networks on the family', in W. R. Burr, R. Hill, F. I. Nye and I. L. Reiss (eds), *Contemporary Theories about the Family*, Volume 1 – *Research-Based Theories*, New York, The Free Press.

LEE, T. (1968), 'Urban neighbourhood as a socio-spatial schema', *Human Relations*, vol. 21, no. 3, pp. 241–267.

LERNER, R. M. and SPANIER, G. B. (eds) (1978), *Child Influences on Marital and Family Interaction: A Life-span Perspective*, London, Academic Press.

LEVINE, S. and SCOTCH, N. A. (eds) (1970), *Social Stress*, Chicago, Aldine Publishing Company.

LEVY, D. M. (1947), *Maternal Overprotection*, New York, Columbia University Press.

LEWIS, M. and FEIRING, C. (1978), 'The child's social world', in R. M. Lerner and G. B. Spanier (eds), *Child Influences on Marital and Family Interaction: A Life-span Perspective*, London, Academic Press.

LEWIS, M. and ROSENBLUM, L. (eds) (1974), *The Effects of the Infant on its Caregiver*, New York, J. Wiley and Sons.

LEWIS, M. and ROSENBLUM, L. (eds) (1975), *Friendship and Peer Relations*, New York, J. Wiley and Sons.

LEWIS, M., YOUNG, G., BROOKS, J. and MICHALSON, L. (1975), 'The beginnings of friendship', in M. Lewis and L. Rosenblum (eds), *Friendship and Peer Relations*, New York, J. Wiley and Sons.

LIEGLE, L. (1974), 'Sozialisationsforschung und Familienpolitik', *Zeitschrift fur Padagogik*, pp. 427–445.

LIGHT, P. (1980), 'The social concomitants of role-taking', in M. V. Cox (ed.), *Are Young Children Egocentric?*, London, Batsford.

LIJLESTROM, R. (1978), 'Sweden', in S. B. Kamerman and A. J. Kahn (eds), *Family Policy: Government and Policy in Fourteen Countries*, New York, Columbia University Press.

LITTMAN, R. A., MOORE, R. C. A. and PIERCE, J. (1957), 'Social class differences in child-rearing: A third community for comparison with Chicago and Newton', *American Sociological Review*, vol. 22, pp. 694–704.

LITWAK, E. and SZELENYI, I. (1969), 'Primary group structures and their functions: Kin, neighbours and friends', *American Sociological Review*, vol. 34, no. 4, pp. 465–481.

LLEWELLYN, C. (1981), 'Occupational mobility and the use of

the comparative method', in H. Roberts (ed.), *Doing Feminist Research*, London, Routledge and Kegan Paul.

LOTHIAN REGIONAL COUNCIL (1984), *Position Statement of Services to Under-fives in Lothian Region* (Joint report by the Directors of Education and Social Work), Edinburgh, Lothian and Regional Council.

MCARTHUR, C. (1956), 'Personalities of first and second children', *Psychiatry*, vol. 19, pp. 47–54.

MCCANDLESS, B. C., BILOUS, C. and BENNETT, H. L. (1961), 'Peer popularity and dependence on adults in pre-school age socialization', *Child Development*, vol. 32, pp. 511–518.

MCCORMACK, G. (1976), 'Reciprocity', *Man*, vol. 11, pp. 89–103.

MCFADYEN, I. (1977), *Planning locally*, Edinburgh, paper presented to the Craiglockart Conference.

MCGRATH, J. E. (ed.) (1970), *Social and Psychological Factors in Stress*, New York, Holt, Rinehart and Winston Inc.

MCGREW, W. C. (1972a), 'How children react to newcomers', *New Society*, pp. 55–57.

MCGREW, W. C. (1972b), 'Aspects of social development in nursery children with emphasis on introduction to the group', in N. Blurton-Jones (ed.), *Ethological Studies of Child Behaviour*, Cambridge, Cambridge University Press.

MCKEE, L. and O'BRIEN, M. (eds) (1982), *The Father Figure*, London, Tavistock.

MACCOBY, E. E. and JACKLIN, C. N. (1980), 'Psychological sex differences', in M. Rutter (ed.), *Scientific Foundations of Psychiatry*, London, Heinemann.

MACKIE, L. and PATULLO, P. (1977), *Women at Work*, London, Tavistock.

MALINOWSKI, B. (1922), *Argonauts of the Western Pacific*, London, Routledge.

MANNERINO, A. P. (1980), 'The development of children's friendships', in H. C. Foot, A. C. Chapman, and J. R. Smith (1980), *Friendship and Social Relations in Children*, New York, J. Wiley and Sons.

MARCUS, J., CHESS, S. and THOMAS, A. (1972), 'Temperamental individuality in the group care of young children', *Early Child Development and Care*, vol. 1, pp. 313–330.

MARSDEN, P. V. and LIN, N. (eds) (1982), *Social Structure and Network Analysis*, Beverly Hills, Sage.

MARSH, A. (1979), *Women and Shiftwork*, London, Office of Population, Censuses and Surveys, HMSO.

MATZA, D. (1964), *Delinquency and Drift*, New York, John Wiley and Sons.

MATZA, D. and SYKES, G. M. (1961), 'Juvenile delinquency and subterranean values', *American Sociological Review*, vol. 26, pp. 712–719.

MAUSS, M. (1954), *The Gift* (translated by Ian Cunnison), London, Cohen and West.

MAYALL, B. and PETRIE, P. (1977), *Minder, Mother, and Child*, London, University of London: Institute of Education.

MAYALL, B. and PETRIE, P. (1983), *Childminding and Day Nurseries: What Kind of Care?*, London, Heinemann.

MAYO, M. (ed.) (1977), *Women in the Community*, London, Routledge and Kegan Paul.

MILLER, N. and MARYAMA, G. (1976), 'Ordinal position and peer popularity', *Journal of Personality and Social Psychology*, vol. 33, no. 2, pp. 123–131.

MINTURN, L. and LAMBERT, W. W. (1964), *Mothers of Six Cultures*, London, John Wiley and Sons.

MITCHELL, A. (1985), *Children in the Middle*, London, Tavistock.

MITCHELL, J. C. (ed.) (1969), *Social Networks in Urban Situations*, Manchester, The University Press.

MORGAN, D. H. (1975), *Social Theory and the Family*, London, Routledge and Kegan Paul.

MORSBACH, G., KERNAHAN, P. and EMERSON, P. (1981), 'Attitudes to nursery school', *Education Research*, vol. 23, no. 3, pp. 222–223.

MOSS, H. A. (1967), 'Sex, age, and state as determinants of mother-infant interaction', *Merrill-Palmer Quarterly*, vol. 13, pp. 19–36.

MOSS, P. (1976), 'The current situation', in N. Fonda and P. Moss (eds), *Mothers in Employment*, London, Brunel University.

MOSS, P. (1978), *Alternative Models of Group Child-care for Pre-school Children with Working Parents*, Manchester, Equal Opportunities Commission.

MOSS, P. (1980), 'Parents at work', in P. Moss and N. Fonda (eds), *Work and the Family*, London, Temple Smith.

MOSS, P. and PLEWIS, I. (1976), 'Who wants nurseries?', *New Society*, vol. 36, p. 188.

MOSTOW, E. and NEWBERRY, P. (1975), 'Work role and depression in women', *American Journal of Orthopsychiatry*, vol. 45, no. 4, pp. 538–548.

MOSTYN, B. (1985), 'The content analysis of qualitative research data: A dynamic approach', in M. Brenner, J. Brown and D. Canter (eds), *The Research Interview*, London, Academic Press.

MOUNT, F. (1982), *The Subversive Family*, London, Jonathan Cape.

MURRAY, A. D. (1975), 'Maternal employment reconsidered', *American Journal of Orthopsychiatry*, vol. 45, pp. 739–791.

NAHEMOW, L. and LAWTON, M. P. (1975), 'Similarity and propinquity in friendship formation', *Journal of Personality and Social Psychology*, vol. 32, no. 2, pp. 205–213.

NEUGARTEN, B. L. and WEINSTEIN, K. K. (1964), 'The changing American grandparent', *Journal of Marriage and the Family*, vol. 26, pp. 199–204.

NEW, C. and DAVID, M. (1985), *For the Children's Sake*, Harmondsworth, Penguin.

NEWLYN, W. T. (1962), *Theory of Money*, Oxford, Oxford University Press.

NEWSON, J. and NEWSON, E. (1963), *Patterns of Infant Care*, Harmondsworth, Penguin.

NEWSON, J. and NEWSON, E. (1970a), *Four Years Old in an Urban Community*, Harmondsworth, Penguin.

NEWSON, J. and NEWSON, E. (1970b), 'Concepts of parenthood', in K. Elliott (ed.), *The Family and its Future*, University of London, CIBA Foundation Symposium.

NICHOLSON, J. (1984), *Men and Women*, Oxford, Oxford University Press.

NIE, N. H., HULL, C. H., FRANKLIN, M. N., JENKINS, J. G., SOURS, K. S., NORUSSIS, M. J. and BEADLE, V. (1980), *SCSS – A user's guide to the SCSS Conversational System*, New York, McGraw-Hill.

NISSEL, M. (1980), 'Women in government statistics: Basic concepts and assumptions', in Equal Opportunities Commission, *Women and Government Statistics*, Manchester, EOC.

NURSERY CONCERNED (1983–5), *Newsletters*, Edinburgh, Nursery Concerned.

OAKLEY, A. (1974a), *Housewife*, Harmondsworth, Penguin.

OAKLEY, A. (1974b), *The Sociology of Housework*, Bath, Martin Robertson.

O'DONNELL, L. (1983), 'The social world of parents', *Marriage and Family Review*, vol. 5, no. 4, pp. 9–36.

OFFICE OF POPULATION, CENSUSES AND SURVEYS (1980), *Classification of Occupations*, London, HMSO.

ORGANISATION FOR ECONOMIC CO-OPERATION AND DEVELOPMENT (1975), *Child Care Programmes in Nine Countries*, Washington, Report of the Working Party on the Role of Women in the Economy, US Department of Health, Education and Welfare.

OSBORN, A. (1981a), *Measures of ability, behaviour and maternal depression*, University of Bristol, unpublished paper.

OSBORN, A. (1981b), 'Under-fives in school in England and Wales', *Educational Research*, vol. 23, no. 2, pp. 96–104.

OSBORN, A. (1984), 'Maternal employment, depression and child behaviour', in Equal Opportunities Commission, *Work and the Family*, Manchester, EOC.

OSBORN, A. F., BUTLER, N. R. and MORRIS, A. C. (1984), *The Social Life of Britain's Five-year Olds*, London, Routledge and Kegan Paul.

OSBORN, A. F. and MORRIS, T. C. (1979), 'The rationale for a composite index of social class and its evaluation', *British Journal of Sociology*, vol. 30, no. 1, pp. 39–60.

OTTO, L. B. (1975), 'Class and status in family research', *Journal of Marriage and the Family*, vol. 37, pp. 315–332.

PACKMAN, J. (1968), *Child Care Needs and Numbers*, London, George Allen and Unwin.

PACKMAN, J. (1973), 'The incidence of need', in J. Stroud (ed.), *Services for Children and their Families*, London, Pergamon Press.

PAHL, R. E. and PAHL, J. M. (1971), *Managers and their Wives*, Harmondsworth, Allen Lane – The Penguin Press.

PARKE, R. D. (1981), *Fathering*, Glasgow, Fontana.

PARKER, R. (1974), 'Social administration in search of generality', *New Society*, pp. 566–568.

PARSONS, T. and BALES, R. F. (1956), *Family, Socialization and Interaction Process*, London, Routledge and Kegan Paul.

PEDERSEN, F. A. (ed.) (1980), *The Father-Infant Relationship*, New York, Praeger.

PEDERSEN, F. A., YARROW, L. J., ANDERSON, B. J. and CAIN, R. L. Jr. (1979), 'Conceptualization of father influences in the infancy period', in M. Lewis and L. Rosenblum (eds), *The Child and its Family*, New York, Plenum Press.

PENN, H. (1982), 'Who cares for the kids?', *New Statesman*, vol. 103, pp. 6–8.

PHILLIPS, M. (1976), 'What kind of care?', *New Society*, vol. 36, p. 420.

PINKER, R. (1971), *Social Theory and Social Policy*, London, Heinemann.

PINKER, R. (1979), *The Idea of Welfare*, London, Heinemann.

PLATT, J. (1969), 'Some problems in measuring the jointness of conjugal role-relationships', *Sociology*, vol. 3, pp. 287–297.

PLOWDEN REPORT (1967), see Central Advisory Committee for Education.

POPAY, J., RIMMER, L. and ROSSITER, C. (1983), *One-Parent Families*, London, Study Commission on the Family.

POPPER, K. (1974), *Conjectures and Refutations*, London, Routledge and Kegan Paul.

PRINGLE, M. K. (1975), *The Needs of Children*, London, Hutchinson.

PRINGLE, M. K. (1983), 'The needs of children and their implications for parental and professional care', in A. W. Franklin (ed.), *Family Matters*, Oxford, Pergamon.

PRINGLE, M. K. and NAIDOO, S. (1975), *Early Child Care in Britain*, London, Gordon and Breach.

RADCLIFFE-BROWN, A. R. (1952), 'Joking relationships', in J. Goody (ed.), *Kinship*, Harmondsworth, Penguin.

RADCLIFFE-BROWN, A. R. (1960), 'Introduction to the analysis of kinship systems', in N. W. Bell and E. F. Vogel (eds), *A Modern Introduction to the Family*, New York, The Free Press of Glencoe.

RAPOPORT, R. and RAPOPORT, R. (1976), *Dual Career Families Re-examined*, Oxford, Martin Robertson.

RAPOPORT, R. and RAPOPORT, R. N. (eds) (1978), *Working Couples*, London, Routledge and Kegan Paul.

RAPOPORT, R., RAPOPORT, R. and STRELITZ, Z. (1977), *Fathers, Mothers and Others*, London, Routledge and Kegan Paul.

RAPOPORT, R. N., FOGARTY, M. P. and RAPOPORT, R. (1982), *Families in Britain*, London, Routledge and Kegan Paul.

RAPOPORT, R. and RAPOPORT, R. (1982), 'British families in transition', in Rapoport, R, Fogarty, R. N. and Rapoport, R. (eds), *Families in Britain*, London, Routledge and Kegan Paul.

RAVETZ, J. R. (1971), *Scientific Knowledge and its Social Problems*, Oxford, Oxford University Press.

REICH, B. and ADCOCK, C. (1976), *Values, Attitudes and Behaviour Change*, London, Methuen.

REIN, M. (1976), *Social Science and Public Policy*, Harmonds-worth, Penguin.

REISS, P. J. (1962), 'The extended kinship system: Correlates of and attitudes on frequency of interaction', *Marriage and Family Living*, vol. 24, pp. 333–339.

RICHARDS, M. P. M., DUNN, J. F. and ANTONIS, B. (1977), 'Caretaking in the first year of life: the role of fathers and mothers' social isolation', *Child: Care, Health and Development*, vol. 3, pp. 23–36.

RICHARDSON, C. J. (1977), *Contemporary Social Mobility*, London, Frances Pinter.

RICHMAN, N. (1978), 'Depression in mothers of young children', *Journal of the Royal Society of Medicine*, vol. 71, pp. 489–493.

RICHMAN, N., STEVENSON, J. E. and GRAHAM, P. J. (1975), 'Prevalence of behaviour problems in three-year-old children: An epidemiological study in a London borough', *Journal of Child Psychology and Psychiatry*, vol. 15, pp. 277–287.

ROBERTS, H. (ed.) (1981), *Doing Feminist Research*, London, Routledge and Kegan Paul.

ROBERTS, R. E. and O'KEEFE, S. J. (1981), 'Sex differences in depression reexamined', *Journal of Health and Social Behaviour*, vol. 22, pp. 394–400.

ROBERTSON, J. and ROBERTSON, J. (1970), *Young Children in Brief Separation*, London, Tavistock Child Development Research Unit.

ROBERTSON, J. F. (1975), 'Interaction in three generation families: toward a theoretical perspective', *Aging and Human Development*, vol. 6, no. 2, pp. 103–110.

ROBERTSON, J. F. (1977), 'Grandmotherhood: A study of role conceptions', *Journal of Marriage and the Family*, vol. 39, pp. 165–173.

ROBY, P. (ed.) (1973), *Child Care – Who Cares?*, New York, Basic Books.

ROKEACH, M. (1973), *The Nature of Human Values*, New York, The Free Press.

ROLLINS, B. C. and GALLIGAN, R. (1978), 'The developing child and marital satisfaction of parents', in R. M. Lerner and G. B. Spanier (eds), *Child Influences on Marital and Family Interaction: A Life-span Perspective*, London, Academic Press.

ROSSER, C. and HARRIS, C. C. (1961), 'Relationships through

marriage in a Welsh urban area', *Sociological Review*, vol. 9, pp. 293–321.

ROSSER, C. and HARRIS, C. C. (1965), *The Family and Social Change*, London, Routledge and Kegan Paul.

ROSSI, A. (1984), 'Gender and parenthood', *American Sociological Review*, vol. 49, no. 1, pp. 1–18.

ROSSI, P. H. (1955), *Why Families Move*, Glencoe, Illinois, The Free Press.

ROSSITER, C. and WICKS, M. (1982), *Crisis or Challenge?*, London, Study Commission on the Family.

ROWE, J., HUNDLEBY, M., CAIN, H. and KEANE, A. (1984), *Long Term Foster-care*, London, Batsford/BAAF.

RUBENSTEIN, J. L., HAWES, C. and BOYLE, P. (1981), 'A two year follow-up of infants in community-based day care', *Journal of Child Psychology and Psychiatry*, vol. 22, no. 3, pp. 209–218.

RUBIN, Z. (1980), *Children's Friendships*, Glasgow, Fontana.

RUTTER, M. (1980a), *Maternal Deprivation Reassessed* (2nd edition), Harmondsworth, Penguin.

RUTTER, M. (1980b), 'The Long-term effects of early experience', *Developmental Medicine and Child Neurology*, vol. 22, pp. 800–815.

RUTTER, M., TIZARD, J. and WHITMORE, K. (1970), *Education, Health and Behaviour*, London, Longmans.

SAHLINS, M. D. (1965), 'Exchange-value and the diplomacy of primitive trade', *Proceedings of the American Ethnological Society*, Spring 1965, pp. 95–129.

SAMEROFF, A. (1975a), 'Transactional models in early social relations', *Human Development*, vol. 18, pp. 65–79.

SAMEROFF, A. J. (1975b), 'Early influences on development: fact or fancy?', *Merrill-Palmer Quarterly*, vol. 20, pp. 267–294.

SCARR, S. (1969), 'Social introversion-extraversion as a heritable response', *Child Development*, vol. 40, pp. 823–832.

SCHAFFER, H. R. (1971), *The Growth of Sociability*, Harmondsworth, Penguin.

SCHAFFER, H. R. (1977), *Mothering*, London, Open Books.

SCHAFFER, H. R. (1985), 'Making decisions about children', *Adoption and Fostering*, vol. 9, no. 1, pp. 22–28.

SCHAFFER, H. R. and EMERSON, P. (1964), *The Development of Social Attachments in Infancy*, Chicago, Monographs of the Society for Research in Child Development, 29, no 3, University of Chicago Press.

SCHAPERA, I. (1971), *Married Life in an African Tribe*, Harmondsworth, Penguin.

SCHMUTZLER, K. H-J. (1976), 'Mutter oder Tagesmutter? Ein neuer Streit um die Vorschulerziehung', *Sozialpadagogische Blatter*, vol. 27, pp. 74–83.

SCHORR, A. (1974), *Children and Decent People*, New York, Basic Books.

SCHWARTZ, H. and JACOBS, J. (1979), *Qualitative Sociology*, New York, The Free Press.

SCHWARTZ, J. C., STRICKLAND, R. G. and KROLICK, G. (1974), 'Infant day care: Behavioural effects at pre-school age', *Developmental Psychology*, vol. 10, no. 4, pp. 502–506.

SCOTT, M. B. and LYMAN, S. M. (1968), 'Accounts', *American Sociological Review*, vol. 33, pp. 46–62.

SCOTTISH EDUCATION DEPARTMENT (1980), *Statistical Bulletin*, Edinburgh, SED.

SEABROOK, J. (1967), *The Unprivileged*, Harmondsworth, Penguin.

SEARS, R. R. (1950), 'Ordinal position in the family as psychological variable', *American Sociological Review*, vol. 15, pp. 397–401.

SECOMBE, W. (1974), 'The housewife and her labour under capitalism', *New Left Review*, vol. 83, pp. 3–26.

SEELEY, J. R., SIM, R. A. and LOOSLEY, E. W. (1956), *Crestwood Heights*, Toronto, University Toronto Press.

SEGAL, L. (ed.) (1983), *What is to be done about the family?*, Harmondsworth, Penguin.

SHARP, C. (1980), *The Economics of Time*, Oxford, Martin Robertson.

SHEFFIELD DEPARTMENT OF EMPLOYMENT AND ECONOMIC DEVELOPMENT (1986), 'Women's work and childcare', *Women in Sheffield*, no. 5.

SHINMAN, S. M. (1981), *A Change For Every Child?*, London, Tavistock.

SIEGEL, A. E. and HAAS, M. B. (1965), 'The working mother: a review of research', *Child Development*, vol. 34, pp. 513–542.

SILVERSTEIN, L. (1981), 'A critical review of current research on infant day care', in S. B. Kamerman and A. J. Kahn (eds), *Child Care, Family Benefits and Working Parents*, New York, Columbia University Press.

SIMPSON, A. E. and STEVENSON-HINDE, J. (1985), 'Temperamental characteristics of three- to four-year-old boys and girls and child-family interactions', *Journal of Child Psychology and Psychiatry*, vol. 26, no. 1, pp. 43–54.

SINFIELD, A. (1980), 'Meeting client need; an ambiguous and precarious value', in D. Grunow and F. Hegner (eds), *Welfare or Bureaucracy*, Cambridge, Mass., Oelgeschlager, Gunn and Hain.

SMITH, P. K. (1979), 'How many people can a young child feel secure with?', *New Society*, pp. 504–506.

SMITH, P. K. (1980), 'Shared care of young children: Alternative models to monotropism', *Merrill-Palmer Quarterly*, vol. 26, no. 4, pp. 371–387.

SNOW, M., JACKLIN, C. N. and MACCOBY, E. E. (1981), 'Birth order differences in peer sociability at thirty-three months', *Child Development*, vol. 52, pp. 589–595.

SOCIAL WORK SERVICES GROUP (1976), *Scottish Social Work Statistics*, Edinburgh, HMSO.

SPANIER, G. B., LERNER, R. M. and AQUILINO, W. (1978), 'The study of child-family interactions: A perspective for the future', in R. M. Lerner and G. B. Spanier (eds), *Child Influences on Marital and Family Interaction: A Life-span Perspective*, London, Academic Press.

SPENCER, L. and DALE, A. (1979), 'Integration and regulation in organisations: A contextual approach', *Sociological Review*, vol. 27, no. 4, pp. 679–702.

STACEY, M. (1969), 'The myth of community studies', *British Journal of Sociology*, vol. 20, pp. 134–147.

STACEY, M. (1981), 'The division of labour revisited or overcoming the two Adams', in P. Abrams *et al.* (eds), *Practice and Problems: British Sociology 1950–1980*, London, George Allen and Unwin.

STANWORTH, M. (1984), 'Women and class analysis: A reply to J. Goldthorpe', *Sociology*, vol. 18, no. 2, pp. 159–169.

STATISTICS (1984), 'Children in care in England and Wales, March 1982', *Adoption and Fostering*, vol. 8, no. 3.

STEVENSON, J. and ELLIS, C. (1975), 'Which three year-olds attend pre-school facilities?', *Child: Care, health and development*, vol. 1, pp. 397–411.

STEWART, R. B. (1983), 'Sibling attachment relationships: Child-infant interactions in the strange situation', *Developmental Psychology*, vol. 19, no. 2, pp. 192–199.

STOKES, R. and HEWITT, J. P. (1976), 'Aligning actions', *American Sociological Review*, vol. 41, pp. 838–849.

STOLZ, L. M. (1967), *Influences on Parent Behaviour*, London, Tavistock.

STONE, E. (ed.) (1981), *Women and the Cuban Revolution*, New York, Pathfinder.

STRATHCLYDE REGIONAL COUNCIL (1985), *Under Fives*, Final Report of the Member/Officer Group, Glasgow.

STREIB, G. F. (1958), 'Family patterns in retirement', *Journal of Social Issues*, vol. 14, pp. 46–60.

SUNDSTROM, G. (1983), *Caring for the Aged in Welfare Society*, Stockholm, Liber Forlag.

SUTTON, A. (1981), 'A new movement in preschool provision', *Early Childhood*, vol. 2, no. 1, pp. 10–11.

SUTTON-SMITH, B. and ROSENBERG, B. G. (1970), *The Sibling*, New York, Holt, Rinehart and Winston Inc.

SWEETSER, D. A. (1968), 'Intergenerational ties in Finnish urban families', *American Sociological Review*, vol. 33, no. 2, pp. 236–246.

SWIFT, J. (1982), 'Minding children in Germany', *Early Childhood*, vol. 2, no. 9, pp. 4–10.

TAYLOR, LORD and CHAVE, S. (1964), *Mental Health and Environment*, London, Longmans.

TAYLOR, P. H., EXON, G. and HOLLEY, B. (1972), *A Study of Nursery Education*, Schools Council working paper 41, London, Methuen.

THOMAS, A. and CHESS, S. (1977), *Temperament and Development*, New York, Brunner/Mazel Inc.

THOMPSON, B. (1975), 'Adjustment to school', *Educational Research*, vol. 17, pp. 128–136.

THOMPSON, B. and FINLAYSON, A. (1963), 'Married women who work in early motherhood', *British Journal of Sociology*, pp. 150–163.

TIMMS, E. (1983), 'On the relevance of informal social networks to social work intervention', *British Journal of Social Work*, vol. 13, pp. 405–415.

TITMUSS, R. (1970), *The Gift Relationship*, London, George Allen and Unwin.

TITMUSS, R. (1976), *Essays on the Welfare State* (3rd edition), London, George Allen and Unwin.

TIZARD, B. (1974), *Early Childhood Education*, Windsor, NFER.

TIZARD, B. (1977), *Adoption: a Second Chance*, London, Open Books.

TIZARD, B., PHILPS, J. and PLEWIS, I. (1976), 'Play in pre-school centres – II. Effects on play of the child's social class and of the educational orientation of the centre', *Journal of Child Psychology and Psychiatry*, vol. 17, pp. 265–274.

TIZARD, J. (1976), 'Effects of day care on young children', in N. Fonda and P. Moss (eds), *Mothers in Employment*, London, Brunel University.

TIZARD, J, Moss, P. and PERRY, J. (1976), *All Our Children*, London, Temple Smith.

TIZARD, J. and TIZARD, B. (1971), 'The social development of two-year-old children in residential nurseries', in H. R. Schaffer (ed.), *The Origins of Human Social Relations*, London, Academic Press.

TOOMEY, D. M. (1971), 'Conjugal roles and social networks in an urban working class sample', *Human Relations*, vol. 24, no. 5, pp. 417–431.

TOWNSEND, P. (1957), *The Family Life of Old People*, Harmondsworth, Penguin.

TOWNSEND, P. (1979), *Poverty in the United Kingdom*, Harmondsworth, Allen Lane and Penguin Books.

TRADES UNION CONGRESS (1977), *The Under Fives*, London, TUC.

TROLL, L., BENGSTON, V. and MCFARLAND, D. (1979), 'Generations in the family', in W. R. Burr, R. Hill, F. I. Nye and I. L. Reiss (eds), *Contemporary Theories about the Family*, volume 1 – *Research-Based Theories*, New York, The Free Press.

TROST, J. (1983), 'Parental benefits – A study of men's behaviour and attitudes', *Current Sweden*, no. 306.

TURNER, C. (1967), 'Conjugal roles and social networks – A re-examination of a hypothesis', *Human Relations*, vol. 20, pp. 121–130.

TURNER, C. (1969), *Family and Kinship in Modern Britain*, London, Routledge and Kegan Paul.

UNGERSON, CLARE (1982), *Women and caring: Skills, tasks and taboos*, paper to the BSA Conference on 'Gender and Society'.

UNGERSON, C. (1983), 'Why do women care?', in J. Finch and D. Groves (eds), *A Labour of Love*, London, Routledge and Kegan Paul.

UTTLEY, S. (1980), 'The welfare exchange reconsidered', *Journal of Social Policy*, vol. 9, pp. 187–205.

VANDELL, D. L. and MUELLER, E. C. (1980), 'Peer play and friendship during the first two years', in H. C. Foot, A. C.

Chapman and J. R. Smith (1980), *Friendship and Social Relations in Children*, New York, J. Wiley and Sons.

VAN DER EYCKEN, W. (1977), *The Pre-school Years* (4th edition), Harmondsworth, Penguin.

VAN DER EYCKEN, W. (1982), *Home-Start*, Leicester, Home-Start Consultancy.

VAN DER EYCKEN, W., MITCHELL, L. and GRUBB, J. (1979), *Pre-schooling in England, Scotland and Wales*, Report for a Conference of the Council of Europe.

VON CRANACH, B. V., HUFFNER, U., MARTE, F. and PELKA, R. (1976), 'Einschatzskala zur Erfassung gehemmter Kinder im Kindergarten', *Praxis der Kinderpsychologie*, pp. 146–155.

WADSWORTH, M. E. J. (1981), 'Social class and generation differences in pre-school education', *British Journal of Sociology*, vol. 32, no. 4, pp. 560–585.

WALDROP, M. F. and HALVERSON, C. S. (1975), 'Intensive and extensive peer behaviour: longitudinal and cross-sectional analysis', *Child Development*, vol. 46, pp. 19–26.

WALKER, A. (ed.) (1982), *Community Care*, Oxford, Basil Blackwell and Martin Robertson.

WARREN, D. I. and ROTHMAN, J. (1981), 'Community networks', in M. E. Olsen and M. Micklin (eds), *Handbook of Applied Sociology*, New York, Praeger.

WARREN, J. R. (1966), 'Birth order and social behaviour', *Psychological Bulletin*, vol. 65, no. 1, pp. 38–49.

WARREN, N. and JAHODA, M. (eds) (1973), *Attitudes*, Harmondsworth, Penguin Books.

WATSON, D. (1980), *Caring for Strangers*, London, Routledge and Kegan Paul.

WATT, J. S. (1976), *Pre-school Education and the Family*, London, Social Science Research Council.

WATT, J. S. (1979), *Co-operation in Pre-school Education*, University of Aberdeen, PhD thesis.

WEBB, R. A. (1977), 'Introduction', in R. A. Webb (ed.), *Social Development in Childhood: Day-care programs and research*, Baltimore, J. Hopkins University Press.

WEINRAUB, M. and LEWIS, M. (1977), *The Determinants of Children's Responses to Separation*, Monographs of the Society for Research in Child Development, vol. 42, no. 4, Chicago, University of Chicago Press.

WEISNER, T. S. and GALLIMORE, R. (1977), 'My brother's keeper:

Child and sibling caretaking', *Current Anthropology*, vol. 18, no. 2, pp. 169–190.

WEITMAN, S. R. (1978), 'Prosocial behaviour and its discontents', in L. Wispe (ed.), *Altruism, Sympathy and Helping*, London, Academic Press.

WHITBREAD, N. (1972), *The Evolution of the Nursery-Infant School*, London, Routledge and Kegan Paul.

WHITE PAPER (1972a), *Education: A Framework for Expansion*, London, HMSO.

WHITE PAPER (1972b), *Education in Scotland: A Statement of Policy*, Edinburgh, HMSO.

WHYTE, W. H. (1960), *The Organization Man*, Harmondsworth, Penguin.

WICKS, M. (1983), 'Enter right: The family rights group', *New Society*, p. 297.

WIDLAKE, P. (1971), 'Does nursery education work?', *Child Education*, vol. 48, pp. 23–28.

WILBY, P. (1980), 'An advocate for children', *New Society*, vol. 53, pp. 126–127.

WILLIAMS, C. T. and WINSTON, K. T. (1980), *Mothers at Work*, New York, Longmans.

WILLMOTT, P. and CHALLIS, L. (1977), *The Groveway Project*, London, Department of the Environment.

WILLMOTT, P. and YOUNG, M. (1960), *Family and Class in a London Suburb*, London, Routledge and Kegan Paul.

WILSON, B. (1981), 'Lothian's stand', *New Society*, p. 263.

WILSON, R. S., BROWN, A. M. and MATHENY, A. P. (1971), 'Emergence and persistence of behavioural differences in twins', *Child Development*, vol. 42, pp. 1381–1398.

WISPE, L. (ed.) (1978), *Altruism, Sympathy and Helping*, London, Academic Press.

WOODHEAD, M. (1976), *Intervening in Disadvantage*, Windsor, NFER.

WRIGHT MILLS, C. (1970), *The Sociological Imagination*, Harmondsworth, Pelican Books.

WRONG, D. (1961), 'The oversocialized conception of man in modern sociology', *American Sociological Review*, vol. 26, no. 2, pp. 183–193.

YARROW, L. J. (1964), 'Separations from parents during early childhood', in L. W. Hoffman and M. L. Hoffman (eds), *Review of Child Development Research*, New York, Russell Sage Foundation.

YARROW, M. R., CAMPBELL, J. D. and BURTON, R. V. (1970),

'The reliability of maternal retrospection', in K. Danziger (ed.), *Socialization*, Harmondsworth, Penguin.

YOUNG, F. (1983), 'Concerned about nursery cuts', *The Scotsman*, Tuesday, 24 January 1983, p. 6.

YOUNG, K. and MILLS, C. (1978), *Understanding the 'Assumptive Worlds' of Government Actions: Issues and Approach*, Bristol, Report to the SSRC Panel on Central/Local Government Relations.

YOUNG, M. and WILLMOTT, P. (1957), *Family and Kinship in East London*, Harmondsworth, Penguin.

YOUNG, M. and WILLMOTT, P. (1973), *The Symmetrical Family*, London, Routledge and Kegan Paul.

YUDKIN, S. (1967), *0–5: A Report on the Care of Pre-school Children*, London, George Allen and Unwin.

YUDKIN, S. and HOLME, A. (1963), *Working Mothers and their Children*, London, Michael Joseph.

ZIGLER, E. and CHILD, I. L. (eds) (1973), *Socialization and Personality Development*, Reading, Mass., Addison-Wesley Publishing Company.

ZIGLER, E. F. and GORDON, E. W. (1982), *Day Care*, Boston, Massachusetts, Auburn House Publishing Company.

Index

adaptability, 240, 274, 300
age of entry to group care, 7, 11, 70–1, 72, 101–2, 118, 193, 254, 255, 274, 296–7
ages of children in sample, 26, 29
aligning actions, 219
altruism, 104–6
anthropology, 23
anxiety, *see* stress
arranging shared care, 115, 213–14, 221
attachment(s), 9, 11, 17, 151, 160, 184–5, 187, 217, 219, 253–5, 272, 273, 374
attendance at group care, 6–7, 71
attitudes, 214, 217, 226, 227, 230, 235, 245, 256, 295; *see also* work, mothers' (attitudes towards); values
aunts, 36, 46, 51, 58, 64, 69, 70, 86, 94, 96, 133, 134, 137, 144, 163–4, 165, 183, 185, 189, 233, 239, 279
au pairs, 60, 62, 68, 69, 89, 129, 190, 205, 232, 234, 253

babies, 81, 95, 130, 133, 138, 195, 238, 240–2, 245, 246, 252, 259, 264
babysitter role, 138, 249
babysitting, 40, 44, 49, 89, 91, 110, 129, 138, 194, 213, 219, 229, 236, 245–6, 266
babysitting circles (groups): book systems, 110–11, 112, 113; care by men in, 63, 130; combined with other carers, 49, 61, 90, 129; and class, 52, 89, 144, 175, 176, 276, 288; definition of, 61; exchange medium systems, 110, 111–12, 114; joining and use of, 44, 61, 110, 129, 176, 232, 249; negative aspects of, 52, 90, 139; positive aspects of, 92, 138, 140; reasons for use of, 34, 49, 140, 181; and reciprocity, 108–15, 288, 289; and social relationships, 151, 181–2, 184, 278
Backett, Kathryn, 215, 225, 237, 275
ballet classes, 75, 118, 134, 296
befriending: by adults, 34, 48, 114, 151, 171–81, 190–1; by children, 53, 82, 101, 120, 135, 177–8, 187–90, 256; children's influence on adult befriending, 177–8, 180, 284, 288; and sharing care, 168, 171, 182, 186, 288, 291, 293, 295; *see also* child-child relationships; friends
beliefs, 214–17, 226, 227–8, 230, 231, 243, 246, 251, 261, 263, 279, 292
benefits of sharing care, 43, 83, 100, 104, 148, 187, 199, 224, 237, 258, 264, 280–2, 297
Bernstein, Basil, 291–2
best friends (of children), 189, 191

For Product Safety Concerns and Information please contact
our EU representative GPSR@taylorandfrancis.com Taylor & Francis
Verlag GmbH, Kaufingerstraße 24, 80331 München, Germany

T - #0050 - 160425 - C0 - 216/138/21 [23] - CB - 9781032438115 - Gloss Lamination